THE COMPLETE MEDICAL SCRIBE

A Guide to Accurate Documentation

EDITION

3

THE COMPLETE MEDICAL SCRIBE

A Guide to Accurate Documentation

DR. KIM D. KWIATEK, MD, DNBPAS

President and Founder, ABC Scribes
Kettering Health Network
Dayton, Ohio

DR. KATERINA M. FLAMM, MD

The Ohio State University Wexner Medical Center
Columbus, Ohio

ELSEVIER

ABC SCRIBES

Elsevier
3251 Riverport Lane
St. Louis, Missouri 63043

THE COMPLETE MEDICAL SCRIBE, THIRD EDITION   ISBN: 978-0-323-81265-8

Previous editions copyrighted 2019 and 2016.

Library of Congress Control Number: 2021941824

Content Strategist: Kristin R. Wilhelm
Content Development Specialist: John Tomedi
Publishing Services Manager: Deepthi Unni
Project Manager: Radjan Lourde Selvanadin
Design Direction: Renee Duenow

Printed in India

Last digit is the print number: 9 8 7 6 5 4 3 2 1

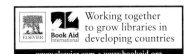

Working together to grow libraries in developing countries

www.elsevier.com • www.bookaid.org

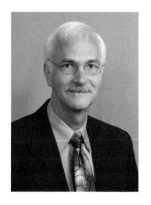

Kim Kwiatek, MD, originally trained as a Family Physician but quickly pivoted to the practice of Emergency Medicine in Dayton, Ohio. His many interests over his 40-year career included the business side of medicine and computerization of the electronic health record. These interests led him to start a medical scribe company that could help him and fellow physicians with more accurate documentation. Aptly named ABC Scribes (for Accurate Bedside Charting), the company started training scribes in its own "Scribe Academy" as well as in area universities. A textbook naturally followed. Now in its third edition, Dr. Kwiatek has collaborated with Elsevier to bring you *The Complete Medical Scribe*. Still actively engaged in medical informatics, Dr. Kwiatek makes time to travel to see his three children and three grandchildren.

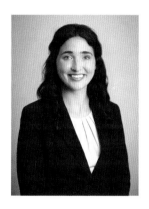

Katerina Flamm, MD, began working for ABC Scribes in 2014. She rapidly mastered the documentation profession and began teaching for the company in her new role as senior medical scribe. Katerina was instrumental in helping to mature the company's curriculum and became its "Director of Education." In that role she collaborated with Dr. Kwiatek in the writing of the first two editions of this text, the first of which was published in 2017, and the second in 2019. In 2021, Katerina graduated from medical school from The Ohio State University College of Medicine. She is starting her residency at The Ohio State Wexner Medical Center and hopes to continue medical documentation education during her residency and beyond.

This book is dedicated first and foremost to Amanda Craycraft, the "ground zero" scribe for ABC Scribes (Accurate Bedside Charting). Amanda is a force of nature who made me believe that I could build a successful scribe program way back in 2010. Without her infectious enthusiasm, our scribe program in Dayton, Ohio and the subsequent college course and textbook would never have happened.

In addition, I want to dedicate this effort to my wife, Candace, who has been the major influence in my life, teaching me by example how much can be accomplished with persistence, patience, and grace.

A shout-out goes to Larry Henry, my small business (SBA) mentor who from the get-go was brutally honest with me as I learned my way in the business world. He helped me to focus on my passion which was quality and innovation as opposed to growth for growth's sake.

Finally, this book is dedicated to the many aspiring healthcare professionals who scribed for ABC Scribes over the years. Their eagerness to learn the art of medical documentation as they began their healthcare careers was my ongoing inspiration in developing a curriculum and creating this text.

ACKNOWLEDGMENTS

Many people contributed to this effort in numerous ways, both large and small. These are but a few.

The original college curriculum that led to this text was written with assistance from Amanda Utendorf Stegemiller. Amanda both scribed for me and cotaught our original course at the University of Dayton (the first college scribing course for credit in the nation). She provided valuable insight into the perspectives of the college student and tackled this new project with professionalism. She enthusiastically shared her scribe expertise with many budding health professionals. Amanda is now a Physician Assistant in Dayton, OH.

Katerina Flamm, MD, my coauthor, deserves special acknowledgement for the countless hours she put in writing this text with me. We collaborated on editions 1 and 2 which we "self-published" on CreateSpace (later Amazon/Kindle). These early editions served as our course text and as certification preparation for many students. The text was used in area colleges and our own "Scribe Academy." I will treasure the memory of the late nights we spent hashing things out in shared documents online, until we both were satisfied. Katerina was a scribe with ABC Scribes and a pre-med student at the time we began work on our first edition. She took a gap year to complete this project with me. We worked on the second edition together over a summer break while she was in medical school at The Ohio State University (OSU). Congratulations Katerina on your graduation from OSU and your acceptance into emergency and internal medicine residencies! You are an exemplar of what a serious scribe experience can produce. There would absolutely be no text without you.

I must particularly acknowledge Rachel E. Evans, RN, who has been by my side almost from Day One in the management of ABC Scribes. She took a chance on me and changed the trajectory of her own career throwing in her lot with ABC Scribes. Rachel has amazing qualities that she invested in our project. Daily she demonstrates how to put personal ethical values into everyday practice and how to be both confident yet humble. Only because of her handling of so many details of running the business did I have the time and energy left to devote to this book. Rachel is now the owner of ABC Scribes, a position that she has earned.

A big thank you goes to Kelly Schulte, longtime employee and manager/director at ABC Scribes, whose expertise in all things technical has been invaluable in getting early editions of this work published. Her range of knowledge is broad and her upbeat, can-do optimism is infectious. I will always be in awe of people who take lemons that life dishes out and make them into great lemonade. Kelly is such a person.

My oldest daughter, Keren Stick, was my proofreader on the first edition. She is a stickler for proper grammar and took the time to go through early versions of the book line-by-line. I will always be grateful that she did this even though it came at a time when she really did not have the time. Keren saved me from many an embarrassment, I am sure.

Finally, John Tomedi, acting as my editor for this edition, deserves special mention for his expertise in editing a medical text and his attention to detail. He was always tolerant of my lack of knowledge of the process, and I hope has succeeded in making me look like I know what I am doing. Most importantly, he tolerated my sense of humor. Thank you, John!

Welcome to the third edition of our text on medical scribing. This edition is called *The Complete Medical Scribe* as it covers the vast landscape of scribing in a thorough fashion. Our intention is to have this serve as your go-to reference for all your scribing questions, both during the course and beyond.

This text has evolved over the years to include not only the technical aspects of scribing, but also elements of the art of scribing with all its nuances. Also, partnering with Elsevier has allowed us to add content and many helpful illustrations that will bring much of the material to life. In addition, the text provides you with opportunities to practice your scribing skills.

The book is divided into four parts. The first introduces the scribe's important role on the healthcare team. Two new chapters have been introduced to this edition to explore the medical-legal and health safety aspects of the job. Part II of the book delves into the heart of scribing, the healthcare note itself, and how it is constructed. Part III reviews each body system with related signs, symptoms, and problems that you, the student, will need to understand to produce accurate healthcare documentation. Finally, the last part of the book offers a practical application of your newly learned skills. Here it guides you to anticipate what may be asked or examined during the medical history and physical and what constitutes required documentation for a given problem. There is also a chapter with sample scenarios for you to practice, with answers and explanations of why we recommend the documentation as we do.

We are pleased to provide as a companion to this book several online resources for the benefit of both students and instructors. For students, this platform offers the opportunity to further practice scribing skills by observing and documenting video provider/patient encounters. There are also online templates for use throughout the course. Additionally, there are self-directed quizzes with answers and rationales explaining those responses.

For the instructor, resources include Lesson Plans and PowerPoints for classroom use and guidance for presenting the information to the class. We also are providing a test bank of over 500 questions mapped to the learning objectives in each chapter.

Good luck as you go through this course and through your scribing career. Medical scribing was born of the need to improve provider documentation to meet the needs of the many parties with an interest in the patient chart. As documentation needs have grown, the provider often has had to decide between spending time with the patient or with the chart. Neither is a perfect choice. Enter the medical scribe who is trained to create a great medical document. The provider wins. The patient wins. The other parties who use the chart win. And the scribe has created a valued spot on the healthcare team. Our hope is that you will find that spot for yourself and enjoy your time scribing while recognizing the valuable contribution that you are making.

CONTENTS

PART IV **Practical Application**

PART I

The Medical Scribe in Healthcare

CHAPTER 1

Healthcare Providers and the Role of the Medical Scribe

KEY TERMS

Acuity

Certification

Consultant

Disposition

Electronic health record (EHR)

Electrophysiology

Hard-stop

History of the present illness (HPI)

Hospitalist

Interventional cardiology

Interventional radiology

Medical scribe

Order

Physical exam (PE)

Primary care

Provider

Review of systems (ROS)

Specialty medicine

Treatment plan

Providers and the Practice of Medicine

In the delivery of healthcare there are distinct and defined roles for the variety of professionals who work together to care for patients. **Providers** are at the center of patient care. These professionals are understood to have the education, experience, and demonstrated competency to practice medicine, meaning that they can recommend and perform treatments to cure a health problem or maintain health. The legal authority to practice medicine is granted by each state. The provider examines and diagnoses patients, prescribes medications, and performs surgeries and other procedures according to the **treatment plan** he or she has developed for the patient. Every aspect of the patient's care is documented.

For the sake of simplicity, there are two types of providers: physicians and nonphysician providers (NPPs), also called advanced practice providers (APPs). By law, the physician is the only professional who is permitted to practice medicine *independently*. This is because only physicians are considered to have enough training and experience to safely treat patients and to understand when the patient requires more advanced care. That being said, physicians may delegate many responsibilities to NPPs. NPPs include nurse practitioners, physician assistants, clinical nurse specialists, and more. Depending on the laws of each state, these providers work under varying levels physician supervision; many work independently and consult with physicians when needed.

Providers may work in a variety of areas in medicine. They may work in primary care, which requires one to know a little about all areas of medicine. **Primary care** is the area of medicine that is generally considered to be the first point of contact for the patient in caring for their general needs (Table 1.1). Alternatively, they may work in **specialty medicine**, which requires expertise within a specific area of medicine. Although not a complete list, Table 1.2 describes many of the providers included in the area of specialty medicine.

Specialty medicine includes those providers who have in-depth training of one specific body system. Often these providers will have completed a residency program in a generalized area (like internal medicine or general surgery), and then complete fellowship training in their chosen specialty (like cardiology or pulmonology).

Specialists often work in the combined settings of the hospital, office, and surgery. Many specialists also may act as consultants. A **consultant** is someone who evaluates a patient and provides recommendations for a treatment plan. A specialist acting as a consultant only documents on active problems within his or her area of expertise. For example: a general surgeon might only

TABLE 1.1 ■ Primary Care Providers

Provider	Description
General Practitioner (GP)	Antiquated term for the doctor who "did it all." No specialty residency was required. These providers used to deliver babies, perform common surgeries, and provide care for everyone.
Family Physician (FP)	This is the "newer" general primary care practitioner. A residency in family medicine is typically completed. They may or may not deliver babies and assist in surgeries. They may take care of pediatric patients as well as adults. Family physicians generally work in offices as part of the outpatient setting.
Internist or Internal Medicine (IM)	This is a general practice physician similar to the family physician, but who usually has not trained to care for pediatric or Ob/Gyn problems. Internists typically work in an office but often also in the hospital setting (some are also called **hospitalists** if they work exclusively within a hospital; see below).
Obstetrician/ Gynecologist (Ob/Gyn)	Gynecologists are trained to care specifically for women, and are experts in women's health. Obstetricians are experts in pregnancy, and care for both the mother and the prenatal baby. Obstetrics/gynecology is one combined specialty.
Pediatrician	Specializes in the care of infants, children, and adolescents. There are many subspecialties in pediatric medicine (like pediatric cardiology, pediatric gastroenterology, etc.). Often when an individual turns 18 they must transition to a family physician for their healthcare needs.
Gerontologist	Focuses on providing care to elderly patients. This is a relatively new specialty that is now caring for a continually growing population.
Emergency Medicine (EM)	Providers are trained to care for higher **acuity** emergent issues—health problems that need to be addressed quickly or immediately—and provide lifesaving intervention if needed. Emergency medicine physicians also function as the gatekeepers of the hospital: they decide which patients are ill enough for inpatient admission, and which can be safely discharged home to follow-up in outpatient primary or specialty care.
Urgent Care	Provides urgent care for lower acuity issues (like common colds, skin infections, minor trauma, and other nonlife-threatening conditions). If a patient needs a more in-depth work-up, they are sent to the emergency department.

TABLE 1.2 ■ **Specialty Medicine**

Specialist	Description
Anesthesiologist	Cares for the patient undergoing surgery and requiring anesthesia. May also deal in pain management for patients who have chronic pain problems.
Cardiologist	Manages diseases of the cardiovascular system. Can also subspecialize into other branches of cardiology, such as **interventional cardiology** (to perform procedures using a catheter) or **electrophysiology** (to treat and manage diseases of the heart's electrical system), among others.
Dermatologist	Deals with issues related to the skin. May do in-office procedures like biopsies and excisions.
Gastroenterologist	Manages and treats diseases of the gastrointestinal tract. Can perform procedures in an office setting or in the hospital.
General surgeon	A surgeon who has not subspecialized into other types of surgery. The types of surgeries that are performed depend on the surgeon's level of training.
Hematologist/ Oncologist	Treats cancer patients and blood diseases.
Hospitalist	A branch of internal medicine which takes care of patients in the hospital only (usually after admissions from the emergency department). A hospitalist will only document on any problem that requires close monitoring or intervention while the patient is hospitalized. They will not generally address stable or old problems. After discharge, the patient will return to their primary care provider for their healthcare needs.
Nephrologist	Specializes in diseases of the kidneys, including caring for dialysis patients.
Neurologist	Provides medical care of neurological problems.
Otolaryngologist (ENT)	Provides office and surgical care relating to the ears, nose, and throat.
Ophthalmologist	Provides office and surgical care of eye problems.
Physical Medicine and Rehabilitation (PM&R)	Rehabilitates the injured, stroke victims, and others.
Plastic Surgeon	Performs reconstructive and/or cosmetic procedures.
Proctologist	Takes care of diseases in the rectal area.
Psychiatrist	Cares for patients with behavioral health problems.
Pulmonologist	Specializes in diseases of the lung. Pulmonologists may also practice critical care medicine.
Radiologist	Reads and interprets various types of imaging studies. May also subspecialize into **interventional radiology** and perform image-guided procedures.
Rheumatologist	Monitors and treats the rheumatologic autoimmune diseases (those dealing with muscles and joints, primarily). Autoimmune disease tends to have a multi-system overlap, so rheumatologists often consult with other specialists to manage autoimmune disease (like dermatology and gastroenterology, for example).
Urologist	Manages diseases of the urinary system. This would include the urinary bladder, ureter and ureters, as well as surgical conditions of the kidneys.
Vascular (Thoracic) Surgeon	Performs invasive surgeries of the heart, lungs, and blood vessels.

comment on the surgical procedure that he or she performed, and any perioperative complications. Things like hypertension or pulmonary disease would be managed by specialists on the treatment team (perhaps cardiology and pulmonology, respectively).

Many providers in different areas of medicine may participate in one patient's care. This is because they each have the training necessary to meet one or more of that particular patient's needs. For example, one patient may be following with a urologist for their recurrent urinary tract infections, a cardiologist for their hypertension, and a rheumatologist for their lupus. Generally, the primary care provider acts as a quarterback of sorts, and coordinates patient care amongst all of the other providers.

> **NOTE**
>
> It is always important to document the names of the providers with whom the patient follows, along with their areas of specialty. This allows the medical scribe's supervising provider to consult the other providers who are familiar with that patient. The scribe should translate the lay verbiage that the patient may use when describing a provider's area of medicine to the appropriate medical term. For example, substituting cardiologist for "heart doctor," and nephrologist for "kidney doctor" and so forth.

The Medical Scribe

A **medical scribe** is a documentation assistant to the medical provider (most commonly a physician). Documentation is recorded in the **electronic health record (EHR)**, which is a computerized healthcare platform to organize patient care information and workflow (Fig. 1.1). The EHR stores all the information about the patient and the medical care he or she receives, including the provider's **orders**, which are the directions about how to care for the patient. The scribe enters patient medical information into the EHR on behalf of the provider. Nurses and other healthcare professionals help to execute the treatment plan by following the provider's orders from the EHR.

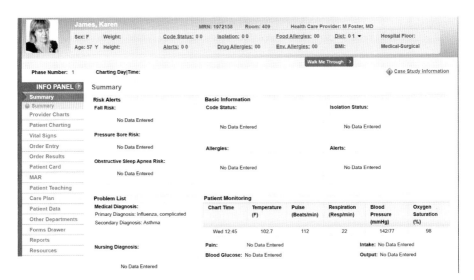

Fig. 1.1   The electronic health record (EHR) is a computerized platform to store and share patient information and to organize the work of providing patient care. (© SimChart for the Medical Office, 2021, Elsevier, Inc.)

The primary responsibility of the medical scribe is to create the **history of the present illness (HPI)** by listening to the provider while he or she is obtaining the patient's medical information (Fig. 1.2). The HPI is a coherent story, usually chronologic, describing the patient's illness or injury from the first sign or symptom to the present. The scribe may also complete the **review of systems (ROS)** after the HPI has been taken. This is a review of the symptoms that a patient may have, which is also obtained by the medical provider. A scribe may do other things if specifically told by the provider. These include recording the **physical exam (PE)**, which consists of the provider's physical findings during that patient encounter. The scribe may also enter orders for diagnostic labs, tests, or imaging into the EHR. At the provider's request a scribe may also document procedures, the results of certain tests (like electrocardiograms [ECGs]), or complete the "paperwork" for the patient's **disposition** and follow-up instructions.

Scribes are one of several solutions that allow the provider to document more accurately, more thoroughly, and more efficiently in the EHR. As an example, a provider may require 5 minutes to document on a single patient encounter. If they see 30 patients in a day, that would amount to roughly 150 minutes (or 2.5 hours) of time lost to documentation. With a scribe, the chart should be completed more or less when the provider exits the patient's room. Time and money are saved, and the chart that the scribe completes will likely be more thorough and accurate than the one the provider would create based on memory alone.

A medical scribe is the provider's partner in documentation. The scribe may have to ask questions to clarify what they did not understand, and prompt the provider to give elements of the history and physical exam that were not heard or observed (Fig. 1.3). A scribe should never be afraid to do this—at an appropriate time. This ensures accuracy and is a part of the scribe's value to the provider. A scribe should also help the provider meet billing requirements. Scribes are expected to inform the provider if billing requirements are not met, and prompt them to obtain all elements needed to complete the chart.

At the end of the day, the scribe helps to improve patient outcomes. Scribes allow the provider to spend more time with the patient and less time with the computer. They create an accurate document for other providers to consult by performing immediate documentation so details are not forgotten. They ensure that the document they create is billable to all standards so the provider will be paid. Lastly, they document details that are necessary for audits that ensure quality care.

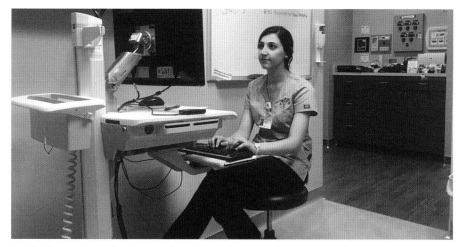

Fig. 1.2   The medical scribe listens to the patient and provider, documenting patient care into the electronic health record (EHR). (© ABC Scribes, Inc. Used with permission.)

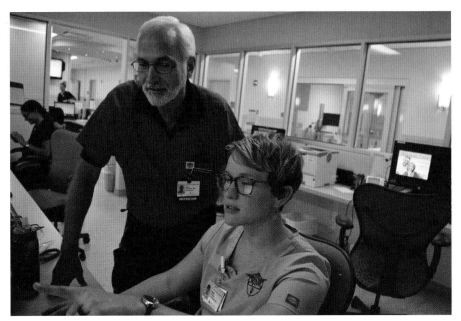

Fig. 1.3 The medical scribe works with the provider to ensure the documentation in the health record is complete and accurate. (© ABC Scribes, Inc. Used with permission.)

> **NOTE**
>
> What does it mean to be certified or to have a **certification**? In healthcare, it is important to have proof that the people working for the organization have met certain professional qualifications. A process of certification verifies that an individual has competence in a given area, and can be relied on to perform a skill. While a certification is usually voluntary, many employers prefer or require new hires to be certified by an agency or professional organization. Becoming a certified medical scribe conveys to the prospective employer that you have been trained, tested, and can be counted on to perform the job with competence.

WHAT IS A SCRIBE NOT TO DO?

A scribe is considered *nonclinical personnel*, meaning that there are a variety of clinical activities in which a scribe may not participate. The scope of a scribe's practice may vary between locations. Therefore, prior to working in a new location the medical scribe should always clarify the facility-based policies and procedures regarding limitations and expectations for a scribe. There are also things that a scribe may never do, regardless of place of employment. These will be discussed in detail.

A scribe both observes and listens to the provider prior to completing any element of the health record listed in the section above. This is because a scribe is prohibited from eliciting the HPI or ROS from the patient themselves, nor can the scribe perform a physical exam. A scribe is also not allowed to assist in performing medical procedures (other than the documentation). They also may not assist other healthcare providers in gathering supplies or administering medications. Only if the scribe has additional training or certifications that allow for it, may they be able to perform those additional functions that they are trained for.

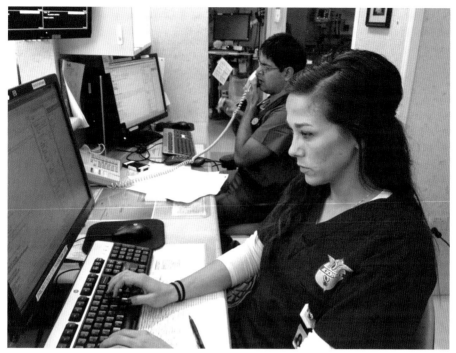

Fig. 1.4 The medical scribe's expertise is in populating the electronic health record (EHR) with the details of the patient encounter to present the most accurate record of care. (© ABC Scribes, Inc. Used with permission.)

The EHR has certain safeguards that are always in place that allow the scribe to work in the record as nonclinical personnel. These safeguards include **hard-stops** that appear after a scribe places orders or creates prescriptions. The hard-stops prevent the order or prescription from being acted upon unless the provider has reviewed, approved/amended, and signed the scribe's work. In addition to the hard-stops, the EHR should also send notifications and alerts to the provider (like medication contraindications such as allergies or drug-drug interactions), even if the scribe is the individual who entered the order.

Considering the restrictions in the EHR which are placed on a scribe, logging onto the computer using the physician's badge or user ID is never acceptable, and in fact constitutes fraud. Each individual working in the EHR must have separate login information, and different user roles and securities that depend on that individual's qualifications and required level of access. Chapter 2 will explore the security features of the EHR in detail.

A scribe must be both an excellent listener and an excellent communicator in order to be a successful part of the healthcare team. Most of the scribe's communication is written and done by documenting the encounter in the EHR (Fig. 1.4). A scribe may also communicate with other members of the healthcare team, but with certain limitations. A scribe may not call other providers to give them patient information, or transmit verbal orders to other healthcare providers. However, they can answer simple questions, such as whether the provider has been in to see a patient, or identify the provider's current location in the department or medical facility.

Occasionally the scribe may interact with patients: the patient may ask for a warm blanket or a drink, or ask questions about their healthcare. The scribe may almost always get patients warm blankets, but must ask the provider if the patient is allowed to have any oral intake ("po," or "per os," intake). There are a variety of reasons why this may not be allowed, including concerns for stroke (choking hazard), or the patient may be a surgical candidate (vomiting hazard). If a patient asks any questions that are medically related, the scribe should politely defer to an appropriate member of the healthcare team to provide an answer. Since a scribe is a nonclinical part of the healthcare team, they are not trained to answer these kinds of questions.

In summary, there are two general rules to heed: (1) a scribe may not touch anything that would be construed as engaging in a medical procedure or participation in a patient's care other than through documentation, and (2) a scribe should keep their communications limited to non-medical topics (other than open communication with their provider). Always use common sense, but when in doubt, ask: "is this a clinical or nonclinical function?"

Others Performing the Role of the Scribe

Although medical scribing is a nonclinical role, it can also be performed by any appropriately trained clinical personnel.

An obvious and common example of a clinical scribe would be the provider acting as his or her own scribe by "scribing" their encounter with the patient. Providers generally have extensive training and experience in this documentation. They generally know how best to convey the patient's clinical condition for later reference either by themselves or another member of the healthcare team who may need this information for aiding them in future care decisions. Often the provider is not quite as adept at documenting for other "customers" of the EHR. These customers include insurance companies, governmental bodies, quality review agencies, and legal entities.

Scribe training and certification is meant to prepare a cohort of professional scribes who are experts in documentation for all of these "customers."

Certified Nurse Assistants (CNA), Licensed Practical Nurses (LPN), and Medical Assistants (MA) are all good candidates for learning to scribe. Often even Registered Nurses (RN) are utilized as scribes in certain circumstances. Usual patient flow in an office or ED setting would, however, make it difficult to perform both scribing and clinical tasks because these generally happen simultaneously in the efficient healthcare setting.

CASE STUDY 1.1

After earning her medical assistant (MA) certification, Shawna worked for several years in a family physician's office. While she enjoyed all aspects of her work, Shawna quickly realized she liked working around the patients much more than doing the administrative tasks in the office. A colleague told her about the demand for medical scribes in all kinds of settings. "With the added skillset," Shawna's colleague said, "providers and practice managers really see the value of utilizing MAs with scribe training during patient care." With that, Shawna made up her mind to obtain certification as a medical scribe.

It turned out to be one of the best decisions she had ever made. Not long after completing her medical scribe certification, Shawna saw a job posting for a Medical Assistant/Scribe at an otolaryngologist's office. She performs all kinds of tasks at the practice, but the bulk of her day is spent with the providers—documenting exams, procedures, and postsurgical follow-ups.

QUESTIONS
1. What does the otolaryngologist specialize in?
2. What type of provider was Shawna's first employer, the family physician, and what type of patients did the office see?
3. When following the provider, Shawna's primary responsibility is to create the _____ by listening to the provider while he or she is obtaining the patient's medical information.
4. Shawna records all the information about the patient's medical care in a computer system called a(n) _____.
5. What are the professional benefits of obtaining certification?

Practice Questions

These questions are included at the end of most chapters as a self-assessment tool to gauge under-standing of the materials presented. For the most benefit, we suggest that you first try and identify the correct answers without referencing the text. After checking the answer key at the back of the book, return to the text and focus on the topics or concepts of the question(s) that were missed.

1. A(n) _____ is a healthcare professional who diagnoses patients, prescribes medications, and performs surgeries and other procedures according to the treatment plan he or she has developed for the patient.

2. To loosen mucus in the patient's lungs, the provider writes a(n) _____ to instruct the nursing staff to perform chest physical therapy on the patient each morning.

3. Which physician is considered a part of primary care?
   a. radiologist
   b. gerontologist
   c. gastroenterologist
   d. proctologist

4. Which healthcare professional is not considered a provider?
   a. surgeon
   b. physician assistant (PA)
   c. unit clerk
   d. nurse practitioner (NP)

5. A(n) _____ is a physician who treats ailments of the brain and nerves.

6. A(n) _____ is a physician who takes care of heart problems.

7. A(n) _____ is a physician who manages diseases of the urinary system.

8. A(n) _____ is a physician who cares for patients with behavioral health problems.

9. A scribe is the last one leaving a patient room and the patient asks them for a drink of water. The scribe should
   a. get the patient a cup of water.
   b. review the patient's test results to ensure it is safe.
   c. politely excuse themselves from the situation.
   d. ask the provider for permission.

CHAPTER 2

Healthcare Law and Ethics*

LEARNING OBJECTIVES

1. Explain the uses of healthcare documentation for legal and compliance purposes.
2. Differentiate criminal law and civil law and explain the role of healthcare documentation in criminal and civil cases.
3. Define consent, list the types of consent, and document patient consent for treatment.
4. Explain patient privacy and confidentiality and document patient care in accordance with the Health Information Portability and Accountability Act (HIPAA).
5. Define fraud and abuse and explain the relationship of fraud and abuse to healthcare documentation.
6. Discuss ethics and ethical concerns in healthcare.

KEY TERMS

Abuse
Accreditation
Assault
Audit trail
Battery
Breach
Business associate
Compliance
Confidentiality
Conscience clause
Consent
Continuity of care
Covered entity
Defendant
Disclosure
Emergency Medical Treatment and Active Labor Act (EMTALA)

Ethics
Explicit consent
Felony
Fraud
General consent
Health Insurance Portability and Accountability Act (HIPAA)
Implied consent
Informed consent
Kickback
Malpractice
Misdemeanor
Negligence
Office of the Inspector General
Patient Self-Determination Act (PDSA)

Plaintiff
Privacy
Privacy Rule
Protected health information (PHI)
Release of information (ROI)
Security Rule
Standard of care
The Joint Commission (TJC)
Tort
Upcoding
Whistleblower

The medical scribe is working in an industry that is heavily influenced by external forces. In healthcare, insurers and government payers have rules to follow; local, state, and federal governments create laws and regulations; accreditation bodies set standards; and professional organizations expect their members to abide by ethical codes. This chapter surveys the legal and ethical landscape as it pertains to the work of the scribe, specifically healthcare documentation.

*The editors wish to acknowledge Elsevier's *Legal and Ethical Issues for Health Professions,* 4th edition, which informs portions of this chapter.

Healthcare Documentation and Compliance

All the information the scribe and other healthcare professionals gather from the patient is recorded. The primary purpose of health record documentation is to communicate what has been done for the patient and what should be done for the patient, so that the providers of healthcare can use this information to provide quality care for the patient. For clinical staff, the health record serves as a reference for decision making and continuing care. It allows for the **continuity of care** of patients by detailing their evaluation, management, and treatments. Using the record, healthcare professionals can reconstruct each patient's medical encounters from the past to the present (Fig. 2.1).

The health record also has great importance as a legal document. Based on a legal principle called the *business record rule*, health record documentation is admissible in court. This means that if there is a dispute over the care the patient received, the health record serves as the documentation to defend the actions of the provider or healthcare facility, or to prove that the provider or facility did something wrong. The law also requires that complete and accurate documentation be kept as a record of the provider's business dealings.

In addition, the practice of medicine is regulated at all levels of government. For example:

- *Federal* agencies (who often serve as the payer on behalf of the patient) have rules about the care that can be offered to their beneficiaries.
- *States* license healthcare facilities, physicians, other providers, nurses, and other allied health professionals, and also mandate reporting of certain findings, such as child abuse or cases of infectious disease.

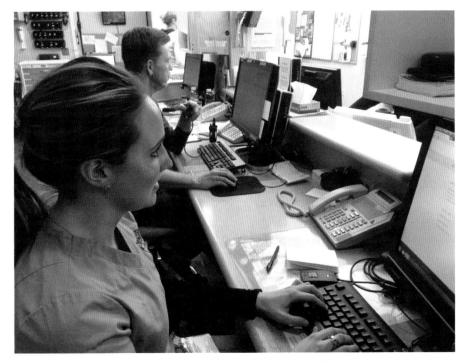

Fig. 2.1   The medical scribe documents in the electronic health record (EHR) so that others can reconstruct each patient's medical encounters from the past to the present. (© ABC Scribes, Inc. Used with permission.)

- *Local* governments can be involved with healthcare when the county facilitates certain services, or when a municipality offers tax savings to a not-for-profit healthcare entity.

At every level, regulators will use health records to monitor *compliance* with their rules. Thus, for the scribe, failure to properly document in the heath record can result in disciplinary action up to and including termination from employment. For the provider, poor documentation can result in fines and loss of licensure.

Compliance, or the adherence to a set of standards, is not only a legal matter. In healthcare, many facilities seek *accreditation* from independent accrediting organizations. **Accreditation** is voluntary, but it is valuable to healthcare facilities because it symbolizes that the organization has achieved a certain level of quality. In addition, earning some types of accreditation satisfies government requirements. There are many accrediting bodies for many different healthcare settings. The most important in the hospital setting is **The Joint Commission (TJC)**, which performs onsite surveys of the facility to monitor whether the facility is adhering to standards. During the visit, TJC surveyors examine patient records to understand how the patient is receiving care, as well as to ensure events are being documented fully and accurately. Hospitals have a *compliance officer* and a *compliance committee* to ensure providers and staff are completing documentation in accordance with regulatory and accreditation standards. Not every hospital will use TJC. There are alternative accrediting bodies such as Healthcare Facilities Accreditation Program (HFAP) that vary somewhat in their approach to ensuring compliance with federal regulations.

Types of Law

In general, there are two main categories of law: civil and criminal. *Civil law* protects the private rights of person or a person's property, whereas *criminal law* protects the rights of society based on government statutes and codes.

CRIMINAL LAW

Violations of criminal laws are called crimes. **Misdemeanors** are lesser crimes punishable usually by monetary fines established by the state, but some misdemeanors may also include imprisonment of 1 year or less. **Felonies** are more serious crimes punishable by larger fines and/or imprisonment for more than 1 year or, in some states, death. In many states, a felony conviction for a healthcare professional also includes the revoking of a license to practice in his or her profession. Two related felonies of interest to the scribe are *assault* and *battery* (Box 2.1). Healthcare professionals are at risk of a charge of assault and battery if they touch a patient without **consent**, or permission. The concept of consent is explored in detail below.

CIVIL LAW

Civil laws are laws that protect the private rights of a person or a person's property. Civil laws include the areas of contracts, property, negligence and malpractice, labor, privacy issues, and family law. A violation of civil law may prompt the supposed victim, the **plaintiff**, to bring a lawsuit to the courts to hold another party, the **defendant**, responsible for a wrongdoing. Civil lawsuits against healthcare professionals often include allegations of failure to provide care that meets the standard of care, resulting in harm or injury to the patient. Penalties in civil law are almost exclusively monetary. The court decides an amount to award for damages. In some cases, the court may order a healthcare professional to stop doing something, such as practicing medicine, to prevent further harm from occurring that money cannot remedy.

A wrongdoing or violation of civil law is called a **tort**. A tort is a private and civil wrong causing an injury. The most common tort against healthcare professionals is for **negligence**, and

---

BOX 2.1 ■ Assault and Battery

An **assault** is the threat of bodily harm that reasonably causes fear of harm in the victim. If the victim has not actually been physically harmed or touched, but only threatened or an attempt was made to harm, the crime is an assault. **Battery** is the unconsented physical contact on another person. For battery to occur, offensive touching is done without permission or consent or in the absence of an emergency situation. Assault and battery are separate crimes, but often occur together, with assault preceding battery.

---

it is the cornerstone of a *malpractice* case. Negligence does not require a specific intent to harm someone and is not a deliberate action, but is the result of an individual or party failing to act in a reasonable way where a duty was owed. **Malpractice** is an act of negligence and describes an improper or illegal professional activity or treatment, often used in regard to a healthcare professional causing an injury to a patient. The negligence might be the result of errors in diagnosis, treatment, postoperative care, or a violation of patient confidentiality. Malpractice requires proof of a breach of a *standard of care*, and the breach must cause damage or harm. In general, the **standard of care** in a medical malpractice case is defined as the type and level of care an ordinary, prudent, healthcare professional, with the same training and experience, would provide under similar circumstances. In other words, the critical question in a medical malpractice case is, "Would a similarly skilled healthcare professional have provided the same treatment under the same, or similar, circumstances?"

NOTE

Scribes are documentarians during the patient encounter, making them natural observers and recorders in the room. The scribe functions as a third-party observer in the room who can verify what the health record says is indeed what was related and what happened.

Some crimes, or violations of criminal law, are also torts, violations of civil law. For instance, a provider who has been accused of the crime of assault and battery may also be sued civilly for assault and battery.

Consent

It is illegal to touch someone without that person's consent. There are many distinct types of consent, but the two primarily related to healthcare are *general consent* and *informed consent*.

GENERAL CONSENT

General consent is an individual's permission to be touched. General consent can be *explicit* or *implied*. **Explicit consent**, also known as express or direct consent, means that an individual is clearly presented with an option to agree or disagree or to express a preference or choice, often verbally or in writing. Explicit consent is usually required when clear, documentable consent is required, and the purpose for which it is being provided for is sensitive, such as the collection, use, or dissemination of personal information. For example, all patients admitted to a hospital are required to sign a general consent form, which grants permission for employees of the hospital to "touch" the patient in order to provide medical care and treatment.

Most of the time, consent is not a formal declaration, but rather implied by the actions of the patient and the provider. This is called **implied consent**. Healthcare professionals routinely obtain implied consent when treating a patient. For example, a provider may ask a patient to roll his sleeve up so an injection may be administered. If the patient rolls his sleeve up, this is implied consent to receive the shot.

INFORMED CONSENT

In healthcare, general consent—even if explicitly given—may not be enough to avoid the risk of a battery charge. A medical battery can be committed in specific situations in which there was consent to perform one particular procedure but a different procedure was performed instead. For example, in the case of *Pizzaloto v. Wilson*, the patient gave consent for the surgeon to perform excisions to remove adhesions and small cysts caused by ovarian endometriosis. During the surgery, the surgeon noted that the patient's reproductive organs had sustained severe damage and determined that the patient was, as a result, sterile. The surgeon proceeded to perform a hysterectomy, removing the patient's uterus and both of her ovaries. When the patient woke up from surgery, she was angry with the actions taken by the surgeon and filed a lawsuit. The court ruled that the patient (plaintiff) was entitled to recover damages and awarded her $10,000 because there was no emergency present and thus the surgeon committed battery because no consent had been given for this specific procedure.

Informed consent is a more formal consent process done before invasive procedures like surgery. In this process, the healthcare provider discusses the reason for the procedure and exactly what it entails so that the patient may make a voluntary choice to accept or refuse treatment. The healthcare provider must detail all possible risks and potential prognoses for having a treatment or procedure performed and the available alternatives. The provider must only perform the procedure as described and within the scope of the informed consent documentation. A signed informed consent form is retained in the patient's health record (Fig. 2.2).

> **NOTE**
>
> In emergency situations, consent—even for invasive procedures—can be implied. The situation must be life-threatening or pose a risk of significant physical injury to the patient if the procedures are not performed. Only those procedures that are absolutely necessary are authorized, and explicit consent should be obtained as soon as possible. Furthermore, only a healthcare provider, such as a physician, can make the determination that a true emergency exists that necessitates proceeding without explicit or informed consent, which will be discussed next.

Privacy and Confidentiality

Careful protection of patient health information has been central to the delivery of healthcare since ancient times. Greek physicians understood that to properly treat the patient, they needed the patient to be honest and complete about the problem and the events that led to it. Of course, the patient would be far less likely to disclose information if he or she thought the physician would tell everyone else about it, especially if the health problem was sensitive or embarrassing. Thus, **confidentiality**, or the careful safeguarding of the patient's health information, has long been a cornerstone of medicine. A similar but distinct concept is **privacy**, the patient's ability to keep health information concealed. The medical scribe is duty-bound to confidentiality, and has a responsibility to protect patient privacy.

In the 1990s, as the healthcare industry began to be computerized, providers started to store certain patient information digitally, and send information electronically to insurance companies and other payers. These new storage and communication methods prompted concerns about the privacy of health information. In 1996, the **Health Insurance Portability and Accountability Act (HIPAA)** was passed in part to address these concerns.

Tingsboro Hospital
Procedure Consent Form

Patient Label

Name

Medical Record #

DOB

Procedure: _____

I,_____, consent to the above treatment procedure as deemed medically necessary by my medical provider. My care provider,_____, has explained to me the nature of my condition, the procedure, the risks and the expected benefits of the above procedure compared with alternative approaches.

My provider has also explained to me the likelihood, and some possible complications of this procedure including, but not limited to, bleeding, infection, loss of limb or organ function, drug reactions or possibly death. I also understand that I may need a blood transfusion during or after this procedure.

I understand that Tingsboro Hospital is a teaching hospital and that students and other trainees may participate in this procedure as permitted by law and hospital policy. I also understand that tissues, blood, body parts or fluid may be removed from the body during the procedure. These materials may be used for diagnostic, therapeutic or research reasons.

Any additional comments:

_____

_____

_____

_____

_____   _____
Signature of Patient   Printed Name

_____   _____
Signature of Provider   Printed Name

Date:_____

Fig. 2.2   Informed consent form. (From Purtilo RB, Doherty RF: *Ethical dimensions in the health professions,* ed 7, St. Louis, 2021, Elsevier.)

HIPAA is a federal law governing all healthcare providers, insurers, and their affiliates. The law has many sections, but its provisions most relevant to the scribe regulate **protected health information (PHI)**, which is any health information that can be linked to an individual. Essentially, HIPAA forbids unnecessarily sharing any health information that can be connected to a person's identity. Furthermore, any patient information that is shared—even among healthcare professionals—is limited to only the information necessary to deliver patient care.

Understanding the HIPAA law is important for anyone who works in healthcare. Healthcare organizations are known as **covered entities**, meaning that the law directly covers their actions. A covered entity must have in place appropriate administrative, technical, and physical safeguards to protect the privacy of protected health information. The law also however extends to other companies that work closely with healthcare organizations, which are called **business associates**. If a covered entity contracts with another company that provides them with a service, and thus may have access to protected health information at any time, the covered entity must have a contract with this other company, the business associate. That contract must state what the business associate will be doing on their behalf, and that the business associate must also comply with HIPAA rules regarding protected health information. An example would be a doctor's office (the "covered entity") which is subject to HIPAA rules, that hires a scribe company (the "business associate") which will have access to protected health information and must sign an agreement outlining their role and responsibilities under HIPAA.

HIPAA legislation has resulted in two rules that are of importance to the medical scribe: the *Privacy Rule* and the *Security Rule*.

PRIVACY RULE

The **Privacy Rule** provides federal protections for any oral, written, or electronic-PHI (e-PHI), and gives patients an array of rights with respect to that information. It limits the **disclosure**, or communication of private information, of this "individually identifiable health information." Health information can be medical history, test and laboratory results, insurance information, demographics, and other data that a healthcare professional collects to identify an individual and determine appropriate care. Patient identifiers include, but are not limited to, the patient's name, birthdate, dates of service, email address, social security number, home address, phone number, and medical record number (MRN). The Privacy Rule limits who gets access to PHI without the patient's express permission. The following scenarios will illustrate this facet of the law.

Example 1: The medical scribe returns home from a long day at work and sits down for dinner with his family. He relates that Ms. Jenkins, a neighbor, was seen in the clinic for a spider bite.

The scribe's actions in this example are a violation of HIPAA, because the scribe is disclosing PHI, health information that can be connected to the identity of an individual. In this case, the health information identified with the patient's name.

Example 2: The medical scribe notices a person who attended her high school in the waiting room of the doctor's office. The scribe is not present for the patient's encounter but is curious about why her high school acquaintance is seeing the physician. The scribe asks a co-worker about the reason for the patient's visit, who tells her it is because the patient has a cold.

In this example, the co-worker is in violation of HIPAA because she disclosed information to the scribe, who did not need to know why the patient was being seen. Similarly, if the scribe had accessed the patient's health record to see why her high school acquaintance was in the office, the scribe would have committed a HIPAA violation. The scribe would have no medical or administrative need to access the patient's health record. All disclosures of PHI must be the *minimum necessary* to deliver patient care.

It is useful to consider an example of how HIPAA would work in an emergency department. A scribe will undoubtedly want to share some of the excitement that occurs in the department when they go home. It is certainly permitted to discuss certain things in a very generic way. For example, if a patient had a collapsed lung and needed a chest tube, then sharing that you got to see a chest tube insertion would be permitted as long as nothing is stated about the patient and only the procedure is discussed. In other words, health information in the absence of patient identifiers is generally not protected information under the law.

On the other hand, if a patient is evaluated for anything that may be reported in the newspapers, then the scribe may not mention anything about the case, lest it be connected with a specific person. A rape case would be an example. This is a forensic or legal case and a public record will be available for that reason, making it very likely that anything a scribe might say about the case could be tied to an individual. A celebrity seen in the emergency department would also be a case that could not be discussed, even indirectly. When in doubt, keep it to yourself.

Example 3: The medical scribe is attending a pool party with friends, and the conversation turns to the use of sunscreen. The scribe relates that he is always careful about sun protection, and that once they had a patient who was so badly sunburned that he had to be hospitalized.

Is Example 3 a HIPAA violation? Because the health information is not connected in any way to an identifier, the scribe has not broken the law.

The patient's privacy may also be violated through carelessness. Even when there is a legitimate need to communicate about the patient, healthcare professionals must be cautious not to reveal health information to others in earshot. When care needs to be discussed, the conversation should happen in private work areas, not in hallways or other public areas where others may overhear. Any printed documentation must not be left unattended. For example, a printout of a patient's laboratory results is, after all, classified as PHI: it will have many patient identifiers at the top of the page, and the rest of the document is health data. Similarly, computer screens should never be left unattended, and the scribe must log out of the system immediately after use. Should a passerby see the information on the computer screen, this would also be a HIPAA violation.

HIPAA protections of PHI extend to the patient's own healthcare providers, and even to the patient's closest friends and family. A blood relationship and even marriage does not entitle a person to the patient's health information (with certain exceptions among parents and their minor children). Of course, patients can choose to have information disclosed to whomever they choose. Patients regularly authorize disclosure to spouses, family, and other physicians. Fig. 2.3 is an example of a **release of information (ROI)** form the patient that they may sign to allow the healthcare organization to disclose his or her health record.

There are some permitted disclosures of PHI that do not require direct authorization from the patient. Some of these circumstances include sharing information in order to obtain payment or reimbursement for healthcare services, or to perform any necessary healthcare activities like the patient's treatment plan or any operation necessary for business. (Treatment, payment, or healthcare operations are collectively known as TPO.) Even though these are permitted disclosures under the law, most facilities will request that the patient sign a consent form authorizing the organization to use and disclose PHI for these purposes (Fig. 2.4).

Researchers are also allowed to access and use protected health information when necessary to conduct research. HIPAA only applies to research if the research is actively being used in patient care in such a way that the researcher is establishing a provider-patient relationship with the patient. In those cases, it crosses the boundary from pure research into the realm of treatment, which is thus covered by HIPAA.

SECURITY RULE

The second important HIPAA provision is the **Security Rule**, which requires all covered entities to enact measures to protect the confidentiality of patient health data. Covered entities must use technical and non-technical safeguards to secure electronic protected health information (ePHI). This includes:

- *Administrative safeguards*—training for employees on HIPAA, confidentiality, and security, and disciplinary actions for employees who violate the law. These include policies for

MEDICAL RECORD	Authorization for the Release of Medical Information

INSTRUCTIONS: Complete this form in its entirety and forward the original to the address below:

NATIONAL INSTITUTES OF HEALTH
MEDICAL RECORD DEPARTMENT
ATTN: MEDICOLEGAL SECTION
10 CENTER DRIVE, ROOM 1N208   TELEPHONE: (301) 496-3331
MSC1192   FACSIMILE: (301) 480-9982
BETHESDA, MD 20892-1192

IDENTIFYING INFORMATION:

Patient Name	Daytime Telephone	Date of Birth

REQUEST INFORMATION: Information is to be released to the following individual or party:

Name	Telephone
Address	

The purpose or need for disclosure (charges will be determined based on purpose of disclosure):

Date Range of Information to be Released: from _____ to _____

Please check specific information to be released:

☐ Discharge Summary   ☐ Radiology Reports   ☐ EKG Reports
☐ History & Physical   ☐ Radiology Films   ☐ Echocardiogram Reports
☐ Operative Reports   ☐ Tissue Exam Reports   ☐ Heart Diagnostic Reports
☐ Outpatient Progress Notes   ☐ Tissue Slides   ☐ Nuclear Medicine Reports
☐ Length of Stay Verification ☐ Lab Results   ☐ Nuclear Medicine Scans

☐ Other (Please Specify): _____

AUTHORIZATION: Permission is hereby granted to the Warren Grant Magnuson Clinical Center to release medical information to the individual/organization as identified above.
(Note: submission of this form authorizes the release of the information specified within one year from date of signature.)

Patient/Authorized Signature	Print Name	Date

If other than patient, specify relationship: _____

Patient Identification	Authorization for the Release of Medical Information NIH-527 (02-01) P.A. 09-25-0099 File in Section 4: Correspondence

Fig. 2.3 National Institutes of Health (NIH) release of information authorization form. (From Clinical Center, National Institutes of Health, US Department of Health and Human Services. In Pepper JK, Beik JI: *Health insurance today: a practical approach*, ed 7, St. Louis, 2021, Elsevier.)

managing user passwords, such as how often they must be changed, and disciplinary actions for sharing passwords with others.

■ ***Technical safeguards***—control of access to electronic systems. Included here are user roles within computer systems that only allow a person access to certain parts of the electronic health record (EHR). Other technical safeguards are automatic logoffs

COLLEGE CLINIC
4567 Broad Avenue
Woodland Hills, XY 12345-0001
Phone: 555/486-9002
Fax: 555/487-8976

CONSENT TO THE USE AND DISCLOSURE OF HEALTH INFORMATION

I understand that this organization originates and maintains health records which describe my health history, symptoms, examination, test results, diagnoses, treatment, and any plans for future care or treatment. I understand that this information is used to:

- plan my care and treatment.
- communicate among health professionals who contribute to my care.
- apply my diagnosis and services, procedures, and surgical information to my bill.
- verify services billed by third-party payers.
- assess quality of care and review the competence of health care professionals in routine health care operations.

I further understand that:

- a complete description of information uses and disclosures is included in a *Notice of Information Practices* which has been provided to me.
- I have a right to review the notice prior to signing this consent.
- the organization reserves the right to change their notice and practices.
- any revised notice will be mailed to the address I have provided prior to implementation.
- I have the right to object to the use of my health information for directory purposes.
- I have the right to request restrictions as to how my health information may be used or disclosed to carry out treatment, payment, or health care operations.
- the organization is not required to agree to the restrictions requested.
- I may revoke this consent in writing, except to the extent that the organization has already taken action in reliance thereon.

☐ I request the following restrictions to the use or disclosure of my health information.

_____

_____   _____
Date   Notice Effective Date

_____   _____
Signature of Patient or Legal Representative   Witness

_____   _____
Signature   Title

Date _____   __ Accepted __ Rejected

Fig. 2.4   An example of a consent form used to disclose and use health information for treatment, payment, or healthcare operations (TPO). This is not required under the Health Information Portability and Accountability Act (HIPAA), but you may find that some healthcare organizations use it. (From Smith LM: *Fordney's medical insurance*, ed 15, St. Louis, 2020, Elsevier.)

when the computer is idle for a certain amount of time, and the encryption of transmitted information.

- *Physical safeguards*—measures taken to protect against unauthorized access and natural and environmental hazards (like floods). Computer hardware is physically locked, and equipment such as data storage servers are kept in locked rooms.

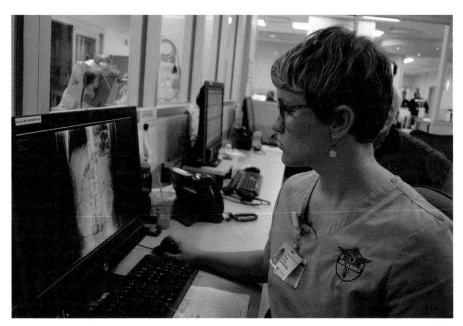

Fig. 2.5 The computer monitor on which this medical scribe is working does not face the hallway; it is oriented toward the work area. This is an example of a physical safeguard preventing others from seeing the information on the computer screen. (© ABC Scribes, Inc. Used with permission.)

Computer monitors are oriented in ways that the screen cannot be seen by others (Fig. 2.5).

Specifically, covered entities must (according to CMS) ensure the "confidentiality, integrity, and availability" of all e-PHI they create, receive, maintain or transmit. In short, the healthcare entity must take all reasonable precautions against any potential violation of the privacy of the patient's medical record that could be anticipated.

BREACHES

If there is ever a **breach** of security of a patient's protected health information, that patient must be notified. Larger breaches, such as hacks into the computer system, require notification of media outlets.

As members of the healthcare team, scribes are always subject to HIPAA laws. Violations of HIPAA may result in large fines and time in jail. Unintentional violations may include an unattended computer that is logged into the EHR, or papers with patient information left in a workspace or discarded in the waste bin (instead of the shred bin). A scribe should also avoid sharing protected health information about a patient unnecessarily, discussing protected health information in a public area, looking-up information about a patient that is not pertinent for the job, browsing through one's own medical records or the records of friends or family, or even sharing that the patient was seen in any medical facility.

PERSONAL PRIVACY

Not only should the scribe follow the rules set by HIPAA, the scribe should also be cognizant of a patient's personal privacy. In the emergency room for example, many patients are asked to change into gowns and stay in rooms separated from the rest of the department by glass doors and/or curtains. Please remember to be considerate of a patient's privacy when entering or exiting a room, and shut the door or curtain. A good rule of thumb in respecting a patient's privacy is to consider how you would like to be treated if you were in their shoes (or wearing their gown)!

Fraud and Abuse

Fraud is the intentional act to misrepresent facts or mislead for financial gain. **Abuse** in healthcare is a reckless disregard or conduct that goes against acceptable business and/or medical practices resulting in greater reimbursement.

Fraud directly relates to medical documentation, because it is an intentional misrepresentation, deception, or act of deceit for the purpose of receiving greater reimbursement. The provider is paid based on the documented services, therefore if the documentation is falsified, a provider can receive higher levels of compensation. Examples of fraud include billing for services not provided, or **upcoding** services to gain larger reimbursement for services provided. Fraud is often obvious, but sometimes it is less obvious and providers or beneficiaries may unknowingly do things that constitute fraud. Therefore, it is important to know some of the pitfalls involved. Some examples of fraud include:

- billing for supplies not used or services not rendered
- providing or billing for unnecessary services
- upcoding, or billing for a higher level of service than that provided
- frequently incorrectly coding a service
- misrepresenting dates or duration of service
- altering medical records to hide something or otherwise falsifying information
- forging prescriptions
- waiving deductibles

It is also fraudulent to document signs or symptoms that a patient does not have in order to obtain insurance coverage for a service.

Violations of key federal fraud and abuse laws can be either civil or criminal offenses. Fraud can lead to, for example, healthcare professionals and medical billing and coding personnel incurring fines, loss of license, and even imprisonment. It is important to note that it is the attempt at deceit that is fraud, regardless of whether it is successful. As an employee in any healthcare organization, it is important to understand that the penalties for committing fraud and abuse are levied not just on the provider but may also be levied on the employer. Staff can also be subject to fines and imprisonment if they take part in a fraudulent activity, even if they were only following the provider's or employer's direction.

> **NOTE**
>
> As we will see in Chapter 4, The Health Record and Notes, each contributor to the EHR has his or her own unique login/credentials. Any actions performed in the EHR under this username is tracked, along with a date and time stamp. In addition, the EHR records the date and time whenever an addendum or other change is made to the record, as well as the changes that were made. Every action leaves an **audit trail**, a record of every individual who accessed the record and what they did. The audit trail is used to help identify fraud, as well as HIPAA violations.

It should be obvious that there are huge sums of money involved in healthcare. Since a large portion of that is administered by the government through Medicare and Medicaid, they have a legitimate interest in safeguarding their investment and that of the taxpayer when it comes to doling out the funds to administer healthcare. Government auditors monitor for inadequate or unnecessary medical procedures and treatments, **kickbacks** to healthcare professionals, and overcharging for Medicare and Medicaid programs.

The job of the government's auditors is to make sure that money is not lost through fraud. The **Office of the Inspector General (OIG)** is tasked with protecting the integrity of Health and Human Services (HHS) programs, like Medicare. They will often take tips from **whistleblowers** who provide the government information about fraud in the medical professions.

Other Federal Legislation for the Medical Scribe

EMERGENCY MEDICAL TREATMENT AND ACTIVE LABOR ACT (EMTALA)

The medical scribe is likely to encounter situations that are influenced by the law known as or the **Emergency Medical Treatment and Active Labor Act (EMTALA)**. This law mostly affects care delivered in the emergency department (ED). It was enacted in 1986 to prevent EDs from refusing to treat patients presenting at the hospital with an emergency medical condition, or transferring unstable patients to another facility. Before EMTALA, some facilities were accused of "patient dumping," transferring a patient based on a potentially high-cost diagnosis, or refusing to treat a patient based on his or her ability to pay.

CASE STUDY 2.1

Devon works for a medical scribe company that has just been contracted to provide scribing services to an ambulatory surgery center. Rather than requiring the patients stay in the hospital overnight, in an ambulatory surgery center, the procedures performed are all completed within a few hours. The physicians at the facility perform many different surgeries, ranging from joint repairs, to vasectomies, to eye surgery. In Devon's job as a medical scribe, he completes the operative reports in the EHR per the physician's instructions, and checks to make sure other documentation is complete and accurate.

Since he began at the surgery center, Devon has worked hard to make sure all his documentation meets compliance standards. The facility's administrators are expecting their biannual survey from TJC any time now, and everyone wants to make sure the records are in excellent shape.

QUESTIONS
1. TJC is a(n)
   a. federal agency.
   b. state agency.
   c. accreditation agency.
   d. professional association.
2. Before undergoing surgery, the provider will explain the procedure, and the patient will be required to sign a(n) _____ form.
   a. general consent
   b. release of information
   c. informed consent
   d. privacy
3. Which is a breach of PHI?
   a. In the office workspace, Devon asks a physician for clarification about the type of suturing used during a surgery.
   b. The nurse yells out a patient's name in the waiting room to call them back for their procedure.
   c. Devon tells his grandmother that he had the chance to witness a cataract surgery a few weeks ago.
   d. One of Devon's coworkers leaves the portable computer station in the exam room without logging off.
4. A patient developed an infection after undergoing a hysterectomy at the surgical center. The patient is taking legal action against the surgeon and the ambulatory surgery center. In the court proceedings, the patient is the _____, while the provider is the _____.
5. During the trial, the patient's attorneys suggest that, although the documentation of the surgical procedure shows no wrongdoing, it is possible that someone altered the record to hide problems. What EHR function would prove that no one altered the health record?

EMTALA requires the facility perform a medical screening exam. The facility must provide stabilizing treatment and ensure the patient is in stable condition before transfer, regardless of the patient's legal status, citizenship, or ability to pay. If the facility cannot adequately treat the patient, a patient (or his or her legal representative) must agree to any intrahospital transfer and be advised as to the reason for the proposed transfer. Whenever a patient is transferred from one hospital to another, there is documentation that is required to ensure compliance with this law. The scribe may well be asked to assist in this documentation. Most hospitals will have a form that they use specifically for this purpose to ensure that all documentation requirements are met.

PATIENT SELF-DETERMINATION ACT (PDSA)

The **Patient Self-Determination Act (PDSA)** requires that adult patients be informed of their right to accept or decline any medical or surgical treatment. It also provides that they be advised of their right to have an **advance directive** describing the care they would like to receive in the event they become *incapacitated*, or unable to understand or communicate in a time of need. With an advance directive, the patient can dictate ahead of time what types of care and services he or she wishes to receive. One type of advance directive is also known as a *living will*, which contains instructions about the types of life-sustaining treatments, such as mechanical ventilation or tube feeding, that should be administered or withheld in the case of a terminal illness. The living will may include a *do not resuscitate (DNR)* indicating the patient does not wish to receive CPR. Another type of advance directive is a *durable power of attorney* in which instead of specifying the care that they want, the patient specifies an alternate person who would be given the responsibility of making these decisions for them, often another family member (perhaps with medical training) or a trusted friend.

These forms often vary state to state. Although it would be unusual for a scribe to be involved in recording these types of documents, being aware of their existence and being able to document that a patient's advance directives were utilized in the medical decision-making process is valuable.

Ethics

Ethics are a belief system about what behaviors are acceptable. A scribe is not considered to be clinical personnel, meaning that they are only responsible for the documentation and should otherwise not function in any clinical manner. However, because the medical scribe is working within a medical environment they should expect to encounter the occasional ethical dilemma.

Some examples specific to the medical community may include end-of-life issues including, physician-assisted death. Religious affiliations may affect healthcare choices and go against the accepted community norms. For example, Jehovah's Witnesses have religious objections to receiving blood transfusions or blood products in treatment. Also there will be different choices surrounding abortion and organ donation. Although it is natural for the medical scribe to have their own opinions regarding these matters, the scribe will never be held responsible for decisions in specific cases.

The **conscience clause**, also known as medical conscience or conscientious objection, is a legislative provision that relieves a person from compliance or duty based on moral or other personal beliefs. In healthcare, the conscience clause is the refusal to perform a legal role or duty because of personal beliefs. It permits healthcare professionals—physicians, pharmacists, nurses, and other healthcare professionals—to not provide certain medical services for reasons of personal beliefs. The conscience clause constitutionally permits private hospitals and healthcare facilities—and physicians, nurses, and other employees—to refuse to perform or participate in medical procedures for "ethical, moral, religious, or professional reasons." However, in public hospitals and healthcare facilities, the conscience clause does not apply. In addition some hospitals may have their own conscience clause where a healthcare professional may refuse to perform or participate in a procedure as long as there is another staff member to take over the duty.

Practice Questions

1. A provider may have committed _____ if he or she did not obtain consent to treat the patient.

2. _____ is an act of negligence and describes an improper or illegal professional activity or treatment, often used in regard to a healthcare professional causing an injury to a patient.

3. _____ consent is neither verbalized nor written, but it is an understood agreement by both parties.

4. The unlawful communication of private information is a(n) _____.

5. Which HIPAA rule requires the organization to construct safeguards to protect the confidentiality of electronic protected health information?
   a. Security Rule
   b. Portability Rule
   c. Patient Safety Rule
   d. Privacy Rule

6. Under HIPAA, a scribe company that is employed by a hospital is considered a(n)
   a. plaintiff.
   b. covered entity.
   c. business associate.
   d. auditor.

7. _____ is a type of fraud where documents are misrepresented to bill for a higher reimbursement than the services actually provided.

8. The _____ is a legislative provision that relieves a person from compliance or duty based on moral or other personal beliefs.

Scribe Safety and Infection Control

1. Describe the measures to ensure scribe safety in the healthcare setting.
2. Discuss infection control measures in the healthcare setting.

Antiseptic

Cough etiquette

Disinfection

Don

Hand hygiene

Isolation

Pathogen

Personal protective
equipment (PPE)

Respirator

Sanitization

Standard precautions

Sterile

Sterilization

Sterile technique

Transmission-based
precautions

Scribe Safety

A scribe may be faced with different types of security challenges in the healthcare setting. The most dangerous area of all would be the emergency department (ED). Violent criminals, their victims, and psychotic patients all tend to come to the emergency department. Many patients have impaired behavior due to alcohol or other substances as well.

Most EDs will have some sort of security personnel present. Security personnel become involved in any dangerous situation. Be aware of your facility's security plan and any role you might be required to play. In theory, your physician will know these things. But in practice, they could be new or a *locum tenens* (temporarily in the area to fill a vacant position), and thus will not be as familiar with that ED as someone who has been there many years.

There are a few general safety rules to which a scribe should adhere. If a patient is known to be potentially dangerous, the physician should excuse the scribe from having to enter that room. As a non-essential person, the scribe ought not be unnecessarily exposed to risk. If the scribe is in a room with a psychotic or otherwise cognitively impaired or potentially violent patient, the scribe should always be standing between the patient and the door. This positioning allows the scribe to avoid "going through the patient" to exit the room. In a trauma or major resuscitation room, the scribe should be unobtrusive while recording the events and avoid being in the way of many essential clinical personnel who will be coming and going.

Infection Control

Safety in the hospital setting encompasses more than just security situations. Working in a medical setting (especially in a hospital), the scribe must be aware of exposure to infectious disease.

Healthcare facilities are home to many viruses and resistant bacterial strains. Medical settings are conducive to the spread of microorganisms because of the many sick people who are treated in them. Controlling the spread of these **pathogens** is important both to protect patients, many of whom are at higher risk because of reduced immunologic function, and also to protect healthcare workers.

STANDARD PRECAUTIONS

Accurate identification of all patients carrying infectious diseases is difficult. However, it is neither practical nor necessary to know whether each and every patient has an infectious disease. Instead, healthcare workers regularly employ **standard precautions**, infection control measures in place when caring for *all* patients. Standard precautions assume that all patients are carrying bloodborne pathogens and are therefore treated as such. The guidelines apply to

- blood
- all body fluids, secretions, and excretions except sweat, regardless of whether they contain visible blood
- nonintact skin
- mucous membranes (such as eyes or mouth)

Measures included in standard precautions are based on creating barriers between the infectious microorganisms that prevent them from entering the body of the healthcare worker, or prevent healthcare workers from transferring them around the facility on their bodies or other objects. Standard precautions use *hand hygiene*, *personal protective equipment (PPE)*, *cough etiquette*, and common-sense behavior to stop the spread of germs.

Hand Hygiene

Hand hygiene is the single most important preventive technique that healthcare workers can use to interrupt the infectious process. Hand hygiene can be traditional handwashing with soap and water, or it can be using alcohol-based foam. Handwashing is recommended when the hands are visibly soiled or after exposure to known or suspected infectious material, but the cleaning of hands with an alcohol-based hand rub or foam is preferred in most situations. This includes when entering and exiting a new patient's room ("foam-in, foam-out"; Fig. 3.1). Healthcare workers also perform hand hygiene immediately after gloves are removed, between patient contacts, and when otherwise indicated to prevent transfer of microorganisms to other patients or environments.

Personal Protective Equipment (PPE)

Standard precautions guide use of **personal protective equipment (PPE)**—gloves, masks, eye protection, and gowns—when in contact with patients. Gloves are **donned** (put on) when there is a potential for touching blood, body fluids, secretions, excretions, and contaminated items. They create a barrier between the potentially infectious material and the healthcare worker's hands. Other types of PPE are donned depending on the type of patient care encounter. For example, a healthcare worker would don a gown and eye protection if she is treating a patient with infectious diarrhea (Fig. 3.2).

Cough Etiquette

Cough etiquette is concerned with containing potentially infectious respiratory secretions. Healthcare workers and patients should cover their mouths and noses with a tissue when sneezing or coughing. Hand hygiene is performed after the hands are used to cover the mouth and nose, including after blowing the nose. If a tissue is not available, one should cough or sneeze into the elbow, remaining aware that there may now be pathogens in that location which could be spread to others.

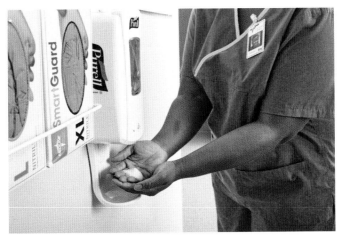

Fig. 3.1 A healthcare worker uses alcohol-based hand rub when entering the patient's room. (Potter PA, Perry AG, Stockert PA, Hall AM: *Fundamentals of nursing*, ed 10, St. Louis, 2021, Elsevier.)

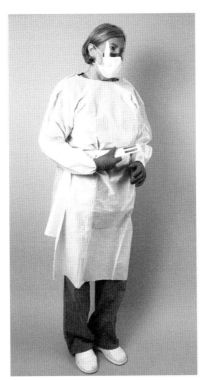

Fig. 3.2 A healthcare worker donning gloves, gown, mask, and face shield. (From Garrels M: *Laboratory and diagnostic testing in ambulatory care: a guide for health care professionals*, ed 4, St. Louis, 2019, Elsevier.)

TRANSMISSION-BASED PRECAUTIONS

Some infectious disease patients may be identified as "higher risk" and have additional safety precautions. **Transmission-based precautions** are used in addition to standard precautions around patients known or suspected to have certain types of infections, resulting in the patient being placed in **isolation**, away from other patients. The disease-specific approach falls into one of three isolation categories:

- *Contact precautions*—pathogens transmitted by direct patient contact or by contact with items in the patient's environment
- *Droplet precautions*—pathogens transmitted by large particle droplets
- *Airborne precautions*—pathogens transmitted by airborne droplet nuclei

Healthcare workers may be required to wear PPE, like a gown, gloves, eye protection, and a mask while in the room. Sometimes they will also need to wear shoe covers and leggings. A **respirator** (air filtration mask) may be required in some cases. Because scribes are considered as nonessential personnel, meaning their presence in the room is not necessary for patient care, there is no reason for a scribe to enter the room of a high-risk patient.

BLOODBORNE PATHOGENS

Because the medical setting is a workplace, the federal government's Occupational Safety and Health Administration (OSHA) has established standards designed protect workers from infectious diseases. OSHA's Bloodborne Pathogen standard requires employers to supply workers with PPE. The rules also require that the employer make available vaccinations against Hepatitis B.

Hospitals will require that anyone working in the facility be vaccinated or tested for some other common illnesses (e.g. tetanus, influenza, and tuberculosis). These requirements vary between healthcare facilities, but OSHA requires that employers offer postexposure evaluation and care to any worker who experiences an exposure incident.

Although a scribe should never have to worry about touching body fluids, there is still a risk of exposure associated with being in any healthcare setting. For example, if body fluids land on intact skin, the area should be washed, but otherwise poses no concern for transmission of infectious disease. If a patient's bodily fluids come into contact with a break in the skin or with mucous membranes (like the eyes or mouth), the scribe should ask their provider or charge nurse what the policy is regarding how to proceed.

INFECTION CONTROL MEASURES

The medical setting uses different terms to describe the level of cleanliness in different areas of the facility. Although the scribe is not responsible for implementing these measures, all healthcare workers are expected to understand them.

Cleaning is the removal of foreign substances, such as soil and organic material, from objects. Generally, cleaning involves the use of water and mechanical action with or without detergents. Another word for cleaning is **sanitization**.

Disinfection is the process of destroying microorganisms. This terminology most often refers to processes that kill pathogens but not their more resistant spores. The agent used is called a *disinfectant*. Usually, when we speak about disinfection we are talking about objects and surfaces.

Antiseptics are a means to destroy or inhibit the growth of microorganisms. An antiseptic agent is applied to the human skin or mucous membrane. Alcohol and chlorhexidine gluconate are antiseptics commonly used in healthcare.

Decontamination is the destruction of microorganisms from an object or surface so that it is safe to handle, touch, or use.

CASE STUDY 3.1

Seibei began training as a medical scribe because of his strong interest in the medical field and a desire to put his organizational skills to work. He studied hard, and it was not long before he landed a position at one of the city hospitals, working in the emergency department. There, he follows the providers in a fast-paced environment, one where people are working together to handle countless situations — including many surprises — with professionalism and flexibility. Seibei thinks he might study nursing someday soon, but for now, he cannot imagine doing anything else!

QUESTIONS

1. A father brings his son into the ED straight from a soccer game with a long laceration along the boy's forehead. Seibei accompanies the provider to collect information about the accident. What will the provider do upon entering the room?
   a. Apply a foam hand rub
   b. Lock the door
   c. Don a gown
   d. Wash his hands
2. The provider will examine the patient and likely clean the wound before suturing it shut. According to standard precautions, what PPE will the provider don before touching the wound?
   a. None
   b. Gloves
   c. Goggles
   d. Gown
3. While Seibei is in the work area finalizing the H&P note, a coworker is complaining that she has a bad cough. Which statement made by the coworker is incorrect?
   a. "I make sure to cover my mouth and nose when I cough."
   b. "I cough into a tissue and then throw the tissue in the trash."
   c. "I wear gloves when I cough to prevent spreading germs."
   d. "I wash my hands after I cover my mouth."
4. Seibei accompanies the provider to examine a patient brought to the hospital by the police. The man crashed his car into a fast food restaurant. When the police explained to the man that he was being arrested, the man said that he wanted to kill himself. Where in the room should Seibei stand while documenting the patient encounter?
   a. Between the patient and the exit
   b. At the head of the patient's bed, opposite the provider
   c. At the foot of the bed
   d. Between the patient and the provider
5. What vaccination did Seibei receive before starting his job at the hospital?
   a. Bacterial pneumonia
   b. Tuberculosis
   c. Shingles
   d. Hepatitis B

Sterilization is the process of destroying all microorganisms and their spores. This can be done chemically or by using intense heat and pressure, such as in an *autoclave*. The **autoclave** is a machine that sterilizes surgical instruments.

STERILE TECHNIQUE

A patient in surgery is especially prone to infectious disease because the body's natural barrier against microorganisms, the skin, is broken. The surgical incision can introduce pathogens into tissues of the body where there are few defenses against them. In the operating room and other areas where invasive procedures are performed, efforts are made to create a **sterile** environment, one that is free of all microorganisms. The methods used to destroy all microorganisms and keep them away from the exposed patient are collectively known as **sterile technique**. For example, sterile gloves, gowns, and drapes are used to create a barrier between the environment (which includes members of the healthcare team) and the patient (Fig. 3.3). All of the surgical instruments used during the procedure are sterile.

The healthcare worker strives to avoid passage of infectious disease agents from the ill patient to the healthcare worker, and also from the healthcare worker to the patient. This is best done by observing and staying clear of areas with instruments and surgical items that are opened from a sealed package, as surgical items are always sterile prior to use (Fig. 3.4). In addition, any area of the patient that is draped in preparation for a procedure is likely to be sterile. The provider will wash hands and use packaged (sterile) gloves before approaching these areas. This should be recognized as another clue to the area and instruments being sterile. Frequently sterile equipment and areas will be identifiable by the color of the drape or packaging, surgical blue, although this is not universal. The scribe should stand back from these areas. He or she should not touch anything on the sterile field (Fig. 3.5), lean over it, or even cough or sneeze in the direction of the sterile field (use "cough and cover").

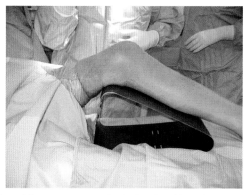

Fig. 3.3   The patient is draped for surgery to repair a broken leg. (From Sheth NP, Lonner JH: *Gowned and gloved orthopaedics: introduction to common procedures*, Philadelphia, 2009, Saunders/Elsevier.)

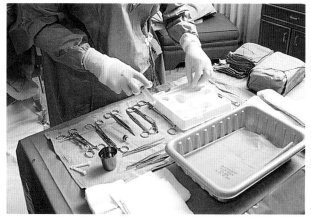

Fig. 3.4   Sterile instruments opened from their packages in preparation for a procedure (in this case, a vaginal birth.) (From Murray S, McKinney E, Holub KS, Jones R: *Foundations of maternal-newborn and women's health nursing*, ed 7, St. Louis, 2019, Elsevier.)

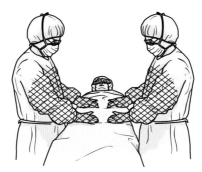

Fig. 3.5   The sterile field. (From Hornacky A, Phillips N: *Berry & Kohn's operating room technique*, ed 14, St. Louis, Elsevier, 2021.)

There are several rules that must be followed during sterile procedures to limit patient exposure to microorganisms while the skin barrier is compromised during the procedure. If a scribe is observing a procedure in which their provider is participating or leading, the scribe must also be adherent to these rules, which include the following:

1. All articles in a sterile field are sterile.
2. Persons who are sterile touch only sterile articles.
3. Persons who are unsterile touch only unsterile articles.
4. Sterile persons avoid leaning over unsterile areas and vice versa.
5. If in doubt, do not touch.

Practice Questions

1. A(n) _____ is a microorganism that causes disease.

2. Gloves, gowns, respirators and facemasks, and eye protection are all types of _____.

3. _____ are used in addition to standard precautions around patients known or suspected to have certain types of infections, resulting in the patient being placed in isolation, away from other patients.

4. The federal agency responsible for the Bloodborne Pathogen standard is the _____ _____.

5. The term _____ refers to the process of destroying all microorganisms and their spores.

6. In the surgical suite, instruments wrapped in packages are considered _____ _____.

PART II

Health Record Documentation

CHAPTER 4

The Health Record and Notes

1. Explain the importance of accurate and complete healthcare documentation and list the uses of healthcare documentation.
2. Define the electronic health record and explain its functions.
3. List and explain the components of a health record.
4. Discuss medical coding and explain the uses of various code sets.

KEY TERMS

Algorithm

Attending note

Centers for Medicare and Medicaid Services (CMS)

Claim

Clinical decision support (CDS)

Coding

Computerized physician order entry (CPOE)

Continuity of care

Current Procedural Terminology (CPT)

Diagnosis

Electronic health record (EHR)

Evaluation and management (E/M) code

Health record

International Classification of Diseases, 10th Revision, Clinic Modification (ICD-10-CM)

Level of service (LOS)

Litigation

Medicaid

Medicare

Objective

Operative note

Order

Outcome

Problem list

Problem-oriented charting

Progress note

Provider note

Quality

Reimbursement

Revenue cycle

Sign

SOAP note

Subjective

Symptom

Therapy

Third-party payer

Trauma note

Treatment plan

Value-based purchasing

Health Documentation and its Uses

As discussed in Chapter 2, medical professionals rely on complete and accurate documentation of patient care. All the data about the patient and the care he or she obtained is documented in the **health record**. The patient's identifying information, medical history, laboratory results, diagnoses, medications, problems, and procedures and other services received are all recorded here. The purpose of the health record is to communicate the services rendered and the plan of care to others.

USE IN PATIENT CARE

Primarily, the health record is used to guide patient care. For example, a physician records his findings in the record so that other physicians, nurses, and the rest of the healthcare team can refer to the patient's health history and execute the provider's plan of care. The provider also documents in the health record so that she can review it during the next patient encounter. The safe and effective delivery of healthcare over time is called the **continuity of care**, which is only possible through complete and accurate documentation.

For the purposes of patient care, the contents of the health record inform the decisions providers and others make about the best way to care for the patient. Without the information in the health record, providers are likely to order duplicate laboratory tests and imaging, or try **therapies** that have already been tried, or administer a medication that causes an adverse reaction. The health record is also the location of the **treatment plan**, containing the provider's instructions for how to care for the patient. The provider's plan guides the activities of nurses and other members of the care team. Nurses use the record to know what to do, and they also document their own activities here. Without the record, a nurse might think someone else already administered a medication to a patient, resulting in a missed dose—or he might not know that another nurse already gave the patient her medication, resulting in a double dose! These examples illustrate that the health record is the cornerstone of the efficient, safe, and effective delivery of healthcare.

USE IN COMPLIANCE

Chapter 2 introduced some of the many legal and accreditation agencies whose rules and regulations govern the delivery of healthcare. Because the health record documents all the information collected during the patient's care, oversight agencies can review the record to understand how healthcare professionals at the facility are delivering care. For example, auditors use the records to see the length of time the patient stayed in the facility, the treatments offered for each **diagnosis** or problem, and whether a patient had to return for treatment of the same issue.

USE IN LITIGATION

The health record is also evidence that can be used on behalf of the patient and the healthcare provider in a legal dispute, called **litigation**. The documentation is admissible evidence in court. It may support the patient's case against the healthcare provider, or defend the healthcare provider's actions (see Chapter 2).

USE IN REIMBURSEMENT

The ways in which providers and facilities are compensated for their services is complicated and beyond the scope of this text. However, because of the key role played by documentation in **reimbursement** (the payment for healthcare services) some background information is appropriate.

In days gone by, paying for healthcare was not all that different from going to an auto mechanic. The physician saw the patient, explained what might be wrong, treated the problem, and billed the patient. The patient paid the bill. Today, very few patients are solely responsible for their medical bills. Instead, most patients have a **third-party payer** who pays the provider for all or part of the services rendered. Insurance companies are one type of third-party payer. Others include federal and state government agencies. In fact, the largest payer in the United States is the **Centers for Medicare and Medicaid Services (CMS)**, which administers **Medicare** and **Medicaid**.

NOTE

The Centers for Medicare and Medicaid Services (CMS) is so large and influential that many of its rules for patient care are also followed by private health insurers.

When a provider or facility has completed a patient care episode, in most instances they work directly with the third-party payer to obtain payment. In a series of processes called the **revenue cycle**, medical billing personnel gather the information about the services provided and submit a **claim** to the payer, requesting reimbursement. The payer reviews the claim and pays all or part of the amount, depending on the payer's agreements with both the provider and the patient. In some cases, the patient is responsible for an additional amount that was not reimbursed by the third-party payer.

Every part of the revenue cycle is dependent on the documentation in the health record. Medical billing staff use the information recorded by the provider and scribe to complete an accurate and comprehensive claim to the payer. The payer may review the health record to ensure the services provided are covered under the patient's policy. Payers also refer to the record to validate the *medical necessity* of the service. As you will learn in Chapter 8, Orders and Disposition Documentation, the payer is only interested in paying for healthcare services that are necessary to treat the patient's problems. Referring to the health record, the payer ensures the diagnostic services and treatments rendered are warranted by the patient's healthcare needs, represented by the diagnosis as determined by the provider. Payers will not reimburse providers for any services that are not completely supported by the health record.

USE IN RESEARCH AND PUBLIC POLICY

The data in the health record is also used for research and to shape public health policy. Medical researchers can use records to see how well treatments are working, compile statistics on risk factors for disease, and gather data to support new therapies. State departments of health monitor the health of the population through documentation. They track births, deaths, and cases of certain infectious diseases, among other things. Much of the data collected is passed on to the Centers for Disease Control and Prevention (CDC). Using the data, policymakers plan initiatives to improve public health, and allocate funding to address specific diseases or populations.

USE IN QUALITY

In recent years, the healthcare industry has placed great emphasis on healthcare **quality**, defined as the rendering of services that follow the most current medical knowledge to achieve health in patients. Chief among quality initiatives is improved patient **outcomes**, or the results of the treatment.

There have been many different quality initiatives over the years, driven by government agencies, accreditation bodies, and various public-private partnerships. All of them rely on healthcare documentation to set goals, track progress, and record results.

One of the more notable quality programs was the ***Physician Quality Reporting System (PQRS)***. This federal program engaged providers to document and report their activities in areas such as care coordination, patient safety, screenings, and services offered. For example, the system encouraged providers to order eye examinations for patients with a diabetes diagnosis, potentially catching eye problems like diabetic retinopathy before they become severe. Different specialties faced different specialty-specific requirements that the government believed would drive quality care. Early in the program there were financial premiums paid for reporting on these measures, which were later replaced with penalties for non-reporting.

PQRS reporting was an early step moving CMS from a ***fee-for-service*** payment model, where providers were paid for the services they rendered, to a ***pay-for-performance*** model, in which reimbursement is based more on patient outcomes. In 2015, Congress passed the ***Medicare Access and Children's Health Insurance Program Reauthorization Act (MACRA)*** which reformed payment methods. The idea was to incentivize practices' participation in a quality incentive program.

In many instances, practices are moving to such programs like the ***Merit-based Incentive Payment System (MIPS)*** which builds on prior programs such as PQRS. On the acute care hospital side of healthcare, CMS has instituted **value-based purchasing** which is an initiative that rewards hospitals with incentive payments for what the government deems to be quality care for Medicare patients. The scribe can help ensure that the appropriate quality measures are documented in the chart so the provider is not penalized for non-reporting.

The Electronic Health Record (EHR)

For many decades, marked file folders stored all the information collected about the patient (Fig. 4.1). While these served their purpose, paper records had limitations. First, anyone who needed to update or refer to the information would need to be in the same physical location as the

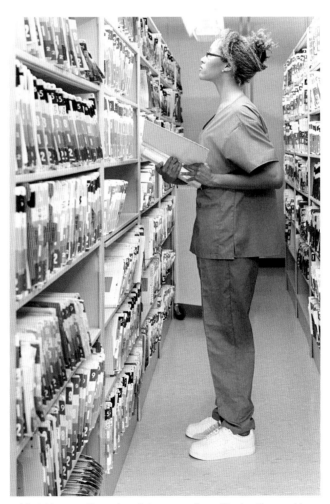

Fig. 4.1   Numbered file folders was the preferred storage medium of the health record for many years. Some practices continue to record patient information on paper, but virtually all hospitals now use electronic health records (EHRs). (© istock.com/XiXinXing.)

file folder, which may have been in the medical records room, with the patient, or somewhere in between. Second, the paper record was mostly handwritten, which could lead to errors related to illegible writing, or misreading what was documented.

Today, almost all healthcare settings use some level of computerization to collect, store, and share patient data. The **electronic health record (EHR)** is a database of patient information that enables information sharing among authorized healthcare professionals, often linked to a knowledge base that can help providers make decisions about patient care. Even when information is initially collected on paper, that information is often scanned, keyed, or otherwise input into the EHR (Fig. 4.2). Using this technology, the health record can be accessed and updated virtually from anywhere. The EHR is also "real time" in the sense that as soon as data is captured—often at the patient's bedside—it is stored and available to others. Because there is not a physical file folder in one geographic location, multiple individuals can access the patient's record at the same time, improving patient care and efficiency.

Data entry into the EHR is simplified through several means. Some information, like body temperature and blood pressure, can be collected directly from the equipment attached to the patient at the point-of-care. When collecting information during the provider encounter, the scribe uses dropdown menus, checkboxes, and other devices to select data values. Even when information is keyed as "free text," the EHR has an advantage over handwriting of varying legibility! Chapter 5 will explore some of these data entry mechanisms in greater detail.

Additional features of the EHR take it beyond simply a tool to store information. For example, in the EHR, the **computerized physician order entry (CPOE)** allows the user to create and send secure provider **orders**, which are the written instructions for therapies such as medications and tests such as labs or imaging. Many EHR systems also have **clinical decision support (CDS)**, which analyzes the information input into the record to suggest to the provider things to do for the patient. For example, the CDS can remind the clinician that the patient is due for certain immunizations, or screening labs, or procedures based on the patient's age or diagnoses. More sophisticated CDS applications can monitor the patient's labs and vital signs, alerting the provider if a patient is deteriorating (sort of an early warning system). Increasingly, the CDS features

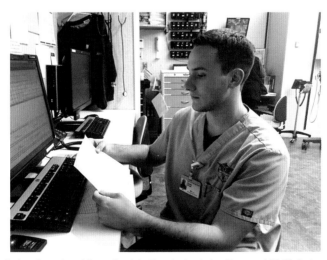

Fig. 4.2 A medical scribe enters information into the electronic health record (EHR) that was originally collected on paper. (© ABC Scribes, Inc. Used with permission.)

complex **algorithms** that, when triggered by patient data, might "pop-up" to make treatment recommendations to the clinician. These will always need to present themselves to the provider, but a scribe could have a role in bringing them to the provider's attention as well.

Health Record Components

The main elements of a health record are usually standard in most healthcare organizations. With few exceptions, the healthcare facility will first collect the patient's basic information, which is often compiled using a patient intake form or patient registration form (Fig. 4.3).

WALDEN-MARTIN
FAMILY MEDICAL CLINIC
1234 ANYSTREET | ANYTOWN, ANYSTATE 12345
PHONE 123-123-1234 | FAX 123-123-5678

Patient Information

Patient Information (Please use full legal name.)

Last Name: *Tapia*	Address 1: *12 Highland Court*
First Name: *Celia*	Address 2: *Apt 101*
Middle Initial: *B*	City: *Anytown*
Medical Record Number: *11012373*	Country: *United States* State/Province: *AL*
Date of Birth: *05/18/1970*	Zip: *12345-1234*
Age: *42*	Email: —
Sex: *Female*	Home Phone: *123-858-1545*
SSN: *857-62-1594*	Driver's License: —
Emergency Contact Name: *Arnold Tapia*	Emergency Contact Phone: *123-200-5006*

Guarantor Information (Please use full legal name.)

Relationship of Guarantor to Patient: *Spouse*	
Guarantor/Account #: *Tapia, Arnold / 12088787*	
Account Number: *12088787*	
Last Name: *Tapia*	Address 1: *12 Highland Court*
First Name: *Arnold*	Address 2: *Apt 101*
Middle Initial: —	City: *Anytown*
Date of Birth: *05/18/1970*	Country: *United States* State/Province: *AL*
Age: *42*	Zip: *12345-1234*
Sex: *Male*	Email: —
SSN: *812-93-1341*	Home Phone: *123-858-1545*
Employer Name: *Anytown String Shop*	Cell Phone: —
School Name: —	Work Phone: —

Provider Information

Primary Provider: *James A. Martin, MD*	Provider's Address 1: *1234 Anystreet*
Referring Provider: —	Provider's Address 2: —
Date of Last Visit: *August 28, 2013*	City: *Anytown*
Phone: *123-123-1234*	Country: *United States* State/Province: *AL*
	Zip: *12345-1234*

Insurance Information (If the patient is not the Insured party, please include date of birth for claims.)

Insurance: *Aetna*	Claims Address 1: *1234 Insurance Way*
Name of Policy Holder: *Arnold Tapia*	Claims Address 2: —
SSN: *812-93-1341*	City: *Anytown*
Policy/ID Number: *CT5487854*	Country: *United States* State/Province: *AL*
Group Number: *41554T*	Zip: *12345-1234*
	Claims Phone: *180-012-3222*

Secondary Insurance

Insurance: —	Claims Address 1: —
Name of Policy Holder: —	Claims Address 2: —
SSN: —	City: —
Policy/ID Number: —	Country: — State/Province: —
Group Number: —	Zip: —
	Claims Phone: —

"I hereby authorize direct payment of all insurance benfits otherwise payable to me for services rendered. I understand that I am financially responsible for all charges not covered by insurance for services rendered on my behalf to my dependents. I authorize the above prociders to release any information required to secure payment of benefits. I authorize the use of this signature on all insurace submissions."

Signature: *Celia Tapia*   Date: *05/06/20XX*

Fig. 4.3   Patient registration form or intake form. (From Proctor DB, Niedzwiecki B, Pepper J, Garrels M, Mills H: *Kinn's the medical assistant: an applied learning approach*, 14th ed, St. Louis, 2020, Elsevier.)

Patient information in a health record should include the following:

- *Demographics*—patient information, including name, contact information, date of birth, occupation, and emergency contact information. In some cases, the Social Security number may be requested.
- *Insurance/financial information*—the name of the insurance provider or payer, and any financial responsibilities, such as a *copayment (copay)*
- *Consent forms*—release of information forms and general consent forms
- *Notes*—clinical detail of the patient's health history problems, medications, physical examinations, diagnostics, treatment plan, and procedures performed.

WHAT IS A NOTE?

A **note** is an entry made by the healthcare worker into medical record that describes the worker's activities as they relate to that patient's care. A **provider note** is any note created by a medical provider. If a scribe creates a note for a provider, it must carry a statement that identifies the scribe who created the note, be "taken over" by the clinician, and include **authentication**—a signed statement that the provider has reviewed the note for accuracy and accepts it as their own. This helps to ensure that the scribe is never legally liable for the content of that note.

If the scribe documents legibly (if on paper) and accurately, times and dates the note (if not done automatically by the EHR), and prepares and completes the note for the provider to authenticate, then the scribe has assisted the provider to meet CMS requirements for a complete health record.

There are many types of notes. The following sections detail some of the most common notes the scribe may encounter.

HISTORY AND PHYSICAL (H&P)

The **history and physical (H&P)** is the main clinical note documenting the patient's explanation of his or her health and health problems, the provider's findings, and the provider's treatment plan. It comprises all of the traditional parts of a medical note, including (but not limited to):

- The *chief complaint (CC)*—the reason for the patient's visit
- The *history of the present illness (HPI)*—the patient's "story" of the illness or problem from the time it started to the present
- The *review of systems (ROS)*—a list of the patient's symptoms organized by body system
- *Additional history*—an account of the patient's past or existing medical problems, medical problems that run in the family, a record of lifestyle behaviors (social history), and surgical history
- *Medications*—current and those taken in the past
- *Allergies*—including medications, foods, and environmental triggers
- The *physical examination*—the provider's observations of the patient's body
- *Laboratory test results and imaging studies* (if any)
- The provider's *assessment* and *plan* (also known as *medical decision making*, or *MDM*).

Most often, the work of the scribe entails documenting the H&P. In particular, the scribe will document the "History" portion of the H&P: CC, HPI, ROS, additional history, medications, and allergies (Fig. 4.4). The scribe may also be responsible for documenting the "physical" portion: the findings of the provider during the physical examination (Fig. 4.5). Documentation of lab results and imaging studies may be imported into a note automatically or the scribe may be involved in making sure this information has been added to the health record. Providers frequently document their assessment and plan independently, but some engage the medical scribe in this task as well. Chapter 5, Anatomy of a Provider Note, will examine each element of the H&P in detail.

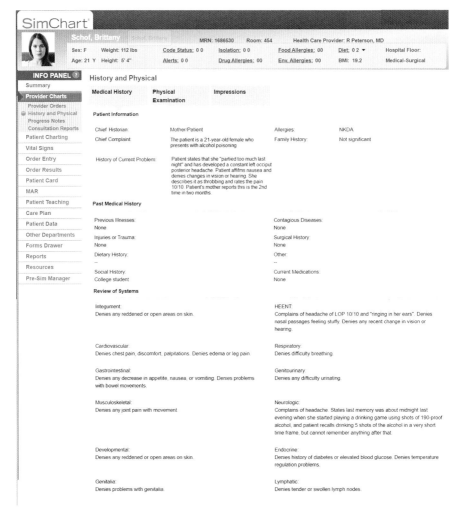

Fig. 4.4 An example of the medical history portion of the history and physical (H&P) note in the electronic health record (EHR). (From SimChart for the Medical Office © 2022 Elsevier, Inc.)

Subjective Versus Objective Information

Note that most of the "history" portion of the H&P is from the point of view of the patient, while the "physical" is the provider's findings. Information that comes from the patient is called *subjective* information. The provider's findings are *objective* information.

Subjective means that something is only able to be felt or valued by the individual experiencing it, and cannot be measured or observed by anyone else. Itchiness is an example of subjective information. The patient can describe a rash as "really itchy," but there is no way for others to measure the patient's itchiness or feel it. We cannot even know the patient is itchy unless he tells us. When we speak of **symptoms**, we are referring to the subjective elements of disease. Other classic examples of subjective information or symptoms include pain, vertigo (dizziness), and tiredness (fatigue). Symptoms are recorded in the CC, HPI, and ROS.

Objective information is observable by others, namely, for our purposes, the provider. Objective findings, called **signs**, are measurable and do not change with the perspective of the observer. *Vital signs,*

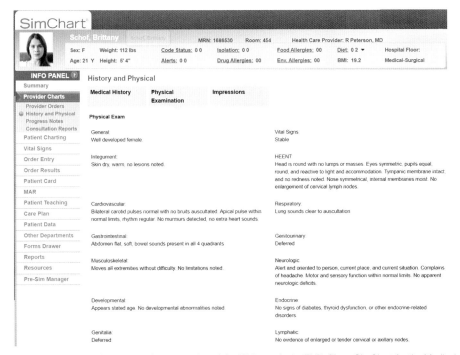

Fig. 4.5 An example of the physical exam portion of the H&P note in the EHR. (From SimChart for the Medical Office © 2022 Elsevier, Inc.)

such as heart rate, blood pressure, and body temperature, are examples of objective signs. To continue the example above, while the provider cannot know that the patient is itchy, a rash is an observable sign, and so is urticaria (hives) and erythema (redness). Objectives signs are recorded during the physical exam.

ATTENDING NOTE

The scribe may complete an **attending note** for the attending physician who is supervising others in the healthcare setting. This is a note that contains the important elements of history and physical, and any discussion that shows that the attending was involved and coordinated the care of this patient along with a resident, physician assistant (PA), or nurse practitioner (NP). It is a more abbreviated version of a complete H&P. If another licensed provider is seeing the patient in conjunction with the attending physician, then a brief note may be all that is needed (also sometimes called an attending note).

A medical student may not create an official note for an encounter. A medical student is not licensed to practice and thus their notes are for educational purposes. If a patient is being seen in conjunction with a medical student, the provider must create a complete H&P of their own. An attending note will not be sufficient, in this case.

BRIEF NOTE

A brief note is a shortened or truncated note that contains only the essential elements for a simpler visit where the entire review of systems and physical exam need not be done. Essentially, a brief note has many of the same elements of a complete H&P, but is a more concise version.

PROCEDURE NOTE

The procedure note documents a medical or surgical procedure. Chapter 7 examines procedure notes in detail.

OPERATIVE NOTE (OP NOTE)

The **operative note** is a very specific type of procedure note that describes the surgery that the patient has undergone. It also has specific elements that should be included. These may vary depending on the type of surgery.

SUBJECTIVE, OBJECTIVE, ASSESSMENT, PLAN (SOAP) NOTE

The **SOAP note** is often used on daily rounds on the floor of the hospital, or in an office setting for a patient's regular follow-up office visits. The "subjective" is equivalent to the history of the present illness, and the "objective" is equivalent to the physical exam. The "assessment and plan" portion is unchanged. This may sometimes be referred to as an *APSO note*, which is essentially the same thing but with the elements arranged in a different order.

PROGRESS NOTE

The **progress note** is written each day, or as indicated by patient's condition, on a patient who is admitted to the hospital or seen in an office. It is important to point out that in progress notes, the time of day the note was taken becomes particularly important because the timing of events can affect a patient's medical course and outcome. Fig. 4.6 shows the record of progress notes in the EHR.

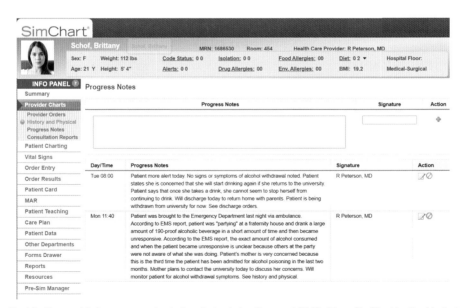

Fig. 4.6 The provider's progress notes in the electronic health record (EHR). (From SimChart for the Medical Office © 2022 Elsevier, Inc.)

TRAUMA NOTE

A **trauma note** is specifically oriented towards trauma cases. It may include all elements of a traditional H&P, in addition to trauma-specific considerations such as whether the patient is up to date on tetanus vaccinations and the timing of their last oral intake.

PROBLEM LIST

The patient's **problem list** is a listing of his or her known medical problems. It may include any combination of diagnoses, symptoms and signs, or clinical impressions (the provider's assessment of the patient's condition). Every patient is different and may have multiple problems in their problem list. Each chapter in Part III of this text, Body Systems for the Medical Scribe, lists examples of the types of problems the scribe may encounter.

The problem list is NOT an exhaustive listing of every medical problem that they have had in the past, but rather (when maintained correctly) a listing of all "active" problems. For example, a patient may have had appendicitis and had surgery to resolve the problem. *Abdominal pain* or *appendicitis* may have been on the problem list while the patient was being seen and treated and followed up for the problem. However, if the patient's surgery went well and they healed up and no longer have an issue with abdominal pain any longer, then this "problem" has been resolved and it should "drop off" of the problem list. Generally, it will be a physician or other medical provider that will "maintain" the problem list to ensure that it is "clean" and current.

Note that a problem can change over time. As with the above example, a patient's problem might start out as "abdominal pain" but then be changed to the more specific "appendicitis" once that diagnosis has been confirmed.

A different example would be hypertension (high blood pressure). This problem should be entered into the problem list and it likely will never be removed from the list, since hypertension is usually a chronic problem that needs to be monitored and treated long term.

Problem lists are used as a reminder for the provider to document on each of the items listed. For example, a patient is admitted with several problems. The hospitalist will likely document on each of these problems individually when writing their progress note for the day: *"hypertension is well controlled, pneumonia is still causing some dyspnea but the patient is on antibiotics, chest pain has resolved."*

The problem list is carried from provider to provider and should be updated appropriately. A specialist might document only on the problems that fall under their area of expertise. For example, the cardiologist on the case will comment on the electrocardiogram (ECG) and the patient's heart enzyme test (troponin). Another example would be a surgeon who might follow-up postoperatively for the surgical incision and any complications (like fevers).

It is the responsibility of the provider to manage the problem list. This often includes "cleaning up the list," which entails removing old problems that have been entered at some time in the past and have lost relevance. When a new problem occurs, it should be added to the list.

A scribe may be asked to assist with maintaining the problem list as a part of their documentation duties. The scribe would never independently decide what should and should not be on the list (although in most instances it is not difficult to figure out which problems are active and which are not). Rather the scribe may perform list maintenance under the direction of their provider. The scribe may even prompt the provider if they see that a problem either does not appear on the list when it should or when the scribe sees a problem on the list that may have been resolved and should perhaps come off of the list or be labeled as "resolved."

Problem-Oriented Charting

Problem-oriented charting is a term that is used for a specific approach to documentation in the patient record. It is a method that breaks down the note into sections that are reflective of the patient's problems from their problem list. This method of documentation is sometimes called the *problem-oriented medical record (POMR)*.

How does problem-oriented charting look?

Any active problems that a patient may have will need to be addressed periodically. Not every provider will need to address every active problem at every encounter. So, a primary care provider may only address certain problems annually while addressing others at every quarterly visit. For example, hypertension will be addressed much more frequently than following a benign mass perhaps. Also, a specialist who uses the problem-oriented charting method of documentation may only address specialty specific problems. The orthopedist is unlikely to get involved in the patient's hypertension but will address the healing fracture or back pain.

Earlier we discussed the SOAP note. It can be applied to the POMR by having multiple SOAP (or APSO) notes follow each other, one for each problem.

Medical Coding

Medical **coding** is the conversion of information into numeric or alphanumeric codes. These short, simple, and distinct expressions are designed to communicate information with the highest accuracy. Codes are a favorable means of sending and receiving information about patient care because they are a universally understood vocabulary, and they are able to be read by computers. Codes are used for diagnoses and problems, procedures, services, treatments, drugs/medications, medical equipment, and more. Medical coding is so important that its use in billing is required by the Health Insurance Portability and Accountability Act (HIPAA).

Although a scribe's involvement in coding is minimal at best, a scribe who is familiar with coding is better equipped to help their provider meet billing requirements to be properly reimbursed for their work.

There are different code sets used in different settings for different reasons. HIPAA mandates which code sets are to be used on billing claims under various circumstances. Table 4.1 shows the code sets the law requires and gives example codes. We will look closely at two code sets of interest to the medical scribe: *ICD-10-CM* and *CPT*.

INTERNATIONAL CLASSIFICATION OF DISEASES, 10TH REVISION, CLINIC MODIFICATION (ICD-10-CM)

The **International Classification of Diseases, 10th Revision, Clinic Modification (ICD-10-CM)** code set is used to record patient problems and diagnoses in all types of medical settings. These codes are 3–7 characters long and consist of a series of numbers and letters. Generally, the longer the code, the more specific it is. As shown in Fig. 4.7, not only the characters, but the positions of the characters in ICD-10-CM have meaning.

Let's look at examples of ICD-10-CM codes. The diagnosis *osteoarthritis* is represented by the ICD-10-CM code M19. The etiologies (origins) of osteoarthritis are represented by the fourth character: primary osteoarthritis is M19.0; post-traumatic osteoarthritis is M19.1; secondary osteoarthritis is M19.2; and unspecified osteoarthritis is M19.9. The body part affected is represented in the fifth character: osteoarthritis in the shoulder is M19._1; in the elbow it is M19._2; when it occurs in the wrist it is M19._3; the hand is M19._4; the ankle/foot is M19._5. The sixth character is representative of the *laterality*: right is M19._ _1; left is M19._ _2; and unspecified is M19._ _9. Putting it all together, the code M19.142 is arguably easier to record and communicate than "*post-traumatic osteoarthritis of the left hand.*" To bill at the highest level, it is always best to use the most specific code possible.

Despite the logical order of ICD-10 codes as explained above, it should be noted that codes are rarely assigned manually, if ever. The EHR program will feature a code lookup tool that can

TABLE 4.1 ■ Health Insurance Portability and Accountability Act (HIPAA) Transaction Code Sets

Coding System	Description	Sample Code	Code Meaning
International Classification of Diseases, 10th Revision, Clinic Modification (ICD-10-CM)	Used for chief complaints and diagnoses in all settings	U07.1	COVID-19 virus infection
International Classification of Diseases, 10th Revision, Procedure Coding System (ICD-10-PCS)	Used for procedures in the inpatient setting	0BJ08ZZ	Bronchoscopy
Current Procedure Terminology (CPT®)	For physicians and other providers to code and describe medical, surgical, radiology, laboratory, and anesthesiology services. The CPT is Level I of the HCPCS	92310	Prescription and fitting of contact lenses
Healthcare Common Procedure Coding System (HCPCS) Level II	Nonphysician services such as ambulance interventions, prosthetics, durable medical equipment, medications, and supplies.	A0021	Ambulance transfer for Medicaid patient out of state
Code on Dental Procedures and Nomenclature (CDT)	Used for dental procedures and treatments	D3348	Retreatment of previous root canal therapy - molar
National Drug Code (NDC)	A product identifier for every medication manufactured and sold for use in humans	50580-170	Children's Tylenol in oral suspension manufactured by Johnson and Johnson

CPT © 2022 American Medical Association. All rights reserved. CPT is a registered trademark of the American Medical Association.

help scribes and clinicians search and select the correct code from a list (Fig. 4.8). Some hospital systems use *computer-assisted coding (CAC)* software that "reads" the health record and generates codes. Medical coders and billers always examine all the documentation in the record and use a combination of bound volumes and computer software to ensure the correct code is chosen.

Since providers must be paid for the work that they have done, coding a record is extremely important. Coding it accurately is equally important to avoid any claims of fraud, as discussed in Chapter 2. Although many individuals (like medical coders) may participate in coding and billing of a chart, ultimately it is the provider who is legally liable for any issues that may arise from any inaccuracies.

CURRENT PROCEDURE TERMINOLOGY (CPT®)

The **Current Procedural Terminology (CPT)** code set is used to code all services rendered by providers in all settings. There are over 10,000 codes in the CPT system and each code is a

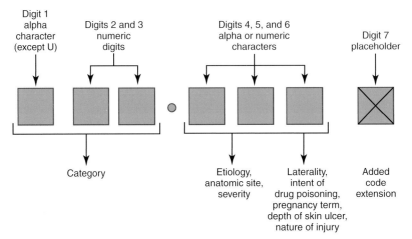

Fig. 4.7   Explanation of the seven character positions in the International Classification of Diseases, 10th Revision, Clinical Modification (ICD-10-CM). (From Smith L: *Fordney's medical insurance*, ed 15, St. Louis, 2020, Elsevier.)

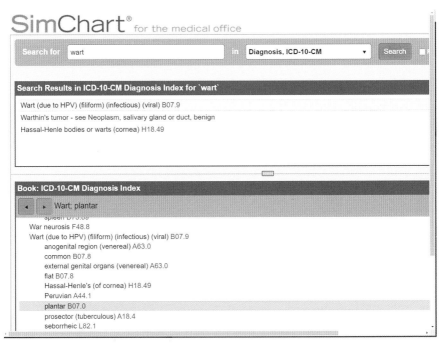

Fig. 4.8   In this electronic health record (EHR) system, the scribe can search for the term "wart" and generate a list of possible International Classification of Diseases, 10th Revision, Clinical Modification (ICD-10-CM) diagnosis codes. (From SimChart for the Medical Office © 2022 Elsevier, Inc.)

five-digit number ranging from 00100 to 99499. Whether a provider sutures (stiches) a bad cut (12002), interprets an ECG, flushes out impacted earwax (69209), counsels a patient on the benefits of quitting smoking (99406), or reattaches a severed thumb (20824), a CPT code is assigned. The CPT code set is owned and maintained by the American Medical Association (AMA). Unlike ICD-10, CPT codes are nonsequential and do not have a decipherable pattern.

Evaluation and Management (E/M) Codes

Evaluation and management (E/M) codes are CPT codes that are used to bill for the provider's **level of service (LOS)**. This is determined by the intensity and extensiveness of the history and physical exam, and medical decision making. Different levels of services include, from the simplest to the most complex:

- Problem-focused
- Expanded problem-focused
- Detailed, and
- Comprehensive

The level of service charge would mandate that a more complex encounter would have a higher rate of reimbursement. For example, a more comprehensive case may require the provider to elicit more history, perform a more in-depth exam, and entail more medical decision making complexity based on the lab tests or imaging tests that are ordered and interpreted. This would require more of the provider's time and energy, thus it makes sense to pay more for this type of encounter.

Initial Versus Follow-Up (Subsequent) Visits. A *new patient* is a patient who has not received any professional healthcare services from that provider, or any other provider of the exact same specialty and/or subspecialty who belongs to the same group practice, within the past three years. Initial visits with new patients are typically more comprehensive, and thus require more of the provider's time and energy. Naturally, these have a higher reimbursement as compared to subsequent visits. E/M codes are used to represent the additional resources it requires to see and treat a new patient.

CASE STUDY 4.1

Miley is a new medical scribe beginning her paid training at Johnson Orthopedics, a large physician-owned practice offering an array of services such as physical therapy, sports medicine, pain management, chiropractic, rehabilitation, and surgery. She is going to shadow one of the billing and insurance specialists, April, for the day—so she can learn the administrative processes before she starts working with the providers. "This is such a great place to work," April said, "and since we offer so many different kinds of care, there's never a dull moment."

Miley and April sit down at one of the computer workstations together. April said, "Let's start by having you log in to the EHR with your username and password. We're going to look at some patient records in order to process the claims from this week."

The first record they look at is for a patient who was seen by one of the physicians for neck pain. The physician discussed the patient's problem, how long he had been experiencing the pain, its characteristics, and asked how it was affecting the patient's life. The HPI in the record states that the patient indicated his pain begins in his neck around the 6th or 7th cervical vertebrae, and radiates down his left arm all the way to his thumb. The ROS further reports that the patient is having difficulty sleeping. During the physical examination, the physician noted "marked slowing and impairment of fine motor coordination in the left hand." The physician ordered x-rays to find out what might be causing the pain. The x-rays were done in-house the same day. The physician believes the patient may have *spinal stenosis of the cervical region* but wants to have a CT scan performed. For now the physician has recorded M54.2, *cervicalgia*, or cervical neck pain. The record shows an order to the pharmacy for gabapentin.

QUESTIONS

1. What is the name of the set of processes April uses to file claims and obtain payment from payers?
2. What are the patient's symptoms?
3. What information in the health record would be objective information, as opposed to subjective information?
4. What type of code will be used to represent the services of the physician?
5. What type of code is M54.2, cervicalgia?
6. Where in the record would M54.2, cervicalgia, be recorded?.
7. If, after the CT scan, the patient is diagnosed with "spinal stenosis of the cervical region," what will happen to the patient's diagnosis of cervicalgia?
8. What EHR component did the physician use to send the order for gabapentin to the pharmacy?

Practice Questions

1. The safe and effective delivery of healthcare over time is called the _____.
2. The provider's official determination of the patient's injury or illness is called the _____.
3. The health record is also evidence that can be used on behalf of the patient and the healthcare provider in a legal dispute called _____.
4. Most patients have a _____, such as an insurance company or government agency, who pays the provider for all or part of the services rendered.
5. In the pay-for-performance and value-based purchasing models of reimbursement, providers and hospitals are paid more on _____, or the results of the treatment, rather than the actual services provided.
6. Medical decision making (MDM) comprises
   a. the assessment and plan.
   b. the review of systems (ROS) and history of present illness (HPI)
   c. medications and allergies
   d. the history and physical (H&P)
7. Which part of the H&P records the physician's objective findings?
   a. review of systems (ROS)
   b. history of present illness (HPI)
   c. physical exam
   d. assessment
8. Which law mandates the use of certain code sets for submitting claims to third-party payers?

Anatomy of a Provider Note

1. Discuss the elements of the history and physical (H&P).
2. Document the history of the present illness (HPI) in accordance with current guidelines for billing and patient care.
3. Document the review of systems (ROS) in accordance with current guidelines for billing and patient care.
4. Document relevant elements of the patient's past medical history, surgical history, family history, social history, medications, and allergies.
5. Document the physical exam and vital signs in accordance with current guidelines for billing and patient care.
6. Explain key concepts in medical decision making (MDM) and provider time as it relates to documentation.

Acuity level
Affirm
Auscultation
Billable element
Blood pressure
Body temperature
Chief complaint
Contraindication
Deny
Descriptor
Differential
Documentation element
Emergent
Hard-stop
Heart rate
History and physical (H&P)

History of the present illness (HPI)
Illicit drug
Inspection
Intercapping
Intolerance
Medical decision making (MDM)
Nature of the presenting problem
Objective
Observable element
Ophthalmoscope
Otoscope
Pack-year
Palpation

Percussion
Pertinent negative
Pertinent positive
Physical exam
Precharting
Respiratory rate
Resuscitation
Review of systems (ROS)
Rule out
Sign
Subjective
Symptom
Tall-man letters
True allergy
Vital sign

The History and Physical (H&P)

As discussed in Chapter 4, the **history and physical (H&P)** is one of the most common notes, documenting the reason the patient is seeking medical service, the patient's medical history, the provider's findings, and the provider's plans to treat the patient. This chapter will focus on dissecting various parts of the H&P, and introduces templates and forms with the elements a scribe may record into the electronic health record (EHR).

Bear in mind that the elements shown in these documentation tools are not universal. Every institution, individual, specialty, and situation will likely require a different template based on the specific needs of the provider, medical practice, or patient encounter. That being said, the American Medical Association (AMA), in partnership with the Centers for Medicare and Medicaid Services (CMS), has developed guidelines for the documentation that supports Evaluation and Management (E/M) coding. This chapter relates the minimum documentation requirements in consideration of these guidelines, which are important for both billing and patient care quality initiatives.

Precharting

Precharting is done by the provider prior to initiating the current patient encounter. This entails reviewing old records for additional information, and populating a new note with prior elements that may be relevant to the current visit. Precharting can be automated. For example, automated links in some EHRs automatically pull forward relevant information. Precharting can also become a scribe function. It is more likely to be some combination of the efforts of the provider and the scribe along with some automated importing of data, depending on the software being used.

Relevant elements from the patient's medical record could include results of tests or procedures that have been performed since the patient's last visit, other provider or consultant evaluations and recommendations, an updated medication and allergy list, updated medical, surgical, familial, and social history. Basically, precharting could include anything else that may have happened to the patient since their last visit.

Forms, Templates, Macros, and Cloning

There are other shortcuts that may be taken by a healthcare provider to improve efficiency in documentation. These include the use of forms, templates, and macros.

FORMS

A *form* is a data collection device with defined fields, prompting the user to input data elements as necessary. Some form fields are spaces in which the user may type freely. Other forms use radio buttons, check boxes, and dropdown menus to give the user limited (but frequent) choices of appropriate entries. Fig. 5.1 is a simple example of using a form with radio buttons, dropdowns, and text entries to complete the patient information portion of a medical record.

TEMPLATES

Templates are blank documents that are preconfigured to show an outline of a standard patient encounter, populated with generic data waiting to be modified to match the current visit. Templates allow for all patient encounters to follow a standardized format, while remaining unique to each patient and condition.

Templates save time by having the sections required for the visit outlined and ready to accept current information, which can be filled in with voice-to-text or by free text to make the template patient-specific. Generally, a provider will use multiple templates and select the one matching the type of visit or encounter at hand. For example, a template for chest pain will have space and

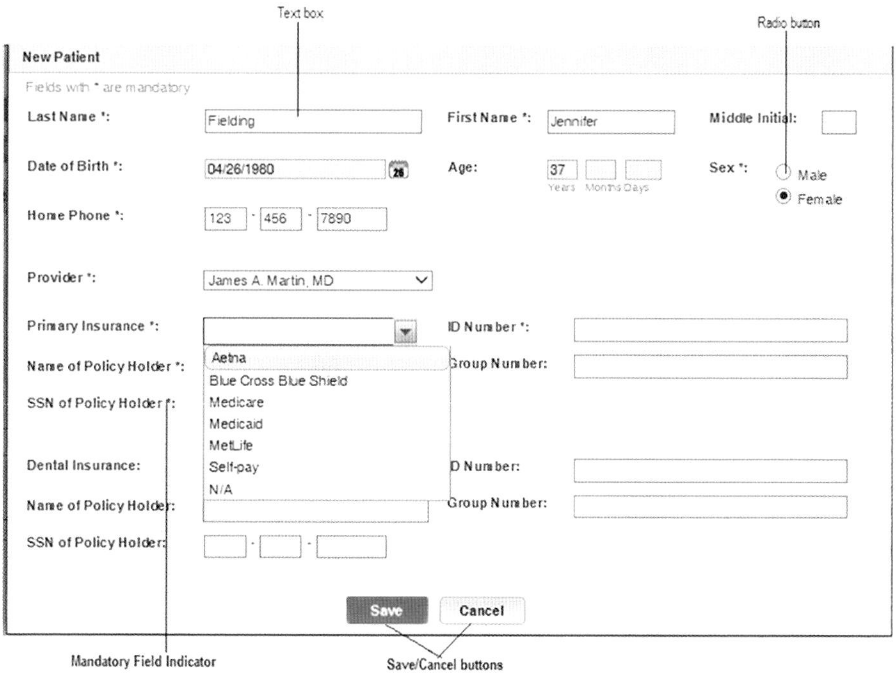

Fig. 5.1 An electronic health record (EHR) screen showing various ways to enter patient information in a form. (From Bonewit-West K, Hunt S: *Today's medical assistant: clinical & administrative procedures*, ed 4, St. Louis, 2020, Saunders/Elsevier.)

options for describing types of chest pain and risk factors for coronary artery disease and other possible causes of the pain. A template for an extended visit will have more sections outlined for completion as compared with a template for a briefer visit, which will have fewer sections marked for completion. Templates are completely customizable to the documentation needs of the provider and the healthcare organization.

MACROS

A **macro** is a computer shortcut that fills in commonly entered data. Macros allow users to create a lot of text with one keystroke, saving time and effort. These are acceptable to use as long as care is taken to modify them to fit the current encounter. Sometimes, the automatic data populated by macros can lead to reporting services not rendered or over-documentation, both of which constitute fraud.

> **NOTE**
>
> Shortcuts should be used with caution, as they can lead to over-documentation that may negatively affect the integrity of the patient's medical record. The only documentation that should be performed is that which justifies the care, treatment, and other services that were provided to that patient.

CLONING (COPY and PASTE)

Plagiarism is never allowed. However, **cloning**, the copying and pasting previously of recorded information from a prior note into a new note, is a permissible keyboard shortcut. Cloning may be used for specific small bits of information that are relevant to the current visit and do not need to be retyped.

Plagiarism is an easy way to ruin a career, and thus care must be taken regarding information that is cloned. One example of an appropriate use of cloning might be if the summary of findings from a recent heart catheterization is copied and pasted (cloned) into a new note because the findings are relevant to current medical decision making. An example of an inappropriate use of cloning would be if a provider copied and pasted (cloned) a resident's H&P into their own note since the resident had a complete note. The attending physician is required to perform their own evaluation and their note should reflect the work that they have done.

Compare the two examples above. In the first, it is clear that the cloned piece of information is a report about a test that is placed in the note because of its importance for the provider's decision making. It does not purport to be the provider's own words. In the second example, the cloned note has an appearance as if it is original to the provider, when in fact it is copied from someone else's work.

Chief Complaint

The **chief complaint** is a short description of a patient's symptom(s), sign(s), or in some instances, diagnosis, that brought the patient to the medical setting. Technically, the diagnosis is not a chief complaint, but a chief complaint could mirror a diagnosis if it is what the patient states is the reason for their visit. The chief complaint is generally recorded in the patient's own words. If the patient is unable to give the reason for their visit for any reason (for example, the patient is incapacitated, or brought in to be seen unwillingly), then the chief complaint is the reason for the visit as given by another party who best knows why the patient has been brought to the provider. An example would be an unconscious patient brought in by emergency medical service (EMS) personnel for "overdose." Here the historian is EMS personnel and they state the reason for the visit as "overdose" which then becomes the chief complaint.

The chief complaint is reflected in the first sentence of the HPI, as seen below:

*The patient is a {age}-year-old {male/female} who presents with {**chief complaint**}.*

In outpatient facilities, the patient is often there to follow up on a previous diagnosis. In those instances, the chief complaint may be that diagnosis which is being followed (e.g., hypertension). If the patient has a new symptom that is to be evaluated, then the chief complaint would be the new symptom or problem as stated by the patient or their representative.

The E/M documentation guidelines allow for the note to record information about the *nature of presenting problem*. A presenting problem is the condition, disease, illness, injury, etc., that brings the patient to see the provider; the presenting problem might be the same as the chief complaint, but it might not be the same. The **nature of the presenting problem** acts as a barometer to measure the risk to the patient of not receiving care. There are five severity levels to this component:

- **Minimal**—The presenting problem may not require the presence of the provider, but care may be rendered under the direction of a provider.
- **Self-limited or minor**—The problem runs a definite and prescribed course, is transient, and not likely to last.
- **Low severity**—The risk of morbidity without treatment is low; the patient will be expected to make a full recovery without further or lasting impairment.

- **Moderate severity**—Without medical treatment, there is moderate risk of morbidity or mortality; the prognosis is uncertain, or there is increased risk of prolonged functional impairment.
- **High severity**—High to extreme risk to the patient without medical treatment of the problem.

In the emergency department, the chief complaint is typically a symptom or sign. The emergency medicine provider does not necessarily try to diagnose, but rather decides if the patient is safe enough to be discharged home to follow-up in an outpatient setting, versus requiring admission to the hospital for additional work-up and treatment.

The emergency department sees patients on a walk-in basis (as opposed to by appointments only, like many offices). Because the emergency department functions as a safety net for potentially life-threatening medical problems, the providers need to know which patients are the sickest and require their attention first.

To address this issue most emergency departments will give a score to each patient: the **acuity level**, based on a scale called the *Emergency Severity Index (ESI)*. Patients are scored according to the triage nurse's assessment of the severity of illness or intensity of services felt to be required, and not entirely upon which patient arrived first to the department.

> **NOTE**
>
> The acuity score given to each patient by the triage nurse is not to be confused with the billing severity scoring (better termed the intensity of service). Determining the level of service for billing depends upon the documentation that is created by the provider.

The Emergency Severity Index is as follows:
- **ESI 1**—Requires immediate life-saving intervention, often including **resuscitation**. Examples include cardiac arrest, severe bleeding, acute stroke, or myocardial infarction.
- **ESI 2**—High risk of deterioration requiring **emergent** evaluation, often indicating that the patient is confused, has severe pain or has abnormal vital signs. Examples might be a severe asthma attack or a seizure.
- **ESI 3**—Stable patients who require attention *urgently*, as they have complaints that likely need multiple resources for evaluation (like labs and imaging) and could indicate a serious medical problem. Examples may include abdominal pain, or COPD with a fever and a cough.
- **ESI 4**—Patients who are stable and *less urgently* need to be seen, requiring only a single resource type to treat or evaluate. Some examples may be a simple laceration or an ankle sprain.
- **ESI 5**—These are *non-urgent* patients with no resources required for their care. Examples include a simple rash or prescription refill.

History of the Present Illness (HPI)

The **history of the present illness (HPI)** is a coherent story, usually chronologic, describing the patient's present illness from the first sign or symptom to the present. The history is the heart of the document and is usually the primary portion of the note where the scribe's work takes place. Creating the history entails:
1. Listening to the history provider, which may be the patient themselves, a family member, a care provider, or someone else such as a paramedic. The history could also come from more than one source.
2. Sorting through the information gathered
3. Creating an accurate and coherent story (the history).

The history should never be pulled from a prior encounter and should be unique to the current visit. Fig. 5.2 shows an example HPI screen in an EHR.

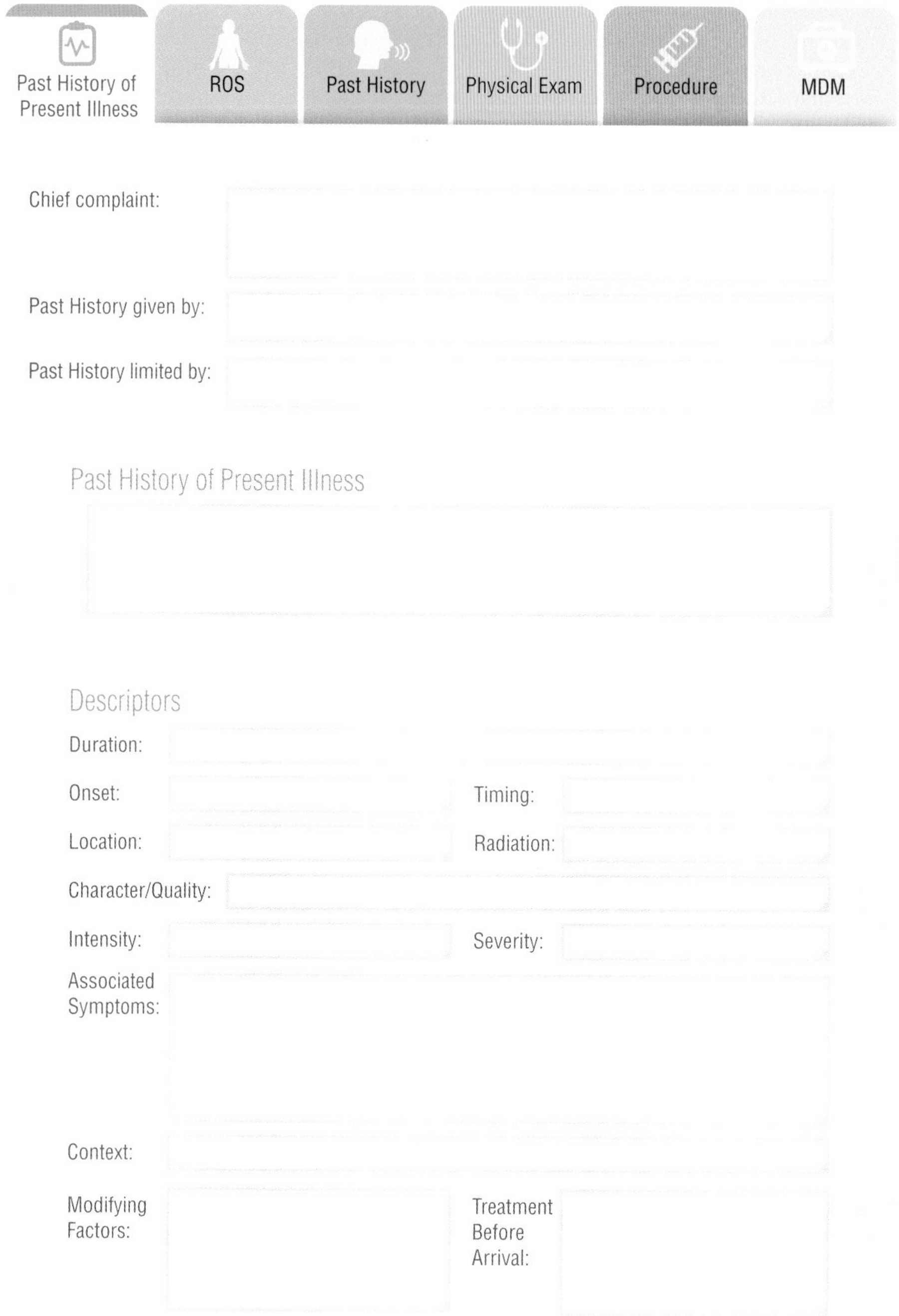

Past History of Present Illness	ROS	Past History	Physical Exam	Procedure	MDM

Chief complaint:

Past History given by:

Past History limited by:

Past History of Present Illness

Descriptors

Duration:

Onset: Timing:

Location: Radiation:

Character/Quality:

Intensity: Severity:

Associated
Symptoms:

Context:

Modifying
Factors: Treatment
                                          Before
                                          Arrival:

Fig. 5.2   A history of the present illness (HPI) form in an electronic health record (EHR).

PERTINENCE

During history taking (whether for the review of systems, past medical history, allergies, etc.), a patient may affirm or deny having any sort of medical problem. *Pertinent elements* are those that are responses to questions related directly to the problem that brought the patient to the visit. **Pertinent positives** are those problems which the patient **affirms** having. **Pertinent negatives** are the problems which the patient **denies** having. The pertinent negatives are equally important as the pertinent positives and absolutely should be documented. This is because they may help to **rule out** a cause of the patient's symptoms or signs. A provider takes all of this into consideration during the medical decision-making process.

The rest of this chapter will review the remaining elements of a provider note. Chapter 6: *Synthesizing a History*, will examine the HPI in further detail.

DESCRIPTORS

Descriptors, also sometimes referred to as **documentation elements** or **billable elements**, are pertinent aspects of the history. These elements are counted and are one factor used to determine the history's level of complexity. It is important to make the distinction that the descriptors are not solely used for billing purposes. They are actually important aspects of the history that are necessary for the provider's assessment of the patient and subsequent plan of care.

The billing requirements differ between locations of service, but the descriptors generally are ubiquitous (again reflecting their necessity in the provider's medical decision making). The E/M guidelines from the CMS and AMA include eight descriptors: *location*, *quality*, *severity*, *duration*, *timing*, *context*, *modifying factors*, and *associated signs and symptoms*. In the example forms and templates used throughout this chapter, the setting, an emergency department, uses 12 descriptors. Based on preference and patient care needs, the providers at this facility want to collect certain aspects of the patient data, such that, in some cases, more than one descriptor contributes to one documentation element. For example: *onset* and *timing* are both descriptors, but count towards one documentation element. One or both can be documented, but only one documentation element will be achieved.

Per the E/M coding guidelines, the number of documentation elements documented in the history HPI will place the encounter into one of two different levels:

- **Low complexity (brief) visit**—1 to 3 of the 8 documentation elements
- **High complexity (extended) visit**—4 (or more) of the 8 documentation elements

Please note that the billing and coding requirements for other facilities (like inpatient and outpatient) differ from the emergency department. For example, according to the 2021 E/M guidelines, outpatient office visits (codes 99202-99215) only require a medically appropriate history. Other evaluation and management codes require the documentation elements above.

Number of Elements to Obtain

Ultimately, the number of documentation elements in the history is considered when calculating the entire chart's level. The scribe will not know how the chart will be billed until after it is evaluated by the billing and coding specialist. However, much of that decision-making depends on the scribe being familiar with the documentation elements and recording them thoroughly. Failure to document an element or two can cause the chart to not be billable at the level otherwise appropriate for the complexity of the case.

To ensure that the chart can be billed at the highest level deemed appropriate for that visit, it is best to try to document enough documentation elements to support the highest billable level. Thus, the recommendation is to **include at least 4 of 8 documentation elements** in the HPI.

Meeting the Billing Requirement

Although generally the scribe will have no trouble finding enough descriptors in the history to complete the chart fully, on occasion this may not be true. This can especially happen in the chaotic emergency department environment where any encounter can be interrupted multiple times due to other emergencies that arise. In any such case, acting as the provider's documentation partner, it is appropriate and helpful for the scribe to get the provider back on track in eliciting the documentation elements. It is important to note here that this will not often be necessary, as most of the descriptors will be discussed during the natural course of history-taking.

Limitations to History

If the history is limited (for any reason) and thus enough documentation elements cannot be obtained, the requirement for billing will be forgiven as long as there is documentation describing the limitation. Some examples could include if the patient is unconscious, has altered mental status, or is an extremely poor historian. If there are historians other than the patient, these should be listed, and if the patient is unable to give an adequate history and no other historians are available, that should be noted as well.

UTILIZING A TEMPLATE

Depending on the facility, the scribe may use a form or a template to collect the data that populates the HPI note. An example of a general template is shown in Fig. 5.3. This template is selected for an undiagnosed patient in the emergency department. The providers at this facility have created this template to make it easier for scribes to record information about the patient during the encounter. In this template, descriptors placed next to one another count as one documentation element (e.g. *onset* and *timing*).

Note that the template in Fig. 5.3 utilizes special characters to offset various textual elements. In this EHR application, data in the fields bracketed by the "<" and ">" signs are automatically populated from other notes in the record. Regardless of the EHR in use at your facility. the parts of the template that import data from other areas will be bracketed in such a way as to clearly indicate their role in automatically filling in the data in question. Since this example is from the ED, the software is aligned to the nursing triage note and pulls the patient's name, age, sex, and room number/bed from the data already entered by the nurses. Fields isolated in curly brackets such as {sudden vs. gradual} act as "stops," where the scribe is prompted to fill in data. In actual practice, the scribe is pressing a specific key on the keyboard to cycle through the bracketed fields in the template quickly and easily.

The descriptors are always included within the HPI narrative but a template may also list them again, together in their own section beneath the history narrative. Reiterating the descriptors in their own section of the history is not required to successfully bill a chart, however, it may help expedite the process for the billing and coding team.

The template is completely configurable by the user and can have fields added or removed. In fact, the template behaves just like a document in a word processing program. The template generally will have all of the categories for documentation in it, and if not used, they will be deleted. Retaining documentation of information that did not occur is falsification and illegal.

If the scribe is documenting in a form without the capability of deleting an unnecessary section, the fields may be left blank, or N/A (or similar language per facility policy) may be entered.

EXPLANATION OF HPI DESCRIPTORS

The following are the descriptors that may be included as part of the history, organized by documentation elements (descriptors placed next to one another count as one documentation element).

```
HPI
<NAME> is a <AGE> <SEX> who presents in <ROOMBED> with <CC>

Specialists:
Dr. {name} ({specialty})
Dr. {name} ({specialty})

Onset: {sudden vs. gradual} / Timing: {frequency of symptoms}
   Location of patient at onset: {automobile, home, other location
                                  location}
   Activity of patient at onset: {injury, exertional chest pain,
                                  syncope}
Duration: {time since symptoms began}
Location: {pain or sensory changes} / Radiation: {movement of pain/
                                                  sensory changes}
Character/Quality: {descriptors}
Intensity: {mild/moderate/severe} / Severity: {x/10}
Associated Symptoms: {positive symptoms other than the chief
                      complaint}
Context: {what the patient was exposed to, what the patient was
doing when the symptom(s) occurred or what was happening around the
patient, at the time the symptom(s) began}
Modifying factors: {things that worsen / Tx before arrival: {tx and
                    or improve symptoms}              with what
                                                      benefit}
```

Fig. 5.3 A template for an undiagnosed patient in the emergency department. In this template, descriptors placed next to one another count as one documentation element (e.g. *onset* and *timing*).

Along with some of the descriptors frequently encountered examples are also listed. These are not comprehensive lists, but can be used as a reference.

Note: The documentation elements are numbered 1 to 8. Descriptors with letters (e.g. "2a" and "2b") count as one documentation element.

1. **Duration**: Length of time the chief complaint has been present.
   Examples: *hours, days, weeks, months, years, since childhood, etc.*
2a. **Onset:** Describes how abruptly the chief complaint began.
   Examples: *abrupt, sudden, gradual*
2b. **Timing:** Frequency that the chief complaint occurs. Multiple descriptors can be used together (e.g. pain is constant and worsening).
   Examples: *constant, intermittent, episodic, chronic, persistent, waxing and waning, worsening, improving, resolving, ongoing, consistent, chronic, etc.*
3a. **Location:** This describes the bodily location of a symptom, and is mostly applicable to pain or other sensory changes (like *paresthesias*, which is described as the sensation of "pins and needles").
   A systems-based approach should not be used for this descriptor because it would be inaccurate for a scribe to try and identify the **etiology** (cause) of a chief complaint or symptom or sign based on history alone. For example: if a patient presents with shortness of breath, "respiratory" is not the location. Shortness of breath can have a variety of causes. It could be cardiac-related (like from a myocardial infarction), a symptom of an allergic reaction, or even from a blood clot in the lungs (i.e. pulmonary embolism).

3b. **Radiation:** Extension of a sensation or pain from the origin to another region. If *location* is not used in the history, then by definition *radiation* will not be used either.

4. **Character (Quality):** Subjective description of how something feels to the patient. Typically, single adjectives are used here (listed below). However, some things cannot be described with a single adjective. In those cases, the patient's words may be recorded in quotations. For example: "The pain feels like being stabbed by a thousand samurai swords."

     Examples: *throbbing, aching, cramping, sharp, dull, stabbing, squeezing, pressure-like, etc.*

5a. **Intensity**: Subjective description of pain on a numerical scale rated 1 through 10, where "1" describes the least amount of pain, and "10" describes the most pain. Sometimes a patient will rate their pain more than once, such as before and after receiving medications, or with waxing and waning pain. In these cases, each pain rating should be documented, and the event which precipitated the fluctuation.

5b. **Severity:** Subjective description of pain on a graded scale comparing mild, moderate, and severe. It should be noted that neither the scribe nor the clinician should rate the patient's severity of symptoms.

6. **Associated symptoms:** All acute symptoms that the patient is experiencing, other than the chief complaint. Although both present and absent symptoms should be documented in the history, only present (or positive) symptoms should be documented here.

7. **Context:** Any circumstances surrounding the present illness. This may include what the patient was doing, where they were, or exposures or activities at symptom onset.

8a. **Modifying factors:** Any alleviating or aggravating factors which make symptoms or signs better or worse. These are typically discovered incidentally.

     Examples: *certain movements, positional changes, or eating or drinking.*

8b. **Treatment before arrival:** Any intentional attempts by the patient or others to alleviate discomfort due to a symptom or sign prior to evaluation.

     Examples: *medications (prescribed or not prescribed), applying ice, heat, pressure, or bandages, or alternative medicines (e.g. acupuncture or herbal supplements)*

     Additional documentation here should include whether or not the treatment provided any relief or benefit.

     Examples: *full or partial relief, transient or temporary relief, no relief*

Review of Systems (ROS)

Review of systems (ROS) is a systematic listing of all symptoms organized by system, which is obtained by asking the patient questions. The body systems are listed in Box 5.1. **Symptoms** are things that a patient experiences and are thus considered to be **subjective**. Symptoms may or may not be associated with the chief complaint. Some symptoms can be appropriately placed into multiple systems, but should only be reflected in the review of systems once.

In the review of systems, symptoms should be documented as either present or absent. Symptoms which are present are designated as "positive" or "+" or "affirms." Symptoms which are absent are designated as "negative" or "−" or "denies." Some electronic medical records may place positive findings in red or bold text. This is not required, but does help the reader to more rapidly identify the pertinent positive findings.

Like the HPI, the review of systems must be documented for the current encounter. If pulled from the health record for a prior visit, they must be adjusted to reflect the current visit. If no changes are made to the cloned review of systems, then comment must be made specifically stating that there is no change from the prior visit. Fig. 5.4 shows an example EHR screen for collecting ROS data.

BOX 5.1 ■ Body Systems

General or Constitutional—A person's *systemic* (overall) health or appearance.
Eyes—Including the eyelid and extraocular muscles
Ears, Nose, and Throat—External, middle and inner ear; nose, nasal cavity; nasopharynx, oropharynx, laryngopharynx
Cardiovascular—Heart and the blood vessels
Respiratory—Nose, mouth, larynx, trachea, and lungs
Gastrointestinal—Digestive tract (mouth, pharynx, esophagus, stomach, intestines, rectum, anus) and accessory organs (liver, gallbladder, pancreas, salivary glands)
Genitourinary—Urinary system (kidneys, ureters, bladder, urethra) and reproductive organs, including genitals
Musculoskeletal—Bones, joints, and muscles
Neurological—Nervous system, including the brain, spinal cord, and nerves
Hematologic/Lymphatic—Blood, lymphatic system (glands, nodes, vessels, lymph)
Psychiatric—Mental health
Endocrine—The hormone-secreting organs and glands
Dermatologic/Integumentary—Skin, hair, and nails
Immunologic/Allergic—Physiological responses to pathogens and other foreign substances

---

BILLING AND CODING

Per the documentation guidelines, as determined by regulation, the review of systems can be billed at five different levels, depending on the number of systems that are documented:

- **Very low complexity visit**—0 systems
- **Low complexity (problem pertinent) visit**—1 system
- **Moderate complexity visit**—2 to 9 systems
- **Moderate complexity but more urgent (extended) visit**—2 to 9 systems
- **High complexity visit (complete)**—10 or more systems

Please note that the billing and coding requirements for other facilities (like inpatient and outpatient) differ from the emergency department. The emergency department documentation guidelines are given here for example. As noted above, for example, certain outpatient visits only require a medically appropriate history and exam.

Number of Elements to Obtain

The number of systems documented in the review of systems is considered when calculating the entire chart's level for reimbursement. To ensure that the chart can be billed at the level deemed appropriate for that visit, it is best to try to document enough systems that appear relevant to that patient's case. If too few systems are documented, the provider will not be compensated for his or her time and efforts. For example, documenting two systems in review of systems for a ESI 2 visit (like an evaluation for a seizure) would be underdocumentation. Documenting too many systems is overdocumentation and not necessarily the best solution. For example, documenting 10 systems in review of systems for a ESI 4 visit (like a minor finger injury) would be over-documentation.

Thus, the recommendation is the following: in the ED for **lower acuity encounters (ESI 4 or ESI 5), aim for 2 to 9 systems**. If an encounter is **higher acuity (ESI 1, ESI 2, or ESI 3), aim for 10 systems**. In other places of service, the number of systems documented depends on whether the visit is for a new patient or an existing patient, an initial visit or a subsequent visit; an E/M Level 3 or 4 visit would require 2–9 systems, while a Level 5 would require documentation of 10

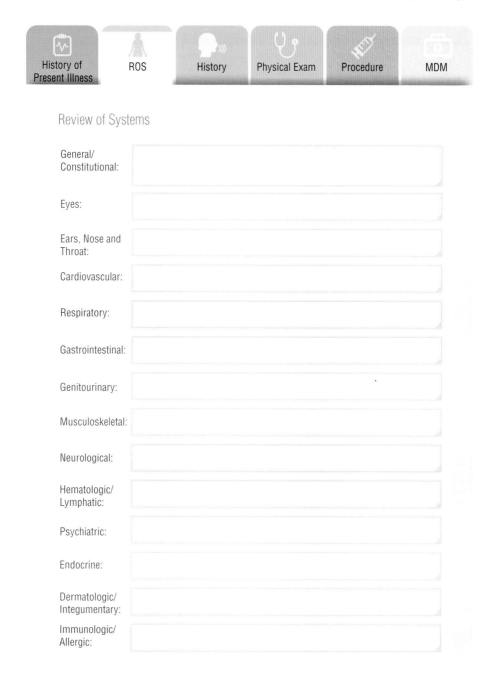

Fig. 5.4 Review of systems (ROS) form in an electronic health record (EHR).

or more. Be aware that the patient's acuity level may change throughout their visit based upon what is elicited during history and exam. If this is the case, your provider will want to elicit (and have you document) adequately for this higher acuity.

Meeting the Billing Requirement

The scribe is acting as the provider's partner in creating the clinical note. As such, the scribe will be expected to assist in making sure that the document is as thorough and complete as possible. This will help the coders and billers have all the information that they need to be able to bill the chart at the level appropriate for the patient's acuity and should accurately reflect the clinician's work in caring for the patient. Tracking the number of documentation (billable) elements for the physician is part of this job.

Limitations to History

If the history is limited (for any reason) and thus enough documentation elements cannot be obtained, the requirement for billing will be forgiven as long as there is documentation describing the limitation. This should be reflected after the review of systems in the form of the following statement (or a statement with a similar effect):

Review of systems is otherwise limited due to _____.

Some examples could include if the patient is unconscious, has altered mental status, or is an extremely poor historian. Be sure to include documentation that states another historian was not available.

UTILIZING A TEMPLATE

The patient's positive and negative symptoms are always included within the HPI, but a template that organizes the symptoms into their respective systems may be included below the HPI.

An example of an ROS template is seen in Fig. 5.5. In this template, all billable systems have been listed but the template has otherwise been left blank. Filling out this template is an easy and quick process. Each symptom should be placed in the proper system and designated as being present or absent. Then the headings of the systems that were not discussed during the ROS should be deleted.

Some providers may choose to offer the scribe an ROS template with prefilled normals (Fig. 5.5A). As the scribe documents the patient encounter, he or she must delete the fields not asked about and change negatives to positives where needed. Retaining documentation of information that did not occur is falsification and illegal.

Additional History

The HPI can also contain additional history felt to be relevant to the chief complaint. **Additional history** includes past medical history, family history, social history, surgical history, the patient's current medication list, and any known allergies (Fig. 5.6).

This information can be found elsewhere in the note (often entered by other members of the healthcare team and automatically imported into the note), and is thus not required to be reiterated in the HPI. However, if additional history is discussed by the provider and the patient, it should be documented in the history because the information likely pertains to the present illness. For example, a patient on many medications recently started a new medication and is now experiencing new symptoms. Since these new symptoms may be related to the new medication, the medication change should be included within the history.

The elements of additional history may be pulled from prior encounters, but must be updated to reflect current realities. A scribe may update these elements. However, they must be specifically

```
ROS
ROS is limited by <LFACTORS>

Constitutional:
Eyes:
ENT:
Cardiovascular:
Respiratory:
GI:
GU:
MS:
Skin:
Neurologic:
Endocrine:
Lymphathic:
Psychiatric:
Allergic:
```

A

```
ROS
ROS is limited by <LFACTORS>

Constitutional: Denies fever. No chills.
Eyes: Denies vision changes.
ENT:  Denies sore throat. No ear pain.
Cardiovascular: Denies chest pain. No palpitations. No swelling.
Respiratory: Denies cough. No dyspnea.
GI: No nausea.  No vomiting. No diarrhea.  No abdominal pain.
GU: No urinary frequency or hematuria.
MS: Denies back pain or other joint pain.
Skin: No rash.
Neurologic: Denies headache.  No extremity weakness.  No paresthesia.
Endocrine:  no excessive thirst or polyuria.
Lymphathic: Denies swollen glands.
Psychiatric:  Denies depression.  No SI/HI.
Allergic: No pruritis or angioedema symptoms.
```

B

Fig. 5.5   Review of systems template. (A) Blank template. (B) Template prefilled with normals.

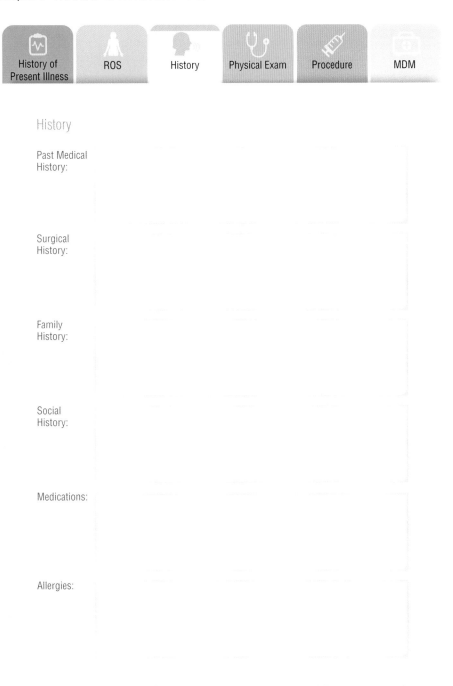

Fig. 5.6 An electronic health record (EHR) form for additional history elements.

told to do so by the provider. Otherwise, the provider or other ancillary staff like nursing or medical assistants should make updates if needed. Finally, the provider must review the elements imported into the note from a previous visit and mark them as reviewed before the note can be completed and signed.

PAST MEDICAL HISTORY (PMH)

All formally documented and verbally relayed medical history should be included within the past medical history. This can include illnesses, injuries, and treatments. It is often obtained by the nurse or brought forward from prior visits. New elements discovered during the current visit may need to be added.

PAST SURGICAL HISTORY (PSH)

This history includes any past procedures or surgeries. It is important to document the type of surgery or procedure, the date it was performed, the name of the surgeon, if there were any complications perioperatively, and the hospital where the surgery took place. Most of the time the patient will be unable to provide all of the specifics for their surgical history, but many patients are at least able to give a year and describe the procedure or surgery in lay terms.

FAMILY HISTORY (FH)

Any major disease that runs in a patient's family is part of the patient's family history. Only blood relatives should be considered. Family history is often used to assess a patient's risk for certain diseases. Typically, family history is recorded for three generations of the family tree. For each family member a list of diseases, if they are living or deceased, and if living their current state of health should all be documented.

SOCIAL HISTORY (SH)

Any social behaviors that may contribute to human health and disease are considered a part of the social history. This includes substance use, occupation, and lifestyle.

Substance use is the use of any substance to achieve a sensory change. Substances may include tobacco, alcohol, and prescription or illegal drugs. Types and quantity of substances may be pertinent to clinical decision making and should be documented. Former substance abuse, the time since last use, and duration of use, and whether a patient is in remission should also be noted. These factors can contribute to addiction and tolerance levels, which may in turn affect the care that the patient needs or receives.

Tobacco can be taken orally (dip or chew), or smoked with pipes, cigars or cigarillos, or cigarettes. Counting **pack-years** is used to quantify an individual's degree of tobacco exposure. This is calculated by multiplying the number of packs a person smokes per day, by the number of years they have smoked. For example, if a patient has smoked one pack of cigarettes a day for thirty years, they have a 30 pack-year history. The use of e-cigarettes is more popular than in the past. Use of e-cigarettes may have its own health-related issues and use of these should be documented here as well.

Alcohol may be used never, rarely, occasionally, or socially. Some may use a certain number of days a week. Others may use alcohol every day. Because different drinks vary in alcohol content, be sure to document the type of drink, amount, and number of drinks during a period of time. This becomes especially important for individuals seen for acute alcohol intoxication, or alcohol related withdrawal.

Illicit drugs are any drug that is illegal to make, sell, transport, or use. These can be snorted, injected, smoked, or ingested orally. The method of intake can pose potential problems or complications, aside from the pharmacologic properties of the drugs. For example, intravenous injection can result in endocarditis (inflammation and infection of the endocardium of the heart) or epidural abscesses (pockets of infection in the space around the spinal cord). Snorting a drug repeatedly can erode the nasal septum and cause frequent episodes of epistaxis (nose bleeds).

The most common illicit drugs include cannabis (marijuana or hashish; legality varies from location to location), amphetamines, cocaine (injected or snorted) or crack cocaine (smoked), MDMA (ecstasy or molly or XTC), and hallucinogenic mushrooms. Opiates and opioids are becoming an area of interest as they continue to grow in popularity. Some, like hydrocodone, hydromorphone, oxycodone, fentanyl, and morphine, are given in the hospital and as prescriptions to treat pain. Heroin is an opioid with no accepted medical uses and is thus classified as an illegal drug. Opioids have high addiction potential and healthcare professionals are now seeing a lot of drug-seeking behavior for these drugs. This means that people are returning to their doctor or coming to the emergency department specifically asking for opioid pain medications for very minor or nonexistent complaints. There are also a rising number of opioid-related drug overdoses, particularly from heroin. In these circumstances a drug called Narcan (naloxone) may be used to reverse the effects of opioids.

Occupation plays a significant role in human health and morbidity and mortality. Different occupations can put an individual at higher risk for certain medical conditions, injuries, or death. For example, black lung disease (also called coal worker's pneumoconiosis) commonly afflicts laborers in coal mines due to prolonged and excessive inhalation of fine coal dust particles. More commonly seen, occupations with a heavy workload (lots of heavy lifting and straining) may result in more musculoskeletal injuries. Sedentary jobs that involve a lot of sitting may be a risk factor for cardiovascular disease (more on this below).

Lifestyle also contributes to human health and morbidity and mortality by altering a person's risk for certain medical conditions or diseases. This can include sexual orientation, exposure to certain environments (e.g. time spent in jail or a nursing home), socioeconomic status and living situation, dietary choices, and activity level. For example, a sedentary lifestyle, which is a combination of inadequate exercise and poor diet, can classify as a risk factor for cardiovascular disease.

MEDICATIONS

Medications are either given "in-house" (on site) or as prescriptions for the patient to take home. A scribe will have to record the names of many medications during documentation. This could include prescribed medications used to treat known disease, over the counter medications, and even medications prescribed to someone else that the patient is taking. In addition to recording the medication name, the scribe should record the dose, form of the drug, and the frequency that the medication is taken or used. This information will likely play a role in the provider's medical decision making. For example, knowing medication dosages is important because too much medication may harm a patient. A provider may need to give a patient their daily medications during their emergency department visit, but should give them the amount that they are currently prescribed to avoid any complications.

Alternative medical supplements are a unique area of interest. There is controversy surrounding the ingredients and possible contraindications (reasons why something is not recommended). Many alternative medicines are unregulated and can have unknown ingredients.

Drug Names

Every drug has a chemical name, a generic name, and one or more trade names. The **chemical/ scientific name** is based on the chemical structure. The **trade name/brand name/trademarked name** is typically a patented drug formulation. One drug can have several manufacturers, each with a different brand name. Brand names always begin with a capital letter. The ***nonproprietary name/generic name*** are drugs with the same drug formulation of a brand name sold at a more affordable cost. Generic names always begin with a lowercase letter.

When recording a patient's medication list, it is always best to be as specific and accurate as possible. For example, if the patient is taking Lipitor (the brand name of atorvastatin), Lipitor should be recorded. If it is unknown whether the patient is taking the brand or generic form of the drug, the generic should be used. In actuality, a scribe does not usually have the knowledge to make this determination. Therefore, the scribe should record what the provider, nurse or other medical personnel has recorded.

There are additional naming conventions used to document medications. **Intercapping** is the capitalization of letters within a drug name. This is sometimes used by companies to make their product distinct. For example, "MiraLAX," where the "LAX" tells the consumer that the drug is a laxative. **Tall-man letters** are a safety precaution in the electronic medical record used to distinguish between similar sounding drugs. For example, these letters are used to highlight the difference between "prednisone" and "prednisoLONE." The scribe need not include these tall-man letters when documenting a medication list. Rather, the scribe should take precautions to document the correct drug and not the similar-sounding one.

Many drugs sound alike but have different functions. For example, naloxone and metaxalone— the former is a reversal agent for opiates, and the latter a muscle relaxant. If there is ever doubt about how to spell a drug name: (1) consult the patient's medication list, (2) put a placeholder next to the drug's name until its spelling can be clarified, (3) ask the provider!

A scribe may be involved in entering a medication or preparing a prescription for signature, so long as they are directed by a provider. There are certain safeguards in place in the electronic medical record that legally allow the scribe to enter medications and prescriptions. These include **hardstops** after a scribe places orders or creates prescriptions. The scribe may pend or save their work, but the hard-stops prevent the order or prescription from being acted upon unless the provider has reviewed, approved, and signed the scribe's work. In addition to the hard-stops, the electronic medical record should send notifications to the provider (such as medication contraindications, which includes allergies and drug-drug interactions), even if they were sent to the scribe first.

ALLERGIES

Allergies may include true allergies, intolerances, or contraindications. Many people have **true allergies** to medications, foods, or after exposure to different environmental triggers. This occurs when the immune system becomes hypersensitive to an innocuous antigen (a protein) and reacts as if the antigen is pathogenic. Allergic reactions may range from mild to severe. Mild allergic reactions may just include a skin rash and redness. Often patients will develop a specific type of welt-like rash called *urticaria* (colloquially known as hives). If it is a simple skin contact allergy, the rash is called a *contact dermatitis*. More severe allergic reactions may cause swelling of the oral mucosa and face (especially the lips and tongue), difficulties breathing, nausea, and vomiting. Other symptoms may also be present depending on the allergen, route of contact with the body, and the type and degree of sensitivity. Over-the-counter medications may cause allergies just like a prescribed medication might.

An **intolerance** differs from an allergy because the symptomatology is not consistent with true allergic reactions. Symptoms oftentimes include known drug side effects listed on the label. Common intolerances include nausea and vomiting. Others may have to do with how a person metabolizes the drug. One example of an intolerance that is not an allergy is muscle pain and inflammation due to use of a group of drugs known as statins (which are used to control high cholesterol).

A **contraindication** is an absolute reason why a certain line of treatment should not be utilized. This could include interactions with other medications or medical conditions in which it is unfavorable to give a certain medication. For example, the use of non-steroidal anti-inflammatory drugs (NSAIDs) in a patient who has renal disease is contraindicated.

Physical Exam (PE)

A **physical exam (PE)** is a list of signs, organized by system, that are elicited by the provider as they are examining the patient. **Signs** are things that a provider finds or observes, and are therefore **objective**. Objective findings can be measured and quantified, and unlike subjective findings, their values do not change with the perspective of the observer. Signs should be designated as present or absent. Some signs may be placed within various systems but should only be reflected in the exam once. An example of this would be the finding of pedal edema (lower extremity swelling) which could rightly be documented under extremities or cardiovascular, as it indicates a circulatory problem.

The provider elicits signs during the physical exam using various techniques. It is worth becoming familiar with the most common of these techniques and findings that the provider might describe for inclusion in the medical record.

The first and most obvious of these techniques is **inspection**. As the name suggests, this is simply looking at the patient and his or her various anatomical areas and describing what is seen. Inspection might reveal a thin or obese patient or a ruddy or pale complexion for example. Inspection might also show skin lesions or some other body deformity. The type of observations that fall under the inspection label would include size, shape, color, location, symmetry, and deviation from normal appearance. The examples are endless and the provider will describe for inclusion in the record any inspection findings he or she deems important for documenting the medical condition of the patient.

A second technique used in the exam is **palpation**. This refers to using the hands with their sense of touch and then describing what is found. Palpation may be used to further describe something that may be inspected/seen, such as a skin lesion, or it may be used to discover and describe a deep structure that may not be seen at all on inspection, such as liver size and consistency during palpation on the abdominal exam. Palpation may also reveal vibrations caused by turbulent blood flow through a partly obstructed blood vessel or valve. This vibration is called a *thrill*.

A third technique the provider will employ is **percussion**. As the word suggests, percussion is tapping on the body to elicit a sound that suggests wellness or pathology in the patient. A common example is chest percussion which will sound different when done over a healthy section of the lungs (which gives a more hollow sound as it is normally air-filled) versus an area of lung that is fluid-filled (a duller sound due to the fluid replacing the air that would normally be within the lung). This finding along with other signs and symptoms (such as cough and fever) could lead the clinician to diagnose pneumonia, for example.

A fourth technique commonly used is **auscultation**. Auscultation is listening, usually employing the stethoscope, and describing what is heard which could have diagnostic significance. The heart, with its various sounds is the usual target of auscultation along with the lungs and their varied breath sounds. The abdomen can also be auscultated for bowel sounds or lack thereof. And auscultating over blood vessels might reveal **bruits** (a swishing or turbulent sound) in areas of restricted or chaotic blood flow.

These are the most common techniques used on physical exam, but they are not the only ones you will encounter. Any of the senses may be used to detect important physical findings. Even the sense of smell (for example, the sweet fruity odor consistent with diabetic ketoacidosis or the bitter almond odor of cyanide poisoning) has its place in the exam. And instruments other than a stethoscope may be used in the physical exam as well. While much can be learned about the patient from **gross** examination, meaning visible with the naked eye, the provider's inspection may be aided with an **otoscope** to look inside the ear canal, and an **ophthalmoscope** is used to look into the eyes. Depending on the specialty, there are potentially many other instruments that you may encounter, which are used to elicit more findings on the physical exam.

The physical exam is typically performed after the history has been collected and may involve one or more organ systems. The extent of the exam and what was examined will depend upon what was elicited during history and review of systems. Thus, the physical exam can be *problem-focused* or *comprehensive*.

Problem-focused exams pertain to one specific minor complaint and attention is given to only one or a few body systems. **Comprehensive exams** are reserved for more complex cases and generally most or all of the body systems are examined. The physical exam should never be pulled from a prior encounter and should be specific to the current visit.

A more experienced scribe will be able to identify specific physical exam elements and may chart the finding without being asked as long as the scribe prompts the provider to confirm the findings **and** asks for any additional findings and clarifications. This will help the provider become more efficient and will result in more accurate and timely documentation. This level of knowledge will come with time and familiarity with the provider.

> **NOTE**
>
> As a partner in documentation, the scribe is assisting the provider to create an accurate chart. As such, it is not only fair but appropriate and desirable that the scribe point out anything that seems inaccurate in order that the provider be able to correct the document that they are creating together.

BILLING AND CODING

Per the documentation guidelines, the physical exam can support five different levels of billing for varying complexities of encounters, depending on the number of systems that are documented:

- **Straightforward complexity visit**—1 system
- **Low complexity visit**—2 to 4 systems
- **Moderate complexity visit**—2 to 4 systems
- **Moderate complexity (but more urgent)**—5 to 7 systems
- **High complexity**—8 or more systems

The billing and coding requirements for other facilities (like inpatient and outpatient) differ from the emergency department. According to the 2021 E/M guidelines, outpatient office visits (codes 99202-99215) only require a medically appropriate exam. (The levels of service in this setting is determined by other factors, such as medical decision making and total time, discussed below.) In other places of service, a Level 2 would require documentation of the physical examination of 2 to 4 systems; a Level 3 or 4 would require 5 to 7 systems; a Level 4 or 5 would require 8 or more body systems.

Number of Elements to Obtain

To ensure that the chart can be billed at the level deemed appropriate for that visit, it is best to try to document enough systems that appear relevant to that patient's case. Document too few systems and the provider will not be compensated for his or her time and efforts. For example, documenting two systems in physical exam for an ESI 2 visit (such as an evaluation for a seizure) is underdocumentation. Documenting too many systems is overdocumentation and not necessarily the best solution. For example, documenting eight systems in physical exam for an ESI 4 visit (like a minor finger injury) is overdocumentation.

Thus, the recommendation is the following: for **very low acuity encounters** (ESI 5), aim for documentation of **one system**. For **low acuity encounters** (ESI 4), **two to four systems** should suffice. If an encounter is **higher acuity** (ESI 1, ESI 2, or ESI 3), **eight systems** should be documented. Be aware that the patient's acuity level may change throughout their visit based upon what is elicited during history and exam. If this is the case, ensure that the billable level of the physical exam changes to reflect the new acuity level.

Meeting the Billing Requirement

Your provider will likely obtain more than enough physical exam elements/systems for the purposes of medical decision making, such that prompting them for more systems to document will be an unusual event. Nevertheless, the provider may not be focused on imparting all of the physical exam observations that he or she is making. Thus, you may need to prompt them for more information to complete your charting to the level needed for a patient of the acuity presenting. A common example of this would be failure of the provider to relate to the scribe what are sometimes called *observable elements*, which are explored in detail below. When your provider (and you for that matter) walks into a room, you already know if the patient is awake and alert. A quick glance may also show that the eyes are tracking normally and have no discharge. These and many other observations satisfy the requirement for a given body system if documented. Your provider may only be focused on certain systems and forget to dictate some obvious findings. This is where the scribe should prompt the provider for completeness. Tracking the thoroughness of the physical exam documentation is part of the scribe's job.

UTILIZING A TEMPLATE OR FORM

A template that organizes physical exam findings into their respective systems, or a form may appear in the facility's EHR software (Fig. 5.7). As you can see, the body systems in the physical exam EHR screen are identical to those in the ROS. A physical exam template with prefilled normals is shown in Fig. 5.8. The provider has included in the template strings of information commonly documented in this setting, but the scribe tailors the template's information as needed for the patient encounter, and deletes any systems not discussed.

The scribe may record the provider's findings in the proper field of the physical exam template. Fields of the descriptors that were not part of the provider's findings should be deleted. Retaining documentation of information that did not occur is falsification and illegal.

If the scribe is documenting in a form with text fields (such as the form shown in Fig. 5.7), the fields may be left blank, or N/A (or similar language per facility policy) may be entered. Many EHR applications allow the user to select common physical examination findings from a menu. The software then populates the note with the items the user has selected (Fig. 5.9).

VITAL SIGNS

Vital signs are external signs that may indicate the functional state of the body. These include **heart rate** (normal range is 60 to 100 beats per minute), **blood pressure** (normal range is 90/60 to 120/80 mmHg), **body temperature** (normal is about 98.6 °F), and **respiratory rate** (normal range is 12 to 18 breaths per minute). Normal ranges given are for an adult and children will have differing normals that change with their age. Vital signs are usually taken by ancillary members of the healthcare team, such as nurses or medical assistants, and are trended in the EHR (Fig. 5.10). If the provider takes the patient's vital signs during their evaluation, the scribe may document these in the physical exam or another appropriate place in the record.

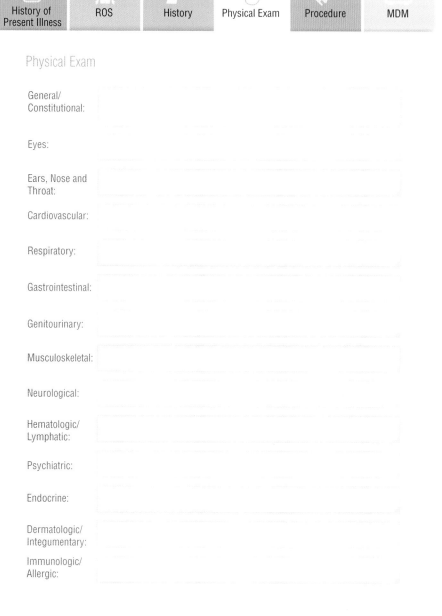

Physical Exam

General/
Constitutional:

Eyes:

Ears, Nose and
Throat:

Cardiovascular:

Respiratory:

Gastrointestinal:

Genitourinary:

Musculoskeletal:

Neurological:

Hematologic/
Lymphatic:

Psychiatric:

Endocrine:

Dermatologic/
Integumentary:

Immunologic/
Allergic:

Fig. 5.7 An electronic health record (EHR) screen for recording the provider's findings during the physical examination.

```
PHYSICAL EXAM
VITAL SIGNS: <EDTRIAGEVITALS>

Constitutional: Well developed. Well nourished. Appearance
 consistent with <BMI>
HENT: Normocephalic. Atraumatic. Bilateral external ears normal.
 Nose normal. Moist mucous membranes.
Eyes: PERRL. EOMI. Conjunctiva normal. No discharge. No scleral
 icterus.
Lymphatic: No lymphadenopathy noted.
Endocrine: No palpable thyromegaly.
Neck: Neck is supple. Normal ROM. No stridor.
Cardiovascular: Normal heart rate. Normal rhythm. No murmurs,
 gallops or rubs.
Thorax & Lungs: Normal breath sounds. No respiratory distress.
 No wheezing.
Abdomen: No masses. No pulsatile masses. No distention. No palpable
 organomegaly. Soft. No tenderness.
GU: No CVA tenderness.
Skin: Warm. Dry. No erythema. No rashes on exposed skin.  Normal
 capillary refill.
Musculoskeletal/Extremities: Good range of motion in all major
 joints as observed. No major deformities noted. No extremity
 tenderness. No edema. No cyanosis. No clubbing.
Back: No tenderness.
Neurologic: Alert & oriented x 3. No focal deficits noted. Normal
 motor function.
Psychiatric: Affect normal. Judgment normal. Mood normal.
```

Fig. 5.8 A prefilled physical examination template.

OBSERVABLE ELEMENTS

There are portions of the physical exam that may be observed about a patient by carefully watching them move and listening to them speak, called **observable elements**. These may be added to the physical exam in addition to the elements that are specifically examined during that encounter. There may be personal or specialty specific preferences regarding which elements will be observed in this manner. Therefore, it is best to clarify with each provider about their preferences regarding these elements. However, the following is a list of a few observable elements that may be used during any encounter, regardless of acuity:

Constitutional: Well developed. Well nourished.

HEENT: Normocephalic. Atraumatic. Bilateral external ears normal. Nose normal. Conjunctiva normal. No discharge. No scleral icterus.

Respiratory: No respiratory distress.

Musculoskeletal: No major deformities noted.

Neurologic: Alert and cooperative. No focal deficits noted. No obvious motor deficits.

Psychiatric: Affect normal. Mood situationally appropriate.

Integumentary: No cyanosis. No clubbing.

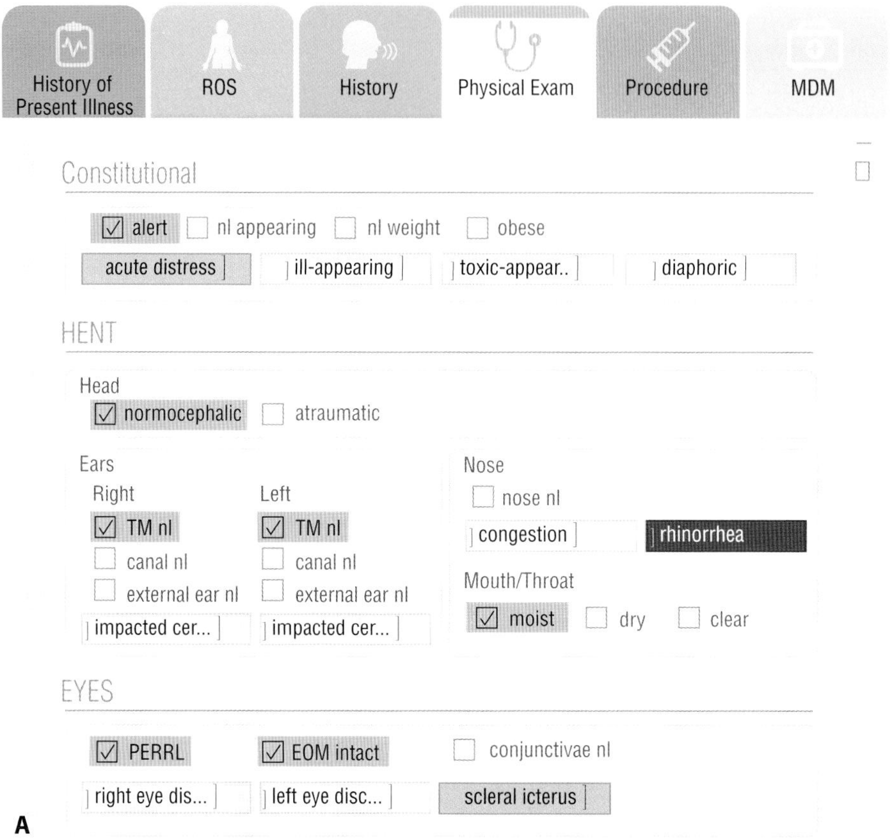

| History of Present Illness | ROS | History | Physical Exam | Procedure | MDM |

Constitutional

☑ alert ☐ nl appearing ☐ nl weight ☐ obese

| acute distress | | ill-appearing | | toxic-appear.. | | diaphoric |

HENT

Head
☑ normocephalic ☐ atraumatic

Ears
| Right | Left | Nose |

☐ nose nl

Right	Left
☑ TM nl	☑ TM nl
☐ canal nl	☐ canal nl
☐ external ear nl	☐ external ear nl
impacted cer...	impacted cer...

Nose
☐ nose nl
| congestion | | rhinorrhea |

Mouth/Throat
☑ moist ☐ dry ☐ clear

EYES

☑ PERRL ☑ EOM intact ☐ conjunctivae nl

| right eye dis... | | left eye disc... | | scleral icterus |

A

Physical Exam

BP (!) 184/90 | Pulse 82 | Temp 96 °F (35.6 °C) | Resp 17 | Ht 5' 4" (1.626 m) |
Wt 167 lb (75.8 kg) | SpO2 98% | BMI 28.67 kg/m^2

```
Physical Exam
Constitutional:
      General: She is not in acute distress.
HENT:
      Head: Tympanic membrane normal.
      Right Ear: Tympanic membrane normal.
      Nose: Rhinorrhea present.
      Mouth/Throat:
      Mouth: Mucous membranes are moist.
Eyes:
      General: No scleral icterus
      Extraocular Movements: Extraocular movements intact.
      Pupils: Pupils are equal, round, and reactive to light.
```

B

Fig. 5.9 The physical exam note being created in the electronic health record (EHR) software from the user's selections on a menu.

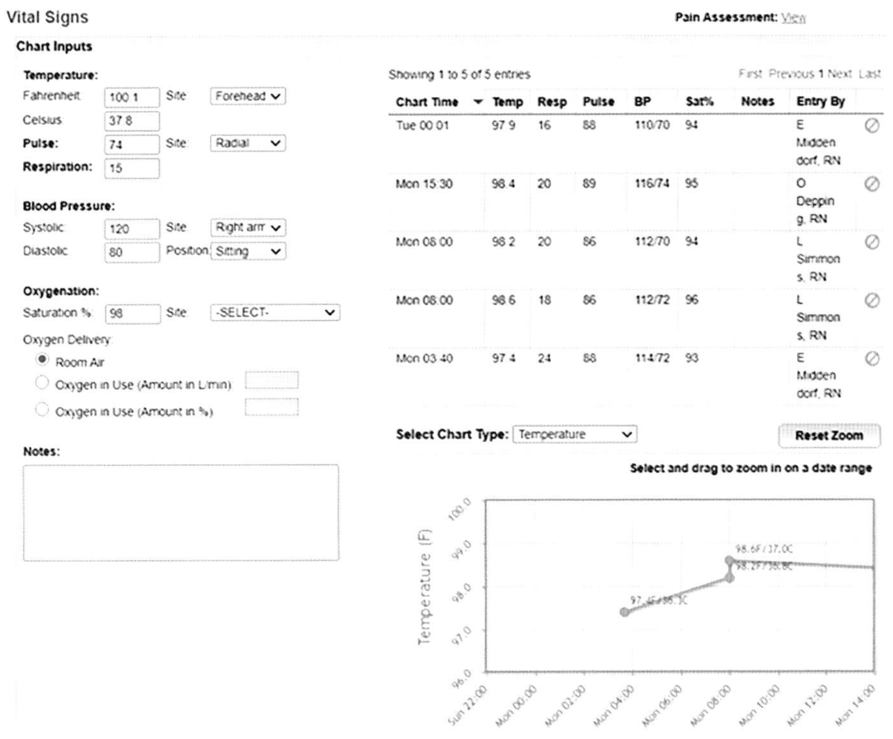
Vital Signs
Pain Assessment: View
Chart Inputs
Temperature:
Fahrenheit 100.1 Site Forehead
Celsius 37.8
Pulse: 74 Site Radial
Respiration: 15
Blood Pressure:
Systolic 120 Site Right arm
Diastolic 80 Position Sitting
Oxygenation:
Saturation % 98 Site -SELECT-
Oxygen Delivery
Room Air
Oxygen in Use (Amount in L/min)
Oxygen in Use (Amount in %)
Notes:
Showing 1 to 5 of 5 entries
First Previous 1 Next Last
Chart Time Temp Resp Pulse BP Sat% Notes Entry By
Tue 00:01 97.9 16 88 110/70 94 E Middendorf, RN
Mon 15:30 98.4 20 89 116/74 95 O Depping, RN
Mon 08:00 98.2 20 86 112/70 94 L Simmons, RN
Mon 08:00 98.6 18 86 112/72 96 L Simmons, RN
Mon 03:40 97.4 24 88 114/72 93 E Middendorf, RN
Select Chart Type: Temperature
Reset Zoom
Select and drag to zoom in on a date range
Temperature (F)
100.0
99.0
98.0
97.0
96.0
Sun 22:00
Mon 00:00
Mon 02:00
Mon 04:00
Mon 06:00
Mon 08:00
Mon 10:00
Mon 12:00
Mon 14:00

Fig. 5.10 An electronic health record (EHR) screen for capturing the patient's vital signs and monitoring trends.

CASE STUDY 5.1

A 29-year-old pregnant woman presents to the emergency room, complaining that she has noticed a dramatic increase in the frequency she has to urinate for the past four days. "The color seems weird, too," she relates. It's sort of hazy." She has had pain in her lower back for about the same amount of time, and she is very worried about the baby. She is a nonsmoker and this is her second pregnancy. "I know I'm at 8 months now so the risks are lower, but I lost my last pregnancy at 20 weeks, and I'm really scared," she says. The triage nurse recorded the patient's blood pressure at 129/68, a temperature of 36.5°C, pulse 79, and respiratory rate 18. The provider orders a urinalysis.

During the patient interview, the woman says she does not have any burning, itching, or pain with urination. When asked whether she has any fever or chills, the patient shakes her head. "I took my temperate a couple times yesterday and right before I came in. It's normal."

"How have you been feeling otherwise during the pregnancy?" the provider asks.

"It's been pretty good," the woman says. The morning sickness went away around 16 weeks, but I did throw up yesterday and today, and I feel kind of queasy. I did have a urinary tract infection (UTI) a few months ago—they helped me at urgent care."

"How did they treat the infection?" asks the provider.

"They gave me an antibiotic, Macrobid I think," the woman replies.

She relates that she has not noticed any vaginal bleeding or leaking of fluid vaginally, and she does not have any abdominal pain.

Continued

The provider uses a stethoscope to listen to the patient breathe and states that both lungs sound clear. He listens to her heart and announces that the rate is normal and rhythm is regular. He palpates the abdomen and asks the patient if anything hurts, noting she is nontender and has a gravid uterus which is normal size for her reported dates (stage of pregnancy). He uses a handheld Doppler ultrasound and counts the fetal heart rate in the 130s. The urinalysis reveals yellow turbid urine with a large amount of white blood cells and bacteria. The provider diagnoses a UTI.

QUESTIONS

1. What is the patient's chief complaint?
2. In which part of the note would the scribe record that the patient is a nonsmoker?
3. What is the *duration* of the chief complaint?
4. The patient says that she has not noticed any vaginal discharge or gushing of fluid. Where and how might the scribe record this in the note?
5. What physical examination technique did the provider use to listen to the patient's chest?
6. Name the four systems that are examined in the physical exam portion of this case.

Medical Decision Making (MDM)

Medical decision making (MDM) is the provider's domain to document their evolving thought processes during the patient's visit. This would include things like the **differential** (a list of possible diagnoses or impressions), consults that were made on behalf of the patient (e.g. cardiology, crisis, home health, etc.), tests ordered and the interpretation of the results, and any final conclusions or impressions with a plan of treatment. An example EHR screen where the provider can record his or her impressions and plan of care is shown in Fig. 5.11.

Medical decision making is ultimately categorized as one of the following complexities by the provider: straightforward, low complexity, moderate complexity, or high complexity. The complexity of the encounter is determined by a combination of factors, including the extent of the work-up and the history required to ascertain a diagnosis.

A scribe generally does not document in this part of the chart, but can add things if a provider explicitly asks. Examples could include consults with other healthcare providers including time-stamps and plan of treatment, or rechecks on patients with the provider's comments, thoughts, or findings. A scribe may also type in the medical decision-making area for a provider who is dictating to them. This may happen if the provider is not proficient or is uncomfortable using electronic medical records.

Time

Time is not a factor in emergency department visits because ED visits are provided on variable levels of intensity, involving multiple encounters over a longer period of time. In the ED it is therefore difficult to determine the time spent with the patient. In other settings, time can be used as an element to determine a level of service. The exception to this ED rule is when there is a *critical care* patient, in which case the critical care rule for billing (see below) is followed.

There are several different types of time. *Floor/unit time* is the time spent on a hospital floor taking care of the patient, writing orders, talking to the patient and/or the patient's family and coordinating care with other healthcare providers,

Face-to-face time is the time spent with patient and/or family directly in their presence.

Total time is the total time spent on the same date of service seeing the patient face-to-face and the non-face-to-face time spent charting, preparing and reviewing the chart, documenting in the

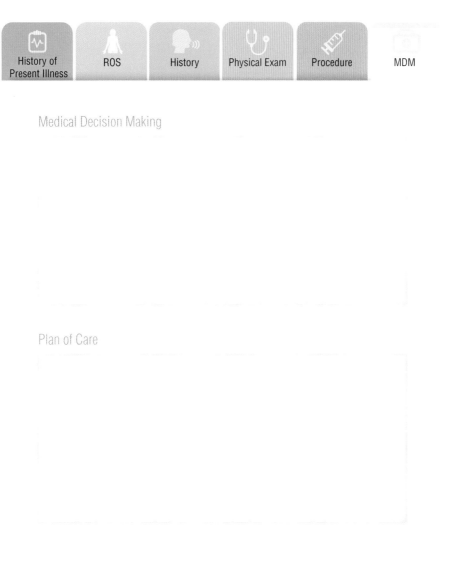

Fig. 5.11 An electronic health record (EHR) screen for medical decision making. (© 2022 Elsevier Inc.)

chart, independently reviewing test results, etc. In office or outpatient settings, the level of service need not be based on the H&P, but rather may be selected based on total time.

For time-based services such as critical care services and for selection of levels of service based on time, time must be documented. Documenting critical care time should however exclude any time that is used performing procedures on the patient, since these are billed separately. The best practice is to record the time that the service began and the time the service ended, so time can be calculated.

Practice Questions

Match the descriptor with its definition.

1. _____ duration   a. makes the complaint better/worse
2. _____ timing   b. where pain/sensation travels
3. _____ location   c. how the complaint came-on
4. _____ modifying factors   d. where pain/sensation originates
5. _____ onset   e. frequency of occurrence
6. _____ radiation   f. time complaint has been present

7. Which can be used as a patient's chief complaint?
   a. Symptoms and signs
   b. A diagnosis
   c. An annual follow-up visit
   d. All of the above

8. Your provider has a full morning schedule and you are falling behind on the notes. While precharting you consider cloning the history from prior encounters so that you do not cause your provider to lose time from your charting. Is this allowed?
   a. No, the history should always be unique to each visit.
   b. No, the scribe does not have privileges to clone the history.
   c. Yes, so long as a new timestamp is noted that is up to date.
   d. Yes, because you created the last history so it is not plagiarism.

9. A patient presents to the emergency department in respiratory distress and requires immediate intubation. There are no other historians. How many systems in review of systems should be documented?
   a. 1 system - this will be a low acuity visit
   b. 2 to 9 systems - this will be a moderate acuity visit
   c. 10+ systems - this will be a high acuity visit
   d. Billing requirements will be forgiven so long as the historical limitation is documented.

10. For each data point, indicate the proper location within "additional history" (e.g. past medical history, medications, allergies, surgical history, family history, or social history).
    a. Hypertension:

    _____

    b. The patient's stepfather's hypertension:

    _____

    c. ACE-inhibitor angioedema:

    _____

    d. Cardiac stenting:

    _____

    e. 30-pack-year smoker:

    _____

    f. The patient's father's heart disease:

    _____

11. A patient is taking metoprolol (Lopressor) for his or her hypertension. Please indicate the generic versus brand name below:
    a. Lopressor: _____
    b. metoprolol: _____

12. Indicate whether each finding is an allergy, intolerance, or contraindication.
    a. Throat swelling after eating peanuts:

    _____
    b. CT scan of the abdomen for a pregnant patient:

    _____
    c. Expected side effects from a medication:

    _____

13. Name four vital signs that can be taken during the physical exam:
    a. _____
    b. _____
    c. _____
    d. _____

CHAPTER 6

Synthesis of a Patient History of Present Illness

1. List the types of historians and their limitations, and document this information in the history of present illness.
2. Document the history of present illness using objective professional language.
3. Utilize a template of documentation elements to relate an accurate and informative history of the present illness.

Differential	History of the present	Action verb
Historian	illness (HPI)	
	Speaking verb	

Historians and Limitations

Now that we have dissected a generic provider note and have discussed each element in detail, let's begin building a **history of the present illness (HPI)**. The HPI is a coherent story, usually chronologic, describing the patient's present illness from the first sign or symptom to the present. Recording this information is the primary responsibility of the medical scribe.

HISTORY GIVEN BY

The HPI may be provided by many sources. It is important to document "who" is saying "what." This may indicate the reliability of the HPI. A space to designate the **historian** is reserved at the very top of the sample template (Fig. 6.1). The historian is not necessarily the patient. Some other examples of history providers are given in Box 6.1. An HPI can have more than one historian, and all historians must be documented. Once the history provider is designated within the HPI, it is assumed that the same speaker is providing the history unless otherwise noted. It is unnecessary to say, "the patient states... the patient reports..." This becomes redundant and difficult to read. If the reported history comes from different sources, however, then this distinction must be made.

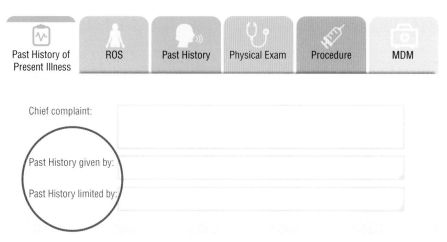

Fig. 6.1 The electronic health record (EHR) software will have a place to record the source of the history of the present illness (HPI) and any limitations to the history provided (circled).

HISTORY LIMITED BY

In the previous chapter, you learned that patients can arrive at the healthcare setting in various states of wellness, many of which can interfere with the provider's ability to gather information. The template offers a space to document any factors that may compromise the reliability of the HPI. This is noted at the very top of the sample template (Fig. 6.1). Some examples of limiting factors to the history are given in Box 6.2.

Documentation of limiting factors is important to achieve billing forgiveness for the documentation elements and review of systems. Basically, if there is an acceptable reason why the HPI is limited, the billing requirements "go away" and a chart can still be billed at the highest otherwise justified level without requiring a certain number of documentation elements or systems in the review of systems.

If the HPI has no limitations, the scribe may be instructed to write words to the effect of "N/A" or "no limitations" in the HPI form, depending on facility policy. The field may also be left blank, or deleted from a template.

BOX 6.1 ■ Examples of Historians

Patient	Nurses
Paramedics	Caretakers
Police	Family

BOX 6.2 ■ Examples of Patient History Limitations

Dementia	Poor historian
Unconscious	Language barriers
Intoxication	Less knowledgeable history providers
Emergent nature	

Language

The language of the HPI should be written with objective terminology. This will make the documentation sound professional and unbiased. For instance, using *"The patient reports..."* to begin a history makes the document sound quite polished and formal. On the other hand, subjective terminology may create a negative perception of the history providers. Using *"The patient complains..."* to begin a history is an example of subjective terminology that makes the history provider appear in a negative light.

The first verbs required when constructing a history are **speaking verbs**. These denote that the historian is actively saying something, and should be written in the present tense. It is important to use objective speaking verbs to make the documentation sound professional and unbiased. Some examples of speaking verb choices are provided in Box 6.3.

It is a good rule of thumb to start the first sentence of the HPI with the type of historian followed by a speaking verb. Using *states* or *reports* are usually the preferred choices for speaking verbs here. This ensures that a historian is designated, and an appropriate and objective verb is used to begin the history.

Example: *"The patient (or other historian) <u>states/reports</u>..."*

The other examples of speaking verbs can be used in different circumstances. Some patients, like certain neurologically impaired patients or small children, cannot speak but can instead *indicate* that they are in discomfort or distress. When reporting quality of a sign or symptom, *describes* can be used. Sometimes a patient will relate their current sign or symptom to a prior episode, or will believe they have identified an inciting factor. In these cases, it can be said that they are *associating* their symptoms. *Affirms* or *denies* may be used when noting positive or negative findings. A concise summary of these alternative circumstances when using speaking verbs are:

- Nonverbal patients or small children: *"The patient indicates..."*
- Reporting quality of a sign/symptom: *"The patient describes..."*
- Identifying inciting factors/prior episodes: *"The patient associates..."*
- Reviewing symptomatology: *"The patient affirms..."* or *"The patient denies..."*

The second verbs required to write an HPI are **action verbs**. These denote that something is happening to a historian, usually the development of signs or symptoms. These can be written in many tenses, though typically they are used to describe past events. It is important to use objective action verbs to make the documentation sound professional and unbiased. Some examples of action verb choices are in Box 6.4. Action verbs should be used after the historian has been designated and the speaking verb has been chosen.

Example: *"The patient (or other historian) states/reports that they <u>developed/began to experience/have had</u>..."*

BOX 6.3 ■ Objective and Subjective Speaking Verbs

Objective (To be Used)	Subjective (To be Avoided)
states	feels
reports	complains
indicates	whines
describes	
associates	
affirms/denies	

BOX 6.4 ■ Action Verbs

developed
began to experience
had

MEDICAL TERMINOLOGY

Medical terminology should be used whenever possible in lieu of the equivalent layman's term. Although the scribe will not be eliciting information from a patient, as a part of the healthcare team it is prudent to consider a patient's level of education. If the patient is unfamiliar with medical terminology, they may describe their medical history in a manner that is familiar to them. It is the scribe's duty to take this information and translate it into medical speak. For example, if a patient says that they had their gallbladder removed, the scribe should document "surgical history includes a cholecystectomy," or something of the like.

Medical terminology is typically taught as its own course (or two courses!) and this text is not intended to teach the subject. However, we will review the construction of medical terms in Chapter 9. Additionally, each of the chapters in Part III, Body Systems for the Medical Scribe, will relate the most essential terms and word roots encountered in the healthcare setting.

Building Blocks

The descriptors are truly the heart of the HPI and are routinely asked by the provider in order to form a **differential**, or a list of possible diagnoses that could explain the patient's symptoms and signs. Descriptors, or combinations of descriptors, also form some of the documentation elements that are used to determine the billing level of the encounter. For reference, an example of an electronic health record (EHR) screen that includes the descriptors/documentation elements is provided in Fig. 6.2. Remember that each field is a descriptor. Fields that share the same line (e.g. *onset* and *timing*) count as a single documentation element. One or either of these elements could be obtained but are counted together regardless.

> *HISTORY OF THE PRESENT ILLNESS: The patient reports that **(duration)** he/she developed a **(onset)** of **(timing)** **(location)** **(chief complaint)** **(radiation)**. He/she describes it as **(character/nature)** and rates it as a **(intensity)**. He/she affirms **(associated symptoms)**. He/she denies **(associated symptoms)**. The patient states that **(context)**. Symptoms are **(modifying factors)**. The patient has **(treatment before arrival)**.*

Let's do an exercise in which we complete this HPI for a fictional patient with a chief complaint of abdominal pain in *Example 1*:

> *EXAMPLE 1: The patient reports that **(2 days ago)** he/she developed a **(gradual onset)** of **(constant)** **(right upper quadrant)** **(abdominal pain)** **(radiating into the back)**. He/she describes it as **(throbbing)** and rates it as a **(5/10)**. He/she affirms **(nausea, vomiting, and diarrhea)**. He/she denies **(hematochezia, shortness of breath, or chest pain)**. The patient states that **(with prior episodes of gallbladder problems they have had similar symptoms)**. Symptoms are **(worsened by eating)**. The patient has **(taken over the counter antacids with little relief)**.*

Although the case content of *Example 1* is quite simplistic compared to what would likely be observed in a real scribing situation, it demonstrates that an organized history that flows well can be created by using the documentation elements fields. Thus, using this template may be a good

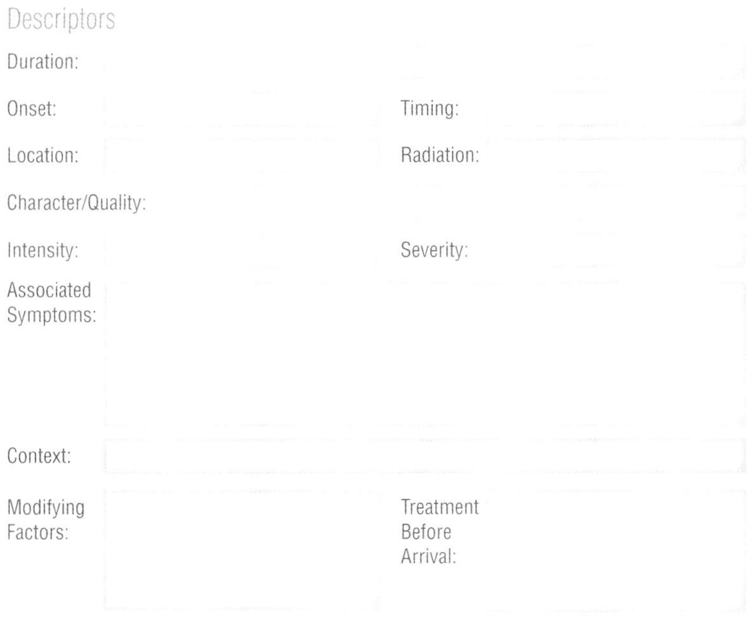

Descriptors

Duration:

Onset: Timing:

Location: Radiation:

Character/Quality:

Intensity: Severity:

Associated
Symptoms:

Context:

Modifying   Treatment
Factors: Before
                                                Arrival:

Fig. 6.2 History of the present illness (HPI) form fields on a templated electronic health record (EHR) screen. Reviewing the documentation elements on the form, notice that many of the elements are ordered in a way that would make sense if telling a story (the history). A free text note of such a history may look like the following:

starting place for a new and inexperienced scribe until they develop more accurate and efficient history writing skills.

A scribe may self-check to assess organization and flow by reading their written history aloud (even if just whispered), as if telling somebody about this patient. If the story is disjointed or does not make sense, then the HPI probably needs to be reorganized.

It is important to state that in a real history-taking situation, neither the provider nor the patient are likely to follow the order given by the documentation elements template or form. The discussion will certainly not be linear, and may even backtrack depending on the provider's evolving thought process and the patient's contributions to the conversation. The scribe should be prepared for this discontinuity, and the ability to process and interpret information given in such an erratic manner certainly improves with experience.

Let's do another exercise in which we complete this HPI for a fictional patient with a chief complaint of shortness of breath in *Example 2*:

*EXAMPLE 2: The patient reports that (**last week**) he/she developed a (**sudden onset**) of (**progressively worsening**) (**shortness of breath**). He/she affirms (**palpitations and lightheadedness**). He/she denies (**chest pain or leg swelling**). The patient states that (**the shortness of breath began after running a marathon**). Symptoms are (**exertionally worsened**). The patient has (**tried relaxing in a spa with little benefit**).*

In *Example 2* notice that several descriptors were not used (location, radiation, character/nature, and intensity). This is because these descriptors should only be used for pain or other sensory changes. Although the documentation elements template may be a good resource for a new and inexperienced scribe, it may not always apply to all situations and the scribe should be aware of this.

There will likely be additional elements of the HPI that will complicate the history-writing process. This may include past medical history, surgical history, family history, and social history. The patient's current medication list and allergies may also be discussed. Although all of these elements are documented elsewhere within the medical record, if the provider is inquiring about them during the history-taking they likely pertain to the patient's current presenting problem and thus should be included in the HPI as well.

There are different opinions regarding the scribe's role when it comes to documentation of these additional historical elements. These opinions are entirely provider-based, and should be clarified with each provider. Some prefer that these additional historical elements be confirmed or updated within their respective places in the medical record. Other providers like to also include the additional history within the HPI of the current encounter.

Let's do an exercise in which we create an HPI for a patient with a chief complaint of chest pain. This time the templated fields will not be used and the content of the HPI will be a bit more complex. While reading this, try to identify the descriptors in the main body of the HPI. Also try to identify the elements of additional history.

> **EXAMPLE 3:** *The patient reports that about 45 minutes ago he was mowing the lawn and developed an acute onset of constant substernal chest pain radiating into his left arm and jaw. He describes the pain as feeling like an "elephant sitting on my chest," and rates it as an 8/10. He is diaphoretic and nauseated with this but denies palpitations or lightheadedness. No dyspnea or increased leg pain/swelling. No recent periods of prolonged immobilization. The patient states that his chest pain feels similar to the chest pain he had with a previous MI. Significant medical history includes CAD status post stenting in the LAD after MI. He also has a history of diabetes, hypertension, and hyperlipidemia. No history of PE or DVT. The patient has a 20 pack-year smoking history. He has a strong family history of CAD at a young age in his father, a paternal uncle, and his paternal grandfather.*

The history in *Example 3* resembles that which a scribe may create. Notice that the HPI begins by describing the acute events, which are the details surrounding the patient's current episode of chest pain, and generally follows the format of the billable elements template. Following the main body of the history is the patient's past medical history including pertinent negatives and positives.

An alternative version of the above history is to include the components of the additional history within the main body of the HPI, as opposed to listing all of the additional history at the end. This style requires a bit more finesse and medical knowledge. Thus for many new scribes, listing the additional history after the HPI (as done above) will result in a better organization and flow.

A common organizational mistake that will confound the content of the HPI is to mix together the different "types" of additional history. The types of history are past medical, surgical, family, and social history. Using the additional historical elements from the last case, *Example 4* shows how an HPI might read if the types of history were to be mixed:

> **EXAMPLE 4:** *Significant medical history includes CAD status post stenting in the LAD after MI. The patient has a 20 pack-year smoking history. He also has a history of diabetes, hypertension, and hyperlipidemia. He has a strong family history of CAD at a young age in his father, a paternal uncle, and his paternal grandfather. No history of PE or DVT.*

Notice that *Example 4* does not have the same organizational flow as compared to *Example 3*. The content is confusing and the HPI is difficult to follow. This example emphasizes the importance of writing the different types of history together, as opposed to mixing them.

CASE STUDY 6.1

Your patient comes to the department with a chief complaint of nosebleed that will not stop, emanating from the right nostril. It started suddenly 3 hours prior to arrival with blood pouring out like a faucet, and he tried putting pressure on it by pinching his nose, without success. In fact, the bleeding has gradually gotten heavier, and he is starting to feel lightheaded. The patient was just started on coumadin, a blood thinner, 2 weeks ago. He just had an INR blood test to check on how thin his blood is, but the results are pending. He has never had nosebleeds before.

Show how you would record the documentation elements from this history.

Duration: _____

Onset: _____ / **Timing:** _____

Location: _____ / **Radiation:** _____

Character/Quality: _____

Intensity: _____ / **Severity:** _____

Associated Symptoms: _____

Context: _____

Modifying factors: _____ / **Tx before arrival:** _____

Practice Questions

1. One of the scribe's primary functions is to record the history accurately. Which of the following is true about recording the history?
   a. The primary historian will always be the patient.
   b. The history is considered objective information.
   c. The history is sometimes very limited, and the scribe should record the reason why.
   d. The history is best copied directly from a prior visit for accuracy.

2. Which sentence from the HPI is written with an objective speaking verb?
   a. "The patient complains that she has not been able to keep food down all day."
   b. "The patient's mother relates that she noticed her son's diaper rash began 2 days ago."
   c. "The patient insists that he has not taken alcohol in 4 days."
   d. "The patient began to have a headache yesterday."

3. A patient seeing the physician in urgent care believes the reason for her diarrhea is that she ate some very old leftovers from the refrigerator. How would the scribe document this in the HPI?

4. You are scribing for an emergency room physician and your shift begins at 10:00 a.m. The first patient you see with your attending physician is a 56-year-old diabetic patient who is brought to the department by the paramedics. They report that the patient was found unconscious in his bathroom. He was noted to be very diaphoretic (sweaty). They administered an ampule of intravenous dextrose and the patient gradually aroused. The patient states that he remembers little about this event but did recall that he had not yet had his breakfast for the day. The patient's wife arrives, and she states that she administered his insulin at his usual time this morning, at 7:00 a.m. Who do you list in your history as the historian in this case?

5. A mother brings in her infant to the office with complaint of a fever for the past 24 hours. She discloses to the doctor that her child has been hitting at his right ear all day. How might you record this in your history?

CHAPTER 7

Documenting Diagnostic Tests and Therapeutic Procedures

1. Explain the electrocardiogram (ECG) and document ECG findings.
2. Discuss types of medical and surgical procedures and document procedure elements.

Anesthetic	Electrocardiogram (ECG)	Repolarization
Atrioventricular (AV) node	Implied consent	Rhythm
Axis	Informed consent	Segment
Bradycardia	Interval	Sinoatrial (SA) node
Cardiac conduction cycle	Laterality	Sterile field
Conduction	Nerve block	Surgical
Depolarization	Normal sinus rhythm (NSR)	Systole
Diagnostic	Precordium	Tachycardia
Diastole	Procedure	Therapeutic
Ectopy	Rate	

There are additional notes that may be created within any other type of note which represent the results or findings or diagnostic testing or procedures that occurred during that patient encounter.

Electrocardiogram (ECG) Notes

The **electrocardiogram (ECG)** is a tracing of the electrical activity of the heart that is recorded as a waveform pattern on grid paper (Fig. 7.1). The duration (x-axis) represents time in seconds (s) or milliseconds (ms). The amplitude (y-axis) represents voltage in millivolts (mV). The configuration/morphology of the wave is also examined.

The ECG tracing is created by the placement of 10 different leads with electrodes in specific locations on the patient's limbs and **precordium**, which is the portion of the chest over the heart (Fig. 7.2). Each of these leads, or combinations of leads, measures the strength and direction of the electrical activity of the heart and translates that information into the waveforms that are seen on the graph.

Each lead is represented by a combination of numbers and letters. The *precordial leads* are designated as V1 through V6, and the *limb leads* are designated as I, II, III, aVR, aVL, and aVF.

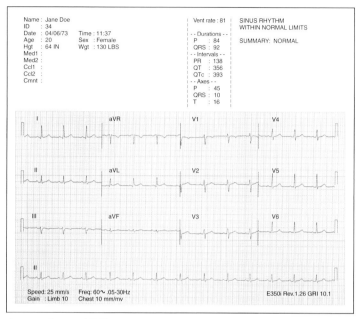

Fig. 7.1 An electrocardiogram (ECG) tracing showing normal sinus rhythm. (From Shiland, BJ: *Medical terminology and anatomy for coding*, ed 4, St. Louis, 2021, Elsevier.)

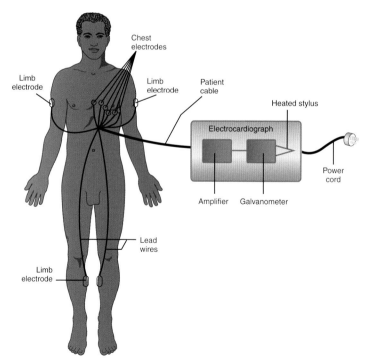

Fig. 7.2 Diagram of the basic components of the electrocardiograph. (From Shiland, BJ: *Medical terminology and anatomy for coding*, ed 4, St. Louis, 2021, Elsevier.)

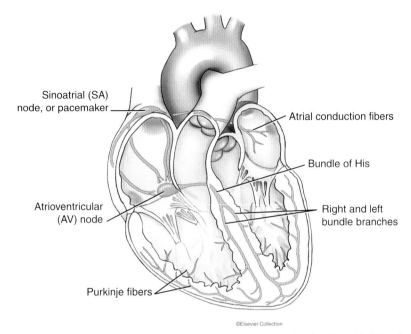

Sinoatrial (SA) node, or pacemaker

Atrial conduction fibers

Bundle of His

Atrioventricular (AV) node

Right and left bundle branches

Purkinje fibers

©Elsevier Collection

Fig. 7.3 Electrical conduction of the heart. An electrical signal is generated at the sinoatrial (SA) node in the right atrium and travels to both atria, down the ventricular septum, and finally to both ventricles. (© Elsevier Collection.)

The *rhythm strip* is an extended version of lead II at the bottom of the ECG that, like its name implies, is the most useful to examine rhythm.

The cardiac conduction system is a collection of electrically excitable myocytes in the heart which generate and conduct the electrical activity that is seen on ECG tracings. This electrical excitement causes the **depolarization** of cardiac myocytes, which is a change in membrane potential between the intracellular and extracellular compartments of the plasma membrane. Without going into too much detail, depolarization of cardiac myocytes results in synchronized contraction of the myocardium. This makes the heart an efficient "pump" which disperses oxygenated blood throughout the body.

In a normal heart the electrical activity is generated in the **sinoatrial (SA) node**, which is located in the right atrium near the entrance point of the superior vena cava (Fig. 7.3). The SA node is known as the pacemaker of the heart, and it is the main determinant of heart rate (which is normally between 60 and 100 beats per minute [bpm]). The electrical activity then travels to the **atrioventricular (AV) node**, which is located inferiorly to the SA node on the posterior wall of the right atrium. If the SA node is not capable of consistently generating electrical activity, the AV node can take over as the heart's pacemaker. Heart rate generated by the AV node will be slower as compared to that generated by the SA node. The electrical signal then travels from the AV node to the *bundle of His*, and then down the *left* and *right bundle branches*. These structures are all located within the ventricular septum. Lastly, the signal travels to the ventricles via the *Purkinje fibers*.

Thus to summarize, an electrical signal is generated at the SA node in the right atrium and travels to both atria, down the ventricular septum, and finally to both ventricles. The following is a depiction of normal electrical flow within the heart:

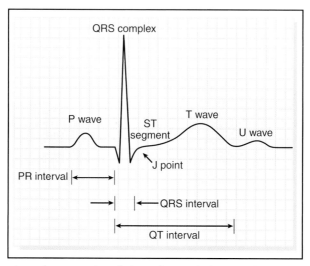

Fig. 7.4 The lines and waveforms seen in a single cardiac conduction cycle (one heartbeat) on a normal electrocardiogram. (From Goldberger AL, Goldberger ZD, Shvilkin A: *Clinical electrocardiography: a simplified approach*, ed 9, St. Louis, 2018, Elsevier.)

SA node → AV node → bundle of His → bundle branches → Purkinje

ECG tracings depict the electrical activity of the heart through a series of waveforms and lines known as intervals and segments (Fig. 7.4). Each of these waveforms, intervals, and segments are normally seen once during a single cycle of the **cardiac conduction cycle** (equivalent to one beat of the heart). One cycle of the cardiac conduction cycle includes **systole** (contraction) and **diastole** (relaxation) of the heart muscle.

The first waveform that should be seen is the ***P wave***, which represents atrial depolarization. The next waveform is actually referred to as a complex (***QRS complex***), because it is made up of three individual waves (the ***Q wave, R wave,*** and ***S wave***) which as a whole represents ventricular depolarization. The last waveform is the ***T wave*** and represents ventricular **repolarization**, which is normalization of the electrical potential gradient between the intracellular and extracellular compartments of the plasma membrane. Notice that atrial repolarization was not discussed here. This is because the signal generated by the repolarizing atria is buried within the very large QRS complex generated by the depolarizing ventricles and is therefore not seen.

The ECG baseline consists of intervals and segments. ECG **intervals** include one or more waveforms within their duration. The ***PR interval*** is the time from the start of the P wave to the beginning of the QRS complex. It represents the total time between the beginning of atrial depolarization to the start of ventricular depolarization (so the time it takes for the atria to completely contract before ventricular contraction). The ***QT interval*** is the time from the start of the Q wave (the first waveform in the QRS complex) to the end of the T wave. It represents the total time between the beginning of ventricular depolarization and the end of ventricular repolarization (so the time it takes for ventricular systole).

ECG **segments** do not include any waveforms within their duration. The ***ST segment*** is the time between the end of the QRS complex and the beginning of the T wave. This segment is particularly useful clinically to identify myocardial infarction (heart attack).

The waveforms and lines of the ECG that were discussed above represent what should be seen on a normal ECG tracing. However, disease of the heart and lungs (and sometimes elsewhere in the vasculature) can produce predictable changes to the ECG—this is what makes the ECG a helpful diagnostic tool.

The scribe will never have to an interpret an ECG, but they may create an ECG note and document the provider's findings. The EHR software may utilize a form or template to populate an ECG note, expediting the note-writing process. An example of such a form is included in Fig. 7.5.

The fields in this form represent categories in which certain ECG findings should be placed. Although a scribe will never be asked to interpret an ECG, they must be able to identify the appropriate heading under which each finding rightfully belongs. Headings for which there were no findings or interpretation should be removed if in a free-text template or left blank if in a form where the headings cannot be modified.

The following is a partial list of ECG findings that may be included in an interpretation. The findings are organized under their respective headings which should be used when creating an ECG note. Each finding is accompanied by a concise description. It is not necessary to memorize specific details about each of these findings, but these descriptions may be used in further understanding of the topic and helping with more efficient and accurate documentation.

TIME

The *time* data point records the time of day the ECG was taken and interpreted. In particular, during acute complaints with a possible cardiac etiology, serial ECGs may be taken and compared to see how the patient's condition is evolving (if it changes at all). Including timestamps within the medical record is important for legal and interpretive reasons.

RATE

Rate refers to how fast the heart is beating on average per minute. A normal rate is between 60 and 100 bpm. An abnormal heart rate may be faster or slower:

- **Bradycardia**—slow heart rate (<60 bpm)
- **Tachycardia**—rapid heart rate (>100 bpm)

RHYTHM

The regularity with which the heart is beating is documented as **rhythm**. An orderly regular progression of beats is called **normal sinus rhythm (NSR)**. Additionally, there are many types of arrhythmias, or abnormal rhythms. Some of the most common rhythms encountered are:

- *Normal sinus*—normal rhythm controlled by the SA node with a normal rate (60–100 bpm; Fig. 7.6)
- *Atrial tachycardia*—tachycardia originating in the atrium
- *Atrial fibrillation*—atrial arrhythmia which causes the atria to fibrillate, causing an irregularly irregular rhythm with or without rapid ventricular response (increased ventricular rate). The ECG will lack distinct P waves (Fig. 7.7)
- *Atrial flutter*—atrial arrhythmia which causes the atria to flutter, causing an elevated atrial rate and characteristic atrial flutter ("sawtooth") waves (Fig. 7.8)
- *Dual Chamber paced (DDD)*—pacemaker that can pace both atrium and ventricle if needed

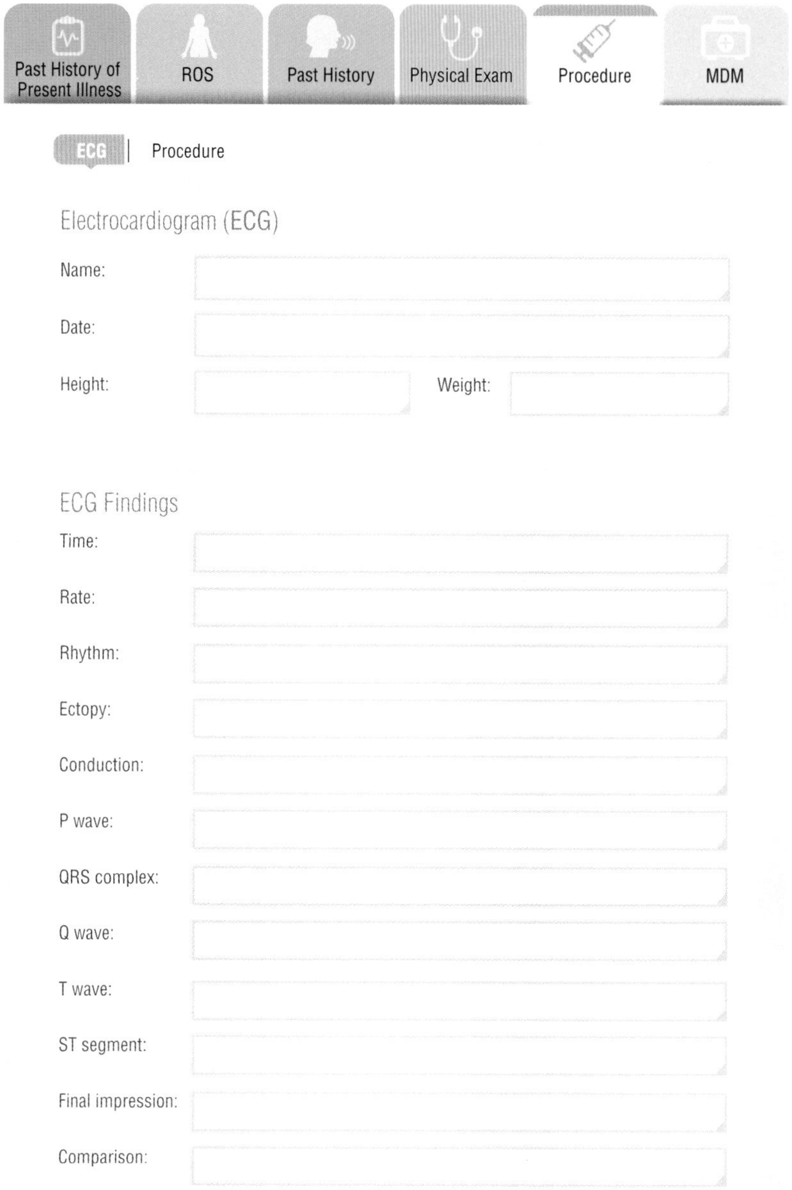

| Past History of Present Illness | ROS | Past History | Physical Exam | Procedure | MDM |

ECG | Procedure

Electrocardiogram (ECG)

Name:

Date:

Height: Weight:

ECG Findings

Time:

Rate:

Rhythm:

Ectopy:

Conduction:

P wave:

QRS complex:

Q wave:

T wave:

ST segment:

Final impression:

Comparison:

Fig. 7.5 Form for the collection of data to create an electrocardiogram (ECG) note.

AXIS

The **axis** is the direction of electrical flow in the heart. In different cardiac conditions, the flow may be altered and can help the clinician to interpret what is happening in the heart. The axis can be imagined as the hands on a clock (Fig. 7.9).

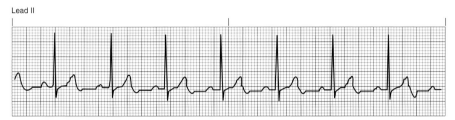

Fig. 7.6   Normal sinus rhythm. (From Skidmore-Roth L, Richardson F: *Introduction to critical care nursing*, ed 8, St. Louis, 2021, Elsevier.)

Atrial Fibrillation with a Slow Ventricular Response

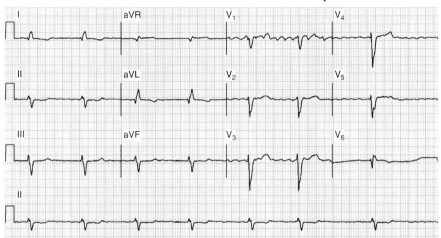

Fig. 7.7   Atrial fibrillation with a very slow ventricular response. The fibrillatory waves are best seen in lead V1. (From Goldberger AL, Goldberger ZD, Shvilkin A: *Clinical electrocardiography: a simplified approach*, ed 9, St. Louis, 2018, Elsevier.)

Atrial Flutter with Variable AV Block

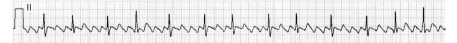

Fig. 7.8   Atrial flutter with its characteristic sawtooth pattern. (From Goldberger AL, Goldberger ZD, Shvilkin A: *Clinical electrocardiography: a simplified approach*, ed 9, St. Louis, 2018, Elsevier.)

- *Normal axis*—electric conduction runs anywhere from about 2 o'clock to 6 o'clock: corresponds to about -30 to +90 degrees off of the 0 degrees (3 o'clock position)
- *Left axis deviation*—electric flow moves in a counter-clockwise direction relative to normal

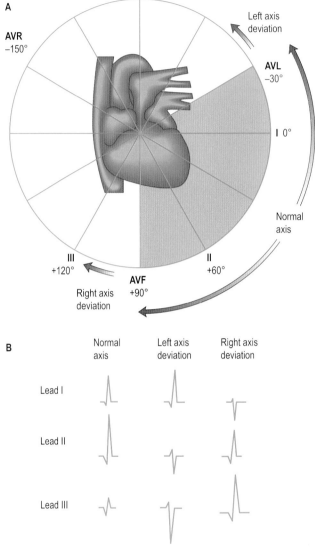

Fig. 7.9   Axial references on the heart (A) and their relationship to the electrocardiogram (ECG) leads (B). (From Waterhouse M, Randall D, Feather A: *Kumar and Clark's clinical medicine*, ed 10, St. Louis, 2021, Elsevier.)

- *Right axis deviation*—electric flow moves in a clockwise direction relative to normal
- *Extreme right axis deviation*—electric flow through the heart is diverted so far clockwise that it may appear to have gone counterclockwise

ECTOPY

The term **ectopy** describes premature beats from the atrium, ventricles, or elsewhere. Some types of ectopy are:

- Premature atrial complex (PAC)—premature atrial beat(s)
- Premature ventricular complex (PVC)—premature beat(s) originating in the ventricles
- Premature junctional complex (PJC)—premature beat(s) originating at the AV junction

CONDUCTION

Conduction is the way in which electricity is conducted throughout the heart. Numerous conditions may alter or disrupt this flow of electricity and disruption can occur at various points along the path. A comparison of how certain conduction blockages manifest on the ECG waveform is shown in Fig. 7.10.

- *Left bundle branch block (LBBB)*—electricity is blocked from the left bundle branch in the septum of the heart and activation of the left ventricle is delayed
- *Left anterior fascicular block (LAFB)*—blockage in the anterior branch of the left bundle branch
- *Left posterior fascicular block (LPFB)*—blockage in the posterior branch of the left bundle branch
- *Right bundle branch block (RBBB)*—electricity is blocked from the right bundle branch in the septum of the heart and activation of the right ventricle is delayed
- *AV block 1st degree (PR interval >200 ms)*—slowed conduction through the AV node
- *AV block 2nd degree*—various subtypes involving intermittent non-conduction through the AV node
- *AV block 3rd degree*—no conduction through the AV node

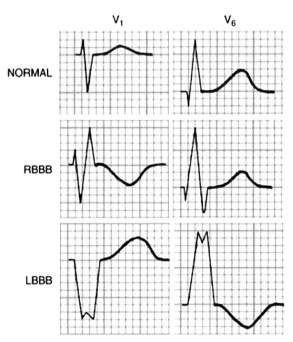

Fig. 7.10 Comparison of patterns in leads V1 and V6, with normal conduction, right bundle branch block (*RBBB*), and left bundle branch block (*LBBB*). (From Goldberger AL, Goldberger ZD, Shvilkin A: Clinical electrocardiography: a simplified approach, ed 9, St. Louis, 2018, Elsevier.)

- *Prolonged QT interval (>440 ms)*—prolonged duration of ventricular systole that may be caused by a variety of reasons

P WAVE

The P wave is the first waveform which represents atrial depolarization. Typically the morphology of these waveforms is examined for changes. Abnormal waves can be inverted, peaked, or ectopic. Common interpretations deduced from these findings include *left atrial enlargement (LAE)* or *right atrial enlargement (RAE)*.

QRS COMPLEX

The QRS complex comprises multiple waveforms (Q wave, R wave[s], and S wave) that represent ventricular depolarization. This is the electrical signature of the heartbeat.

The *QRS width* (normal 70–100 ms) is used to determine the origin of each QRS complex. A *broad waveform* (>100 ms) indicates that the QRS complex originates in the ventricles. A *narrow waveform* (<70 ms) indicates that the QRS originates above the ventricles.

QRS voltage, represented by the height of each QRS complex, can also be indicative of pathological changes. Short QRS complexes are of *low voltage*, while taller QRS complexes are of *high voltage*. *Electrical alternans* is a special situation in which the QRS voltage alternates between low and high.

Q WAVE

The Q wave is the first part of the QRS complex. There can be Q waves that are considered normal, and these are expected to be seen in certain leads. Other Q waves that are larger in amplitude and found in unexpected leads are considered to be *pathologic Q waves*. These can indicate an acute myocardial infarction, or can signify that a myocardial infarction took place at some point in the past.

T WAVE

The T wave represents ventricular repolarization. Abnormalities can indicate evidence of acute cardiac ischemia or infarction, or electrolyte imbalances (especially of potassium).

- *Hyperacute*—broad and uneven T waves that may precede ST changes in an acute myocardial infarction
- *Inverted*—wave is flipped "upside down" across the baseline
- *Biphasic*—T wave splits and one wave deflects positively (above the baseline) and the other negatively (below the baseline)
- *Flattened*—T waves have lost amplitude and appear flattened
- *Peaked*—tall and peaked T waves that may indicate hyperkalemia

ST SEGMENT

The duration of time from the end of ventricular depolarization to the beginning of ventricular repolarization is represented by the ST segment. Abnormalities, including segment elevation or depression, may be indicative of acute cardiac ischemia or infarction, or electrolyte issues.

FINAL IMPRESSION

The overall interpretation of the ECG based on the findings that were observed is recorded as the *final impression*. This can include a summary of all ECG findings and comments about whether they are new or were present on prior ECGs.

COMPARISON

The *comparison* records any changes from a prior ECG that may shed light on what is happening acutely (new onset). Be sure to document what has changed in the new ECG compared with any prior ECG, and note the dates between the comparisons. There could also be no comparison, which should also be recorded if this is the case.

Procedure Notes

In the medical community, **procedure** is an umbrella term used to describe a variety of activities related to patient care. Procedures may include simple and routine activities, such as taking a patient's vital signs or performing components of the physical exam. Some procedures are **diagnostic**, and are used to help confirm a diagnosis. Such an example may be cardiac catheterization which is used to examine the coronary arteries for disease. Other procedures are **therapeutic**, and are part of the patient's treatment plan. An example of this may be phototherapy, used by dermatologists to treat some skin conditions.

Other procedures may be **surgical** in nature. These types of procedures alter or repair the body. An example could be suturing a laceration together to help a wound heal. Surgery is performed in both inpatient and outpatient settings. Often prior to any of these procedures a patient is given an **anesthetic** to diminish the patient's pain. The types of anesthetics are discussed in detail under the Medications heading, below.

A **sterile field** is a microorganism-free area that may be created around the patient prior to a procedure, introduced in Chapter 3. A scribe should be able to recognize a sterile field so that they can avoid contaminating it (Fig. 7.11).

A scribe will be unable to assist in a procedure of any type, however, he or she may be asked to document important elements of the procedure in a *procedure note* for that encounter. The content of a procedure note will change depending on the area of medicine in which the provider is practicing. For example, a gastroenterologist may need to record a colonoscopy, a dermatologist may need a biopsy recorded, and an emergency medicine provider may need to document an intubation. However, there are some procedural items which are included in most (if not all) procedure notes. A form may be used for a procedure note to expedite the note-writing process. An example of such a form is included in Fig. 7.12.

TIME-OUT

Sometimes a time-out will be performed prior to beginning a procedure. This is done by healthcare workers to confirm that they are about to operate on the correct patient, the correct surgical site and procedure, and the correct **laterality**, the side of the body on which the procedure is being performed. The time at which this is performed and the name of the person who did the time-out should be documented.

PROCEDURE NAME

Although the type of procedure can be inferred based on content, the *procedure name* should always be documented regardless for clarity.

INDICATION

The indication is the reason why the procedure is being done. For example, the indication for a chest tube could be *pneumothorax* (collapsed lung). The indication for suturing could be a *laceration*.

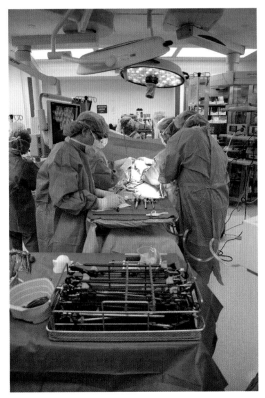

Fig. 7.11   A sterile field at patient bedside. (From Hartman CJ, Kavoussi, LR: Handbook of surgical technique: a true surgeon's guide to navigating the operating room, Philadelphia, 2018, Elsevier.)

CONSENT

For any procedure, consent must be obtained by the patient (or other consenting party if the patient is unable). This is a statement saying that the patient agreed to have the procedure performed. As discussed in Chapter 2, a provider who performs a procedure on a patient who does not consent may have committed the crime of *battery*.

Informed consent is a situation in which the provider gives the patient adequate information about the procedure, including risks and benefits, and allows the patient to make an informed decision. Exceptions to informed consent include the unconscious patient, the patient who is not competent enough to make a rational decision, and the minor (less than 18 years old) who requires emergent care in the absence of an adult representative. **Implied consent** is used for minor procedures for which the patient has sought treatment. Implied consent does not require signed documentation by the patient giving permission to be treated, and is instead based on the actions of the patient and provider.

TIME

The starting time of the procedure should be documented in the medical record. This is mostly done for legal reasons.

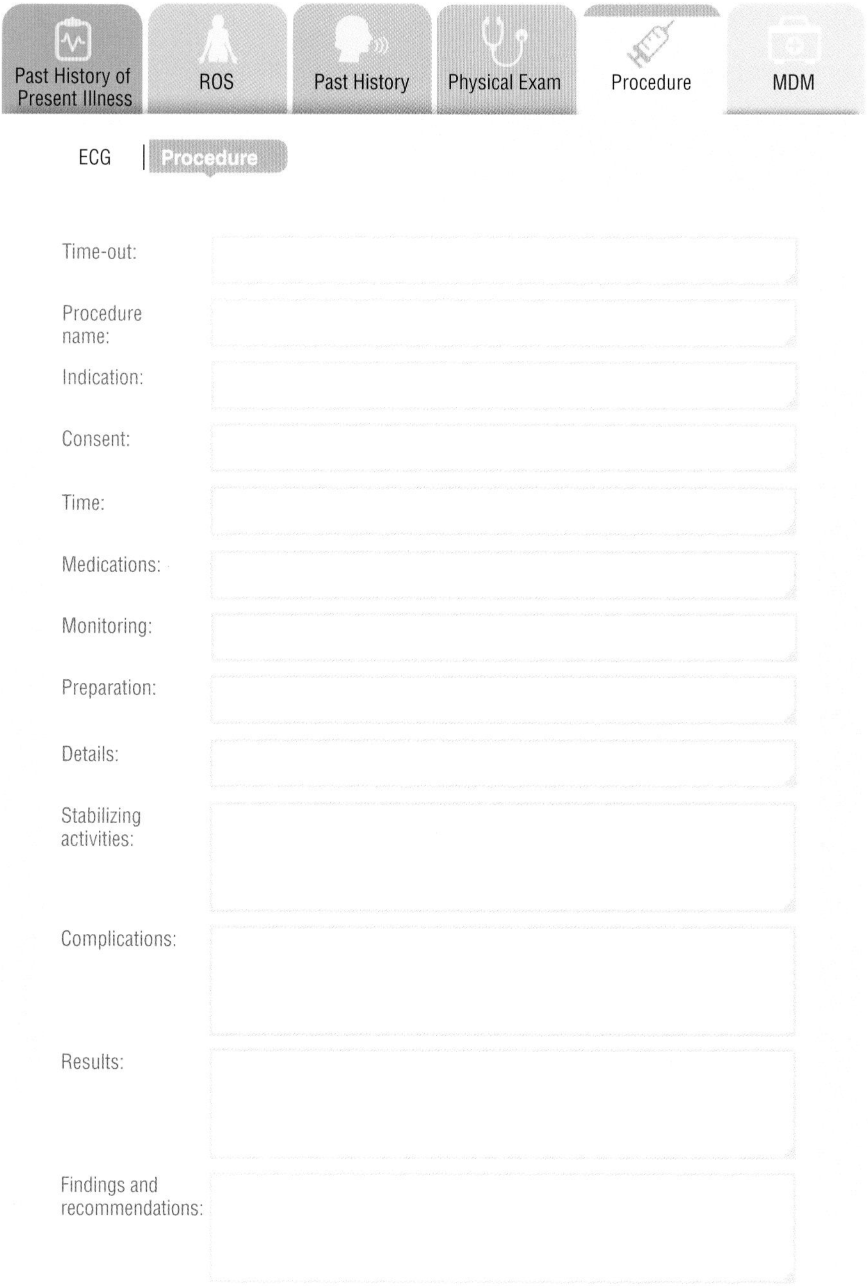

| Past History of Present Illness | ROS | Past History | Physical Exam | Procedure | MDM |

ECG | Procedure

Time-out:

Procedure name:

Indication:

Consent:

Time:

Medications:

Monitoring:

Preparation:

Details:

Stabilizing activities:

Complications:

Results:

Findings and recommendations:

Fig. 7.12 A form used to gather information for a procedure note in the electrocardiogram (ECG).

MEDICATIONS

Any medications used during the procedure, their dosages, the time they were given, and if the patient had any adverse reaction should be documented within the medical record. Some types of medications that are commonly utilized during procedures include topical or local anesthetics, sedatives or amnestics, or analgesics. Other medications may be given to stabilize the patient's vital signs or otherwise support the patient through the procedure. These could be as basic as oxygen or pain medications, or medications that modulate blood pressure or heart rate. Medications for nausea are also frequently administered in the perioperative environment. Other categories of medication frequently used are antibiotics to prevent post-operative infections and anticoagulants to prevent blood clots during the patient's recovery phase.

The administration of anesthesia is in itself a type of procedure. It is important for the scribe to be familiar with some of the many types of anesthetics, which may be either

- *Local*: applied or injected directly into the site requiring anesthesia
- *Regional*: injected into the area around a nerve, giving a wide area of anesthesia
- *Systemic (general)*: to modulate the patient's pain perception pathway or to sedate the patient

The names of some of the more common types of anesthetics are provided in Box 7.1.

A *local anesthetic* numbs a small area where it is injected. This is commonly seen used in numbing up the skin surrounding a laceration in preparation for repair with sutures. Many of the local anesthetics will be recognized by their common ending, "-caine" like novocaine. The provider will want the scribe to record the anesthetic given, the amount given, the concentration, and also whether or not it was given with epinephrine, which is sometimes added to the local anesthetic in order to prolong the effect of the anesthetic and lessen any bleeding by decreasing circulation to the area being treated.

A *regional anesthetic* is also called a **nerve block**. In a regional nerve block, a local anesthetic is injected around a nerve in order to numb up the region that is supplied by the nerve.

Finally, there is the option of using a *general (systemic) anesthetic*. A general anesthetic is an agent that is often given through an IV in order to put the patient completely asleep (or in some cases only partly asleep or in a "twilight sleep") so that they are not aware of the procedure being performed. Major surgeries will almost always require a general anesthetic to be used.

Other types of medication that the scribe may encounter in documenting a procedure are those that are known as *sedatives* and *paralytics*. A *sedative* will dull the patient's senses and make them very drowsy but is not a full unconsciousness as seen with general anesthetic. *Paralytics* keep the patient's muscles from voluntary or involuntary movements during the procedure. Being unable to move one's muscles (including the breathing muscles) is very frightening for a patient. Therefore, your provider will want to be sure that they are able to assist the patient's breathing and that the patient is completely asleep and unaware before administering any of these paralyzing agents.

MONITORING

The patient may require monitoring by specific medical personnel (like a respiratory therapist) if they are given sedatives or anesthetics because many of these drugs can drastically change a patient's vital signs and even cause them to become unstable. Vital signs that are monitored include respiratory rate, pulse oximetry, temperature, and end-tidal CO_2 ($ETCO_2$).

PREPARATION

Any preparation done prior to the procedure should be documented here. Some examples include sterilization or draping of the area of focus for the procedure.

BOX 7.1 ■ Commonly Used Anesthetic Agents

The following are not the only anesthetic types available for use, but serve as a general summary of some of the more common ones you may encounter.

General Anesthesia Agents

methohexital (Brevital)
thiopental (Pentothal)
droperidol (Inapsine)
etomidate (Amidate)
ketamine (Ketalar)
propofol (Diprivan)

Local (and Regional) Anesthesia Agents

procaine (Novocaine)
tetracaine (Pontocaine)
bupivacaine (Marcaine)
lidocaine (Xylocaine)
mepivacaine (Carbocaine)

Paralytic Agents (Also Known as Neuromuscular Blocking Agents)

succinylcholine (Anectine)
rocuronium (Zemuron)

DETAILS

A step-by-step description of the course of the procedure should be documented. By nature, this is the most detailed portion of the procedure note.

STABILIZING ACTIVITIES

This section documents any postprocedural activity that is done to stabilize an area that has been compromised by the procedure. This could include the application of dressings, slings, and splints.

COMPLICATIONS

Any complications encountered during or shortly after the procedure should be documented. Also the time of the complication, its course, and resolution (if any) necessitate documentation as well. Some common complications encountered could include a period of oxygen desaturation, loss of pulse, or unexpected bleeding.

RESULTS

The results field records the end result of the procedure. This could include something like "good approximation of edges" after a laceration repair, or "good alignment of bone with strong pulses" after reduction of a joint.

FINDINGS AND RECOMMENDATIONS

Any postprocedural recommendations for the referring physician (if applicable) are documented in this section.

COMMON PROCEDURES

A given healthcare setting regularly performs the same types of procedures, so the scribe working in a facility will become familiar with the documentation of the diagnostic and therapeutic interventions that providers at the setting tend to perform. The following is a list of the most common procedures that may be encountered in the emergency department, along with some peculiarities for each procedure that may require non-standard documentation. While many of these procedures are performed in an array of healthcare settings, a list of common procedures would look quite different in an orthopedic office, a gastroenterology clinic, a dermatology center, or a hospital surgical suite.

Central Line

Insertion of a large catheter into major veins to rapidly administer fluids or medications.
  Indications: Hemodynamic instability.
  Medications: Local anesthetic (like lidocaine or bupivacaine).
  Monitoring: Telemetry and blood pressure.
  Preparation: Patient placed into Trendelenburg (for subclavian lines) and creating a sterile field with draping.
  Details: Location of insertion and the vein used (e.g. femoral vein in the left groin). Type of central line and the catheter gauge (e.g. #9 French triple lumen Cordis catheter). Special techniques (e.g. Seldinger technique or ultrasound guided). Ease of threading the catheter.
  Results: All lumens are checked for patency and the status of the distal neurovasculature is also observed.

Chest Tube (Thoracostomy)

Tube inserted through the chest wall to remove fluid/pus/air from the pleural cavity.
  Indications: Pneumothorax or hemothorax.
  Medications: Local anesthetic (e.g. lidocaine or bupivacaine).
  Monitoring: Telemetry, blood pressure, and pulse oximetry.
  Preparation: Positioned to expose area to be used as an entry point (usually the 5th intercostal space). Creating a sterile field with draping.
  Details: Location and length of incision. Manner of dissection into pleural space. The presence of air or blood or purulent material from the pleural space. Whether or not a finger was used to guide placement of tube. Tube size and depth of insertion. Kelly clamp use.
  Stabilizing activities: How (and if) the tube was sutured into place. Attachment of the tube to Pleur-Evac and hooked to suction (continuous).
  Results: Estimated blood loss.

Conscious Sedation

Pre-procedural sedation given before other procedures. Conscious sedation is almost always accompanied by another procedure note, which documents the intended procedure for which the conscious sedation was performed.
  Indications: Painful procedures where the patient should be sedated.
  Medications: Sedatives (e.g. ketamine, propofol, etomidate, versed).
  Monitoring: Respiratory therapist or others in attendance. Monitoring of oxygen saturation, heart rate, blood pressure, $ETCO_2$.
  Complications: Any rescue needed, such as bagging or a reversal agent.
  Results: Good anesthesia achieved or the patient was lightly sedated.

Incision and Drainage (I&D)

Using a scalpel to release pus from an abscess or boil.
>*Indications*: Fluctuant abscess.
>*Medications*: Local anesthetics and sometimes narcotic premedication.
>*Preparation*: Antiseptic preparation and infiltration.
>*Details*: What material was drained (serosanguinous, purulent, bloody, clear). Irrigation or packing of the abscess. Breaking-up of loculations.
>*Results*: Drainage of material with culture taken and abscess packed.

Endotracheal Intubation

Placing a tube in the trachea.
>*Indications*: Respiratory failure, airway protection, rapidly deteriorating level of consciousness or respiratory status, cardiac arrest.
>*Monitoring*: Heart rate, pulse oximetry, respiratory rate.
>*Details*: Patient's head in "sniffing" position; blade or other technique used (e.g. Macintosh, Miller, Magill, Glidescope); size of tube (e.g. 7.5 or 8.0); Stylet; ease of intubation; comments on balloon inflation; the level that the tube was inserted (e.g. 22 cm at the teeth).
>*Stabilizing activities:* Anchoring of tube in place.
>*Results*: Post-procedure chest x-ray ordered. How placement was verified (e.g. color change, CO_2 meter, auscultation, ease of bagging).

Joint Reduction

Returning a joint back to anatomical position.
>*Indications*: Joint dislocation.
>*Medications*: Sedatives (e.g. ketamine, propofol, etomidate, versed).
>*Monitoring*: Respiratory therapist or others in attendance. Monitoring of oxygen saturation, heart rate, blood pressure, ETCO2.
>*Details*: Patient position. Technique used.
>*Stabilizing activities:* Sling and swathe for shoulders, finger splint for fingers, abduction pillow after hip reduction.
>*Results*: Pre- and post-procedure exam of the distal neurovascular status. Success of maneuver and how this was determined (e.g. exam, imaging, feeling the joint reducing during the procedure).

Laceration Repair

Using sutures or other means to repair a laceration.
>*Indications*: Laceration.
>*Medications*: Topical anesthetic (e.g. lidocaine or bupivacaine). Anesthetic technique (infiltration or digital or regional block).
>*Preparation*: Irrigation with saline, area prepped with antimicrobial, sterile draping.
>*Details*: Any deep structures involved (exploration). Suture or staples or other agent used in closure. Type of suture (e.g. prolene or nylon) and size (e.g. 5-0 or 6-0). Number of sutures or staples and number of layers of closure. Any debridement or revision.
>*Stabilizing activities:* Dressings or immobilizations.
>*Complications:* Any bleeding and how this was controlled.
>*Results*: Wound edges well approximated.

Lumbar Puncture (LP)

A long spinal needle is inserted into the spinal canal to collect cerebrospinal fluid (CSF) for testing.

Indications: Rule-out meningitis or subarachnoid hemorrhage.

Medications: Local anesthetic like lidocaine.

Preparation: Sterile draping.

Details: Patient position (e.g. left lateral decubitus or sitting). Size of needle inserted (e.g. 22 or 24 gauge) and the level of insertion (e.g. L3-L4). Nature of fluid obtained (e.g. clear, purulent, serosanguinous, blood-tinged). Opening and closing pressures. Number of tubes of CSF obtained for analysis.

Stabilizing activities: Post procedure patient placed supine.

Results: Successful or unsuccessful collection of CSF. Number of tubes sent to lab for evaluation.

CASE STUDY 7.1

The patient, Mr. Donald Morse, a 75-year-old man with recurrent angina, is in surgery to treat coronary artery disease. Atherosclerotic blockages are preventing oxygenated blood from reaching the muscles of Mr. Morse's heart. Since the patient has had six cardiac catheterizations in the past 10 years, his physicians believe that a double vessel coronary artery bypass graft (CABG) is necessary to prevent further damage to the tissues of Mr. Morse's heart.

The CABG aims to restore blood flow to the cardiac muscles. During the surgery, the team will perform a sternotomy, sawing down the center of the breastbone to open Mr. Morse's chest. They will free one end of the left internal mammary artery (LIMA) and reattach it to the left anterior descending artery (LAD) of the heart, in a place below the blockage. Simultaneously, the surgical team will make an incision in Mr. Morse's right leg from his thigh to his knee. There, they will harvest the great saphenous vein, which will be used to create a second conduit between the aorta and the right coronary artery.

Before the operation, the surgeon, Dr. Brennan, discussed with Mr. Morse the details of the surgery and the reasons he thought the CABG was the best treatment option. Dr. Brennan also reviewed the risks of the surgery, and provided alternatives to the procedure, including a review of the consequences of doing nothing at all. The patient signed documentation that he understood the procedure, its risks, and the alternatives to surgery.

Mr. Morse was given general anesthesia and had endotracheal intubation and was prepped from his chin to his feet bilaterally. The surgeon used a type of suture called Prolene (size 7-0) to attach the vessels in their new locations, using a single knot technique. The surgeon checked for leaks, placed drains in the patient's chest, and closed the wound in layers, wiring the sternum shut. The patient tolerated the procedure well.

Mr. Morse was monitored with a cardiac monitor for 24 hours post op. At one point the patient showed atrial fibrillation, with a rapid ventricular response (Fig. 7.13), which proved to be transient and benign.

QUESTIONS

1. Which is the indication?
   a. Atherosclerotic heart disease, coronary artery disease with depressed LV function
   b. Atrial tachycardia with rapid ventricular response
   c. General anesthesia
   d. Double vessel coronary artery bypass graft (CABG)
2. What procedure was performed?
   a. Atherosclerotic heart disease, coronary artery disease with depressed LV function
   b. Atrial tachycardia with rapid ventricular response
   c. General anesthesia
   d. Double vessel coronary artery bypass graft (CABG)
3. What is included in the sterile field for this patient?
4. What type of consent was obtained before the operation?
5. Did Mr. Morse receive local or systemic anesthesia?
6. What information might be included in the Results portion of the procedure note form?

Continued

CASE STUDY 7.1   — cont'd

Atrial Fibrillation with Rapid Ventricular Response (Not PSVT)

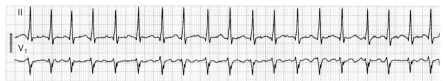

Fig. 7.13   Atrial fibrillation with a rapid ventricular response. (From Goldberger AL, Goldberger ZD, Shvilkin A: *Clinical electrocardiography: a simplified approach*, ed 9, St. Louis, 2018, Elsevier.)

7. The postoperative ECG showed tachycardia, meaning the _____ of Mr. Morse's heartbeat was greater than _____ bmp.
8. What appears at the bottom of an ECG tracing and is helpful for understanding the heart's rhythm?
9. The findings of the physician who interpreted Mr. Morse's ECG would be recorded in which field of the ECG note form?
10. How does the clinical staff know that Mr. Morse is in atrial fibrillation?
    a. The elevation of the Q wave
    b. The length (time) of the QT interval
    c. The depression of the P wave
    d. The lack of distinct P waves and an irregularly irregular rhythm

Practice Questions

For questions 1 and 2, use the following ECG template to correctly place the findings from the interpretation provided.

1. Sinus tachycardia at 110 bpm with narrow QRS complexes. There is a first degree AV block. Occasional premature ventricular complex. Axis is normal. There are no acute ST changes, T waves are normal, and there are no pathologic Q waves. Prior ECG from 3/22/2013 shows similar changes except rate is normal.

ELECTROCARDIOGRAM (ECG)

Rate: _____

Rhythm: _____

Axis: _____

Ectopy: _____

Conduction: _____

QRS complex: _____

Q wave: _____

T wave: _____

ST segment: _____

Final impression: _____

Comparison: _____

2. Narrow complex tachycardia at 140 bpm. There is a new right bundle branch block in V1-V3 and T wave inversions in these leads. Right axis deviation. P wave is peaked in lead II. Diffuse ST segment elevation. These changes are consistent with acute pulmonary embolism and right heart strain. All changes are new compared to prior ECG on 4/26/2021.

ELECTROCARDIOGRAM (ECG)

Rate: _____

Rhythm: _____

Axis: _____

Ectopy: _____

Conduction: _____

P wave: _____

QRS complex: _____

Q wave: _____

T wave: _____

ST segment: _____

Final impression: _____

Comparison: _____

For questions 3 and 4, use the following procedure note template to correctly document the procedure description.

3. Shoulder dislocation on the left with reduction. Respiratory therapist in attendance. Patient placed on heart monitor with oxygenation, blood pressure, and pulse monitored. At 1245 the patient had procedure explained and signed consent. At 1300 the patient and procedure and laterality were reviewed. Versed 5 mg given IV at 1310. When the patient was sedated, reduction achieved using traction/countertraction method. Pulses were checked and good pre-and post-procedure. Axillary nerve tested and intact before and after procedure. Placed in shoulder immobilizer. Post-reduction x-ray shows good alignment. Patient recovered slowly over 25 minutes.

PROCEDURE NOTE

Time-out: _____

Procedure name: _____

Indication: _____

Consent: _____

Time: _____

Medications: _____

Monitoring: _____

Preparation: _____

Details: _____

_____

_____

Stabilizing activities: _____

Complications: _____

Results: _____

4. Patient has 6 cm laceration to left forearm that is full thickness. Distal neurovascular tested and found to be intact. Laceration repair done with 1% plain lidocaine local anesthetic at 15:35. Area cleaned with Shur Clens. Closure with running 5-0 Vicryl in SQ layers followed by #8 5-0 Ethilon sutures on the skin. Good approximation achieved. Dressed with a bacitracin dressing.

PROCEDURE NOTE

Time-out: _____

Procedure name: _____

Indication: _____

Consent: _____

Time: _____

Medications: _____

Monitoring: _____

Preparation: _____

Details: _____

_____

_____

Stabilizing activities: _____

Complications: _____

Results: _____

Orders and Disposition Documentation

- Differentiate the types of provider orders and their significance in patient care.
- Explain the components of a prescription and document a prescription in the electronic health record (EHR).
- List types of laboratory tests, explain their purposes, and document laboratory orders in the EHR.
- Document provider orders for common imaging modalities.
- Document provider orders for nursing care and other health professionals.
- Recognize common order panels.
- Document the disposition of the patient from the healthcare facility.

Admission

Against medical advice (AMA)

Angiography

Clinical impression

Complete blood count (CBC)

Computed tomography (CT)

Computerized physician order entry (CPOE)

Consultation

Contraindication

Contrast medium

Controlled substance

Culture

Diagnosis

Direct admission

Discharge

Dispense as written (DAW)

Disposition

Dose

Duration

ED contact order

Eloping

Formulation

Frequency

Hard-stop

ICD-10-CM

Imaging study

Indication

Intensive care unit (ICU)

Laterality

Leave without being seen (LWBS)

Magnetic resonance imaging (MRI)

Medical necessity

National Provider Identifier (NPI)

Observation

Order

Order panel

Prescription

Problem list

Radiograph

Route

Serum

Signatura (Sig.)

Telemetry

Transfer

Ultrasound (US)

Urinalysis

Ventilation perfusion (VQ) scan

The medical scribe may be asked to perform duties inside the medical record other than strict documentation that are relevant to the patient's stay. These duties may include placing orders for testing and imaging, completing prescriptions for the patient to take home, and completing the patient's end of visit paperwork to send them home and for follow-up.

Because a scribe is a nonclinical person, the provider must specifically ask the scribe to do these things and then review and approve the scribe's work before it is acted upon. The duties which a scribe may legally perform are somewhat subject to interpretation, local customs, changing laws, and also educational parameters and certifications. If uncertain, the local experts at the institution of employment should be consulted.

Orders

Orders are the provider's electronic or written instructions for therapies such as medications, testing such as labs or imaging, or communications that are meant for other healthcare workers. Orders can either be performed on-site, as in the hospital or within some outpatient facilities, or they can be *prescribed* for future use in other settings or at the patient's home. When writing out an order for the patient to take for fulfillment elsewhere, the order is termed a **prescription**. Prescriptions are usually thought of as orders for medications to be filled at a pharmacy, however the term is frequently used for any prescribed treatment or test that is written out for the patient to take with them. Increasingly, the paper prescription is becoming a thing of the past and these types of orders are recorded and transmitted electronically. Nevertheless, the terminology distinction between an order for the patient to fulfill later, prescription, remains as distinct from other orders meant to be done within the clinic or hospital setting during the patient's stay.

In the EHR, the system that documents and sends provider orders is called the **computerized physician order entry (CPOE)**. Fig. 8.1 is an EHR screen showing four provider orders for a patient.

A scribe will never independently decide what should be ordered for each patient. The scribe should be adept at listening to the provider's list of orders and then accurately entering these into the EHR for the provider to review, approve, and sign. Because many tests are ordered by protocol, however, a scribe may anticipate what the provider may order based on the patient's history and exam. For example, if a patient has a cough and fever, the provider will likely order a chest x-ray to rule out pneumonia. This kind of knowledge often comes with experience and makes a scribe more valuable to the provider.

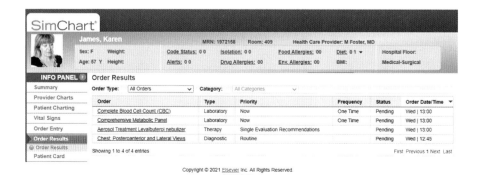

Fig. 8.1 A variety of provider orders for a patient in the electronic health record (EHR). (From SimChart © 2021 Elsevier, Inc.)

MEDICAL NECESSITY

In any setting, justification for any order must be provided for billing and insurance reasons. The **indication** is a valid reason for the provider to order tests, prescribe medications, or perform procedures, including surgeries. Third-party payers, such as insurance companies and government agencies, will not pay for services that do not have a **medical necessity**; that is, the order must be warranted by a patient's condition. The type of justification required may vary depending on the medical facility.

In the emergency department or an inpatient facility, a written reason for an order must sometimes be provided within the medical record. This is typically required for any type of imaging study. For example, the physician cannot order a CT scan of the patient's neck without cause or because the patient requests it. But if the patient is showing signs of a neck injury based on the clinician's professional judgement, the imaging would be considered medically necessary. In the EHR, a blank text box on the order screen prompts the provider to document a written reason.

Generally, a provider's diagnosis or suspected diagnosis assures medical necessity. As you learned in Chapter 4, **ICD-10-CM codes** are used to record the patient's diagnoses and conditions in all settings. In an outpatient facility, ICD-10-CM diagnosis codes should be associated with each order. In the EHR, this usually entails a pop-up box with a grid listing of orders and ICD-10-CM codes (Fig. 8.2). There will be a prompt to check the boxes associating an ICD-10 code with an order.

Prescriptions

A prescription is a provider's order to be fulfilled at a later time. Most commonly it is used to dispense a drug to a patient, generally for their use at home. There are certain safeguards that must be in place in the EHR that allow the scribe to lawfully enter prescriptions for the provider.

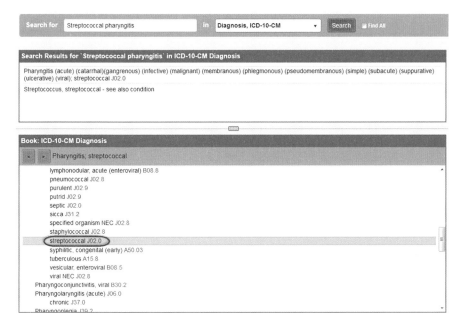

Fig. 8.2 The assignment of the diagnosis code J02.0, streptococcal pharyngitis, provides the medical necessity for the provider to prescribe an antibiotic. (From Elsevier: *SimChart® for the medical office: learning the medical office workflow*, St. Louis, 2019, Elsevier.)

Hard-stops prevent the prescription from being acted upon unless the provider has reviewed, approved, and signed the scribe's work. Fig. 8.3 shows an order for the drug lithium (Lithobid). The order will not be sent or executed until the provider reviews and electronically signs the order. The ability to enter prescriptions is determined by the legal/compliance department. Facility-specific rules and standards should be confirmed at any location.

The CPOE should also send notifications to the provider, such as medication **contraindications** like allergies or drug-drug interactions, even if they were sent to the scribe first. In Fig. 8.4, the CPOE alerts the individual who ordered the prescription of an interaction between the order for the medication glyburide and another medication the patient is already taking, lisinopril.

Although prescriptions may be written for a variety of orders, there is a generalized formatting that is used. Medication prescriptions are the most likely type that a scribe may encounter, and thus will be discussed here. Other prescriptions may require different elements, but the general formatting is the same. Fig. 8.5 shows the elements of a prescription.

NAME

Generally, both the generic and trade name will be listed on the prescription by the medical record. The *generic name* is typically all lowercase, and the *trade name* (or brand name) has an initial capital letter. Sometimes a patient or the provider will specifically request the generic or the brand version for different reasons. The generic is generally cheaper than the brand version, and patients who are trying to save money generally prefer the generic. On the other hand, the brand version has a consistent ingredient list and this seems to be preferred by patients who have allergies or intolerances to some of the inactive ingredients in the generic drugs.

DOSE

The **dose** is the amount of drug to be given. This may be listed in a variety of units depending on the drug and the form of the drug.

Examples of various doses:

- Weight—such as milligrams (mg)
- Volume—such as milliliters (mL), drops
- Number—such as the number of capsules, tablets, patches, puffs, etc.

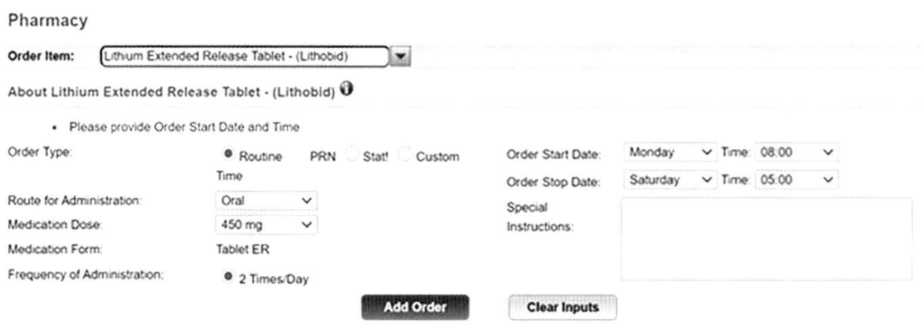

Fig. 8.3 Entering an order in the computerized physician order system (CPOE). (From SimChart © 2021 Elsevier, Inc.)

REVIEW PATIENT - MEDICATION INTERACTIONS

GlyBURIDE
1.25 mg oral tablet

Mark Rogers
M, 42 yrs, 03/05/1970

learn

New interactions

Moderate drug interaction: lisinopril 40 mg oral tablet

glyBURIDE can increase the effects of lisinopril and cause your blood sugar levels to get too low. Symptoms of low blood sugar include headache, dizziness,

more info >

* Reason | Will implement follow-up plan to reassess | ▼ | ☐ Do not show this alert for this patient

Comment

Existing interactions

(i) There are no existing interaction alerts for this medication.

Quick entry: Select a reason and enter comments to apply to all (1) new interaction alerts

Reason | (select a reason) | ▼

Comment

Back | Override

Fig. 8.4 The computerized physician order entry (CPOE) alerts the individual who ordered the prescription of an interaction between the order for the medication glyburide and another medication the patient is already taking, lisinopril. (Courtesy Practice Fusion, Inc., San Francisco, CA.)

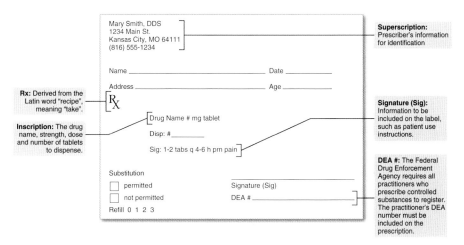

Mary Smith, DDS
1234 Main St.
Kansas City, MO 64111
(816) 555-1234

Superscription: Prescriber's information for identification

Name _____ Date _____

Address _____ Age _____

Rx: Derived from the Latin word "recipe", meaning "take".

℞

Drug Name # mg tablet

Disp: #_____

Sig: 1-2 tabs q 4-6 h prn pain

Inscription: The drug name, strength, dose and number of tablets to dispense.

Signature (Sig): Information to be included on the label, such as patient use instructions.

Substitution

☐ permitted

☐ not permitted

Refill 0 1 2 3

Signature (Sig)

DEA # _____

DEA #: The Federal Drug Enforcement Agency requires all practitioners who prescribe controlled substances to register. The practitioner's DEA number must be included on the prescription.

Fig. 8.5 Example prescription. (© Elsevier Collection.)

FORMULATION

Drugs come in many physical forms depending on the chemical properties and purpose of the drug. Sometimes the same drug comes in multiple **formulations** so that the route of administration can be changed based on the situation.

Examples of formulations:

- Tablet
- Capsule
- Cream
- Ointment
- Aerosol
- Patch

Examples of formulation modifiers:

- Extended release (ER)
- Chewable
- Disintegrating

ROUTE

The manner in which the drug should be administered is the **route**. The decision on route is made based on a variety of factors, such as drug metabolism, the drug's duration of action, the dose, and the patient's condition, to name a few.

Examples of routes:

- Oral (*per os* [PO], meaning by mouth)
- Per rectum (PR)
- Inhalation
- Intranasal
- Topical
- Intravenous (IV)
- Intramuscular (IM)
- Subcutaneous (SQ)
- Via PEG tube or J tube
- Sublingual (SL)

FREQUENCY

The **frequency** is the number of times that a drug should be administered in the prescribed dose within a period of time. The frequency is chosen to keep a certain level of the active drug in the body over time.

Examples of frequency (*abbreviation*):

- Once daily (*qd*)
- Twice daily, or every 12 hours (*bid*)
- Thrice daily, or every 8 hours (*tid*)
- Four times daily, or every 6 hours (*qid*)
- At bedtime (*qhs*)
- As needed (*prn*)

DURATION

The **duration** is the period of a time over which the drug should be taken, written in number of days. There is also an option to modify start and end dates that is often used for controlled substances.

PATIENT SIGNATURA (Sig)

The patient **signatura** (**Sig**) comprises any other written specifications describing "how" a patient should take a drug or "why" they should be taking it. The provider writes the sig for the pharmacist to print on the container.

DISPENSE

This refers to the exact quantity of the medication that should be given to the patient by the pharmacy (e.g. 15 tablets). This is typically used for *controlled substances* or for "as needed" (prn) medications. If a medication is to be taken at a specified frequency for a specified number of days, then the "Dispense" amount is simply the product of the number of times a day multiplied by the number of days. A simple "QS" or "quantity sufficient" entered in the "Dispense" section instructs the pharmacy to do this basic calculation in order to dispense the correct amount.

DAW (DISPENSE AS WRITTEN)

The pharmacist can fill any trade name drug with the generic equivalent unless the prescription explicitly forbids this, designated with **dispense as written (DAW)**, or by otherwise indicating that substitution is not permitted. DAW is typically used in circumstances in which the patient is unable to tolerate anything but the trade name drug, for a variety of reasons.

CONTROLLED SUBSTANCES

The Drug Enforcement Administration (DEA) is a federal agency that is under the auspices of the Department of Justice. It is tasked with enforcing the Controlled Substances Act along with the Federal Bureau of Investigation (FBI) and Immigration and Customs Enforcement (ICE). Although the DEA has a large role in controlling the sale and distribution of illegal drugs, it also regulates the distribution of legal narcotics and other **controlled substances**.

The DEA verifies authorization to write for controlled substances or any drug with abuse potential. This includes but is not limited to narcotics, sedatives, or amphetamine-like substances. The DEA also maintains a registration system for persons and organizations who are permitted to prescribe or otherwise use substances listed as controlled.

When an entity (in our case a provider) applies for a DEA number, they are requesting permission to write prescriptions for certain classes of controlled substances. Different practitioners may have different levels of *prescriptive authority* and may only write for drugs that fall into those categories for which they have been approved. A prescription can be called-in by a designated employee of the provider as long as it is not a medication with high abuse potential.

The DEA number consists of two letters followed by seven numeric digits. There is a formula for these numbers that is not important to know, but it makes it possible for someone (say a pharmacist) to recognize a made-up number in many cases. There are other identifiers like the **National Provider Identifier (NPI),** which is given to every provider by the Centers for Medicare and Medicaid Services (CMS) that pharmacies and others can use to track the prescriber.

When writing prescriptions, it is important to know that they may fall into different DEA categories called *medication schedules* that are based on abuse potential and legitimate use for medical purposes (Table 8.1). *Schedule I* drugs have a high abuse potential and have no accepted medical indications. Heroin or LSD are schedule I drugs that are never legally prescribed. *Schedule II* drugs have a high abuse potential but can be prescribed for certain medical conditions (e.g. oxycodone, an opioid pain medication). *Schedule III* drugs have a lower abuse potential and also have accepted medical uses (e.g. butalbital, a barbiturate). *Schedule IV* drugs have a low abuse potential and accepted medical uses (e.g. tramadol, an opioid pain medication). *Schedule V* drugs have a

TABLE 8.1 ■ **Drug Schedules From U.S. Drug Enforcement Administration**

Schedule	Definition	Examples
Schedule I	No currently accepted medical use and a high potential for abuse.	Heroin, lysergic acid diethylamide (LSD), marijuana (cannabis), 3,4-methylenedioxymethamphetamine (ecstasy), methaqualone, and peyote
Schedule II	High potential for abuse, with use potentially leading to severe psychological or physical dependence	Combination products with less than 15 mg of hydrocodone per dosage unit (Vicodin), cocaine, fentanyl, methamphetamine, methadone, hydromorphone (Dilaudid), meperidine (Demerol), oxycodone (OxyContin), fentanyl, Dexedrine, Adderall, and Ritalin
Schedule III	Moderate to low potential for physical and psychological dependence	Products containing less than 90 mg of codeine per dosage unit (Tylenol with codeine), ketamine, anabolic steroids, testosterone
Schedule IV	Low potential for abuse and low risk of dependence	Xanax, Soma, Darvon, Darvocet, Valium, Ativan, Talwin, Ambien, Tramadol
Schedule V	Lower potential for abuse; generally used for antidiarrheal, antitussive, and analgesic purposes	Cough preparations with less than 200 mg of codeine or per 100 mL (Robitussin AC), Lomotil, Motofen, Lyrica, Parepectolin

Data from United States Drug Enforcement Administration: *Drug scheduling: drug schedules* (n.d.). Retrieved February 19, 2021, from United States Drug Enforcement Administration Website: https://www.dea.gov/drug-scheduling.

very low abuse potential and accepted medical uses (e.g. promethazine with codeine cough syrup). Noncontrolled medications do not require a DEA number on the prescription.

Every prescription for a controlled substance must have the following:

1. Patient's full name and address
2. Provider's full name and address
3. Provider's DEA number
4. Basic elements of a prescription such as drug name, dosage, form, number prescribed, number of refills, sig, etc.
5. Provider's signature

Laboratory Orders

The laboratory performs testing on samples of body fluids including blood, urine, stool, fluids aspirated from joints, cerebrospinal fluid, or samples from wounds, the mouth, and skin lesions. Specimens may be sent to measure certain chemical components (such as electrolytes), to **culture** (see what organisms grow), to obtain cell counts, or to obtain pathology analysis. Fig. 8.6 shows a laboratory order, sometimes called a requisition, for a complete blood count (CBC), a type of test that analyzes the formed elements of the blood.

The following is a list of the most common labs that may be seen. It will be very useful for a scribe to know spellings and abbreviations. A deeper understanding will facilitate efficiency and accuracy.

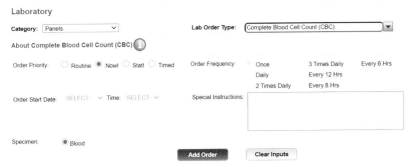

Fig. 8.6   Laboratory order for a complete blood count (CBC). (From SimChart © 2021 Elsevier, Inc.)

HEMATOLOGY

Hematology examines type and quantity of blood cells, and viscosity.
- *Complete blood count (CBC)* w/differential—quantity and size of RBCs, quantity and type of WBCs, and quantity of platelets.
- Prothrombin time/international normalized ratio (PT/INR)—measures various reactions to certain coagulation factors, or how "thin" the blood is; generally done for patients taking the blood thinner Coumadin (warfarin) or those with certain bleeding disorders.

BLOOD BANK

Determines blood type and qualities for transfusion.
- *Type and screen*—blood type (ABO and Rh) and screens for any additional antibodies that may cause a transfusion reaction.
- *Type and crossmatch*—blood type (ABO and Rh) and tests the compatibility of the donor blood with the recipient blood.

CHEMISTRIES

These tests measure electrolyte, hormone, and enzyme levels. They are often performed on the patient's **serum**, the liquid portion of a blood sample after it has been spun in a centrifuge.
- *Comprehensive metabolic panel (CMP)*—electrolytes, glucose, renal function, and hepatic function.
- *Basic metabolic panel (BMP)*—electrolytes, glucose, and renal function.
- *Liver function test (LFT)/hepatic panel*—hepatic function.
- *Lipase*—quantity of the pancreatic enzyme lipase.
- *Human chorionic gonadotropin (hCG)/"beta quant"*—amount of a hormone that is excreted by an embryo after implantation in the uterus; used to monitor pregnancy.
- *Point of care (POC) glucose*—blood strip test measuring blood glucose.
- *Magnesium level*—serum magnesium.
- *Phosphorus level*—serum phosphorus.
- *Zinc level*—serum zinc.
- *Sedimentation rate (sed rate)*—inflammation in the body.
- *C-reactive protein (CRP)*—inflammation in the body.

- *Thyroid stimulating hormone (TSH)*—quantity of serum thyroid hormone secreted by the pituitary gland; used to screen for and monitor thyroid disease.
- *Thyroxine (T4)*—quantity of serum T4 secreted by the thyroid gland.
- *B-type natriuretic peptide (Pro-BNP)*—hormone released by the ventricles of the heart in response to dilation of the ventricles; used to screen for/monitor heart failure.
- *Troponin*—cardiac enzyme released after cardiac muscle cell damage
- *D-dimer*—protein that is released during the process of blood clot degradation; used to screen for thrombosis (blood clots).

BLOOD GASES

Measures the pressures of various gases in the blood.
- *Venous blood gas (VBG)*—partial pressure of gases within venous blood.
- *Arterial blood gas (ABG)*—partial pressure of gases in arterial blood.

URINE TESTS

These examine the quality and content of urine.
- *Urinalysis*—appearance and amount of protein, bacteria, cells, and other molecules in the urine.
- *Point of care (POC) pregnancy*—dipstick urine pregnancy test.

MICROBIOLOGY

Microbiology personnel study samples to understand various pathogens within body fluids. Cultures and other identification means give the provider insight into what medications (if any) will fight the pathogen.
- *Blood culture*—sample of blood that is allowed to culture in order to identify any bacteria present.
- *Urine culture*—sample of urine that is allowed to culture in order to identify any bacteria present.
- *Influenza screen*—identifies different variants of the influenza virus.
- *Sexually transmitted disease (STD) screen*—identifies the most prevalent sexually transmitted infections (STIs).
- *Strep screen*—presence/absence of streptococcus bacteria.
- *Viral pathogen screen*—depending on the sample source, there are screens for different viruses, with respiratory viruses being the most commonly used screen.
- *Wound culture*—sample from a wound that is allowed to culture in order to identify any bacteria present.

TOXICOLOGY

These tests examine various body fluids to identify any toxins such as drugs, controlled substances, and heavy metals.
- *Serum toxicology screen*—identifies toxic substances in the blood.
- *Urine toxicology screen*—identifies toxic substances in the urine.
- *Serum ethanol level*—measures blood alcohol level.
- *Digoxin level*—measures digoxin toxicity (medication level).
- *Other various blood levels*—identifies medications such as lithium, dilantin, tegretol, and many others.

Imaging

Any type of test used to better visualize an interior structure of the body is an **imaging study**. This can include radiographic imaging (x-rays; Fig. 8.7), CT scans, MRI, PET scans, ultrasound imaging (also called sonography), or nuclear medicine studies. The region of the body to be imaged and **laterality** (left, right, or bilateral) must always be specified in an imaging order.

Of special interest in imaging, there are other considerations that providers will likely have in mind prior to placing their imaging orders. The first is costliness. Some forms of imaging can be very expensive and may not be covered by certain insurance companies. Patients of a lower socioeconomic status may not be able to afford some modes of testing and thus may not agree to have them done. An exception to this is in the emergency department where urgency might trump costliness in certain circumstances.

The second consideration is radiation exposure. Many providers monitor the radiation a patient receives, typically from x-rays or CT scans. For perspective: one CT scan emits the same amount of radiation as approximately 250 chest x-rays (depending on the efficiency of the equipment used)! Increased radiation exposure has been positively correlated with an increase in the probability of developing cancer or fertility problems. ***Risk versus benefit analysis*** is a term which refers to an assessment of the potential value of the information obtained by scans (in this example), versus the possible long-term effects of radiation exposure.

The third consideration is possible time constraints. Especially in the emergency department where even seconds to minutes can make a difference in a patient's health outcome during the course of treatment, the type of imaging ordered must be correlated with the acuity of the situation. For example, MRIs are rarely ordered in the emergency department. Although there is no radiation exposure associated with this type of imaging, they are often not immediately available and they take notably longer to perform than CT scans, which are much quicker but cause a degree of radiation exposure.

RADIOGRAPHS

X-rays are directed through part of the body onto a detector. Because different body structures deflect x-rays differently, the x-rays mostly pass through soft tissues like skin and muscle, but bounce off of denser tissues like bone and teeth. The x-rays that make it to the detector produce contrast, creating a **radiograph** or x-ray (Fig. 8.8).

Contrast of softer tissues is also possible with administration of a **contrast medium** prior to in imaging. The medium obstructs the x-rays that would normally pass through the organ or structure, allowing the less dense tissue to be visualized. Sometimes this technique is used to view the hollow organs of the gastrointestinal tract. In other cases, it may be used to view certain vessels (typically arteries), which is called **angiography** (Fig. 8.9).

Diagnostic Tests
Category: X-Ray Examinations
Diagnostic Order Type: Chest w/o Contrast
About Chest w/o Contrast
Order Priority: Routine Now! Stat! Timed
Transportation: Wheelchair
IV Required: Yes No
Oxygen Required: Yes No
Order Start Date: -SELECT- Time: -SELECT-
Special Instructions:
Add Order
Clear Inputs

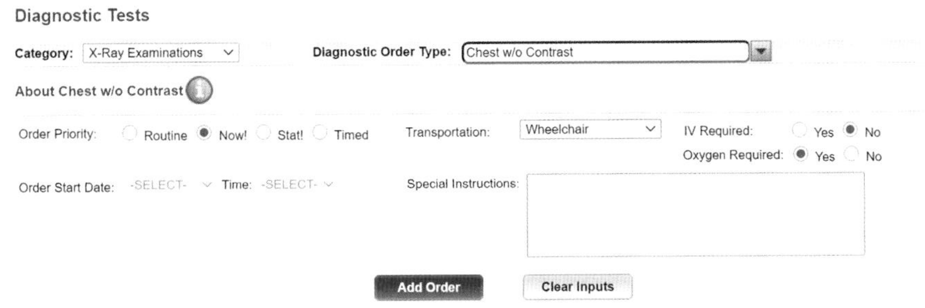

Fig. 8.7 An order for a chest x-ray (CXR). (From SimChart © 2021 Elsevier, Inc.)

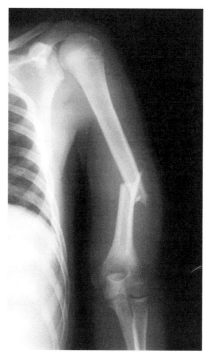

Fig. 8.8 The radiograph shows a fractured arm. The x-rays were blocked by the patient's bones, but most of the rays passed through the skin, muscles, and other structures to reach the detector. (From Long B, Rollins J, Smith B: *Merrill's atlas of radiographic positioning and procedures*, ed 13, St. Louis, 2016, Mosby.)

The use of contrast must be specified within the medical record:

- with (W/) contrast
- without (W/O) contrast
- with and without (W/WO) contrast

How the contrast dye is given must also be specified. Options include orally, intravenously, or both orally and intravenously.

If IV contrast is required, blood chemistries are generally ordered prior to performing the scan to assess renal function. IV contrast dye should only be given after consideration of the risk versus benefit analysis in patients with renal impairment or failure. Additionally, a pregnancy test should be ordered if the patient is a pre-menopausal female—radiation is harmful to a fetus and should be avoided in pregnancy whenever possible. Typically, the provider and other members of the healthcare team will remember to order these extra tests prior to imaging, but this is also an easy thing for a scribe to anticipate as an order.

Radiographs can be taken in different views (Fig. 8.10), which are the direction from which the x-ray is taken. To name a few common examples: AP view (anterior to posterior), PA view (posterior to anterior), lateral and oblique. Because x-rays produce 2D images, most of the time different views are taken of the same body structure.

Standard radiographs are frequently ordered as a "series." When ordering radiographs of the chest, for example, typically it is best to get both a PA and a lateral view for the best diagnostic capabilities. This series is often called a "PA and lateral chest." Other body parts also have standard views which together make a series. So you might have a lumbar series or a knee series. Although a standard series for any given body part will generally be the same from location to location, they could differ somewhat in the views requested based on the preference of the radiologist at each

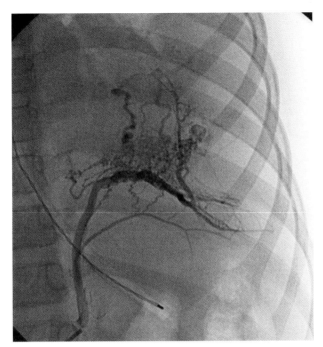

Fig. 8.9   Preoperative angiogram showing aberrant systemic arterial supply. (From Gotway MB, Dawn SK: *An unusual cause of a pulmonary mass. Clin Pulmon Med* 11:266–268, 2004.)

location. The series may also vary depending on the indication so that if the patient is a trauma patient, you may have more or different views than in a non-trauma case with imaging of the same body part. The scribe will not have to know what series is required for any given patient but should be aware that there could be different series available for ordering at any institution and should be careful to select the precise series that the provider is requesting.

COMPUTERIZED TOMOGRAPHY (CT) SCANS

Computed tomography (CT) imaging modality combines radiographs with the help of computer technology. The series of these radiographic images are spliced together to create a 3D reconstruction of a region of the body. Like radiographs, CT scans may utilize contrast media to visualize certain structures.

ULTRASOUND (US)

Ultrasound (US) or sonography produces real-time images by bouncing sound waves of various frequencies off of body structures; the returning signal is used to construct an ultrasound image. This is similar to how dolphins and bats hunt using echolocation. Ultrasounds emit no radiation and are thus the safest imaging modality, especially during pregnancy (Fig. 8.11).

MAGNETIC RESONANCE IMAGING (MRI)

In the **magnetic resonance imaging (MRI)** modality, radiowaves and a magnetic field are used to make a 3D reconstruction of a region of the body. MRI is used infrequently in the emergency department due to time and cost constraints, but this type of imaging is well suited for visualizing

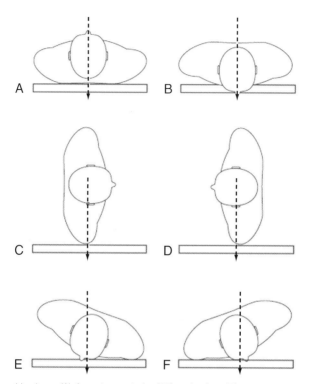

Fig. 8.10 Radiographic views. (A) An anteroposterior (AP) projection; (B) a posteroanterior (PA) projection; (C) indicates a lateral projection in a right lateral position; and (D) indicates a lateral projection in a left lateral position. In (E), the patient is in a left anterior oblique (LAO) position, and in (F), the patient is in a right anterior oblique (RAO) position, both corresponding to PA oblique projections. (From Marchiori DM: *Clinical imaging: with skeletal, chest and abdomen pattern differentials*, ed 3, St. Louis, 2014, Elsevier.)

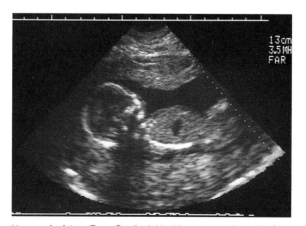

Fig. 8.11 Ultrasound image of a fetus. (From Gerdin J: *Health careers today*, ed 7, St. Louis, 2021, Elsevier.)

tumors and cancerous masses, joint problems, brain and blood vessel abnormalities, problems with the gut, liver disease, and more.

MRI can also be done with or without contrast, and thus the same similar considerations exist as discussed above for CT scans.

NUCLEAR MEDICINE (NM)

In nuclear medicine, radioactive compounds that adhere to certain body areas are used to visualize the metabolism of a region of the body on imaging.

Ventilation-Perfusion (VQ) Scan

The **ventilation perfusion (VQ) scan** examines pulmonary air and blood flow to identify a possible *V/Q mismatch*. A V/Q mismatch is a disturbance of the normal circulation (Q = perfusion) or airflow (V = ventilation) ratio within the lungs. For example, a pulmonary embolism would impair perfusion but not ventilation to a part of a lung.

Other Tests

"Other tests" are a broad category that includes any test used to better understand a disease process or the functionality of certain parts of the body. These would be more concisely described as any additional testing that does not fit within the previous categories.

- *Electrocardiogram (EKG or ECG)*—visualization of the electrical activity of the heart (see Chapter 7).
- *Biopsy (pathological analysis)*—examination of cells that were removed from a suspicious mass or lesion in order to help make a diagnosis.
- *Pulmonary function testing (PFT)*—lung functionality.
- *Electroencephalogram (EEG)*—electrical activity of the brain.

Orders for Healthcare Workers

Provider orders also include any orders to communicate with other members of the healthcare team, such as nurses, technicians, laboratory staff, and other providers. For any order, specific instructions may be entered into the EHR as free text (Fig. 8.12). To name just a couple of examples amongst the many thousands of possibilities, the provider could write an order for a social services consult or an occupational therapy assessment.

NURSING ORDERS

Nurses see to the execution of the provider's orders for medications and other therapies. In addition, some provider orders pertain specifically to nursing interventions. These include requests to apply dressings, perform wound care (Fig. 8.13), facilitate patient ambulation, place the patient on a monitor, perform patient education, position the patient for a pelvic exam, obtain vital signs, and many more.

CONSULT ORDERS

A **consultation** is a formal request by a physician for the opinion or services of another healthcare professional. The consultation may be with a specialist (e.g. cardiology) or with another department (like social services).

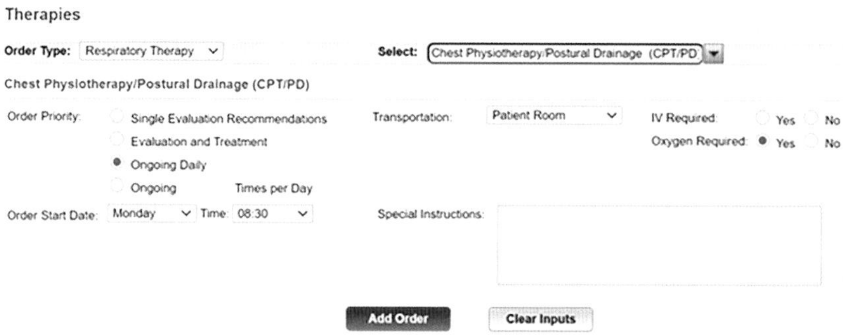

Therapies

Order Type: Respiratory Therapy ⌄   Select: Chest Physiotherapy/Postural Drainage (CPT/PD) ⌄

Chest Physiotherapy/Postural Drainage (CPT/PD)

Order Priority: ○ Single Evaluation Recommendations   Transportation: Patient Room ⌄   IV Required: ○ Yes ● No
                  ○ Evaluation and Treatment   Oxygen Required: ● Yes ○ No
                  ● Ongoing Daily
                  ○ Ongoing   Times per Day
Order Start Date: Monday ⌄ Time: 08:30 ⌄   Special Instructions:

[Add Order]   [Clear Inputs]

Fig. 8.12 An order in the electronic health record (EHR) for chest physiotherapy services from a respiratory therapist. (From SimChart © 2021 Elsevier, Inc.)

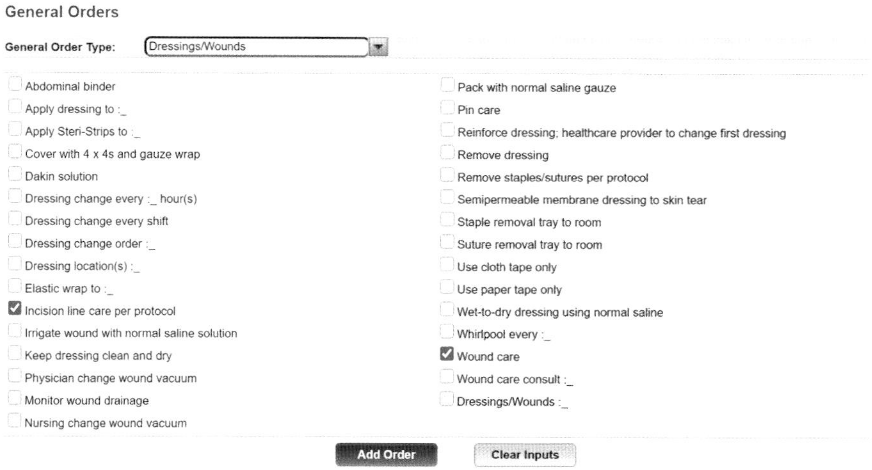

General Orders

General Order Type: Dressings/Wounds ⌄

☐ Abdominal binder   ☐ Pack with normal saline gauze
☐ Apply dressing to :_   ☐ Pin care
☐ Apply Steri-Strips to :_   ☐ Reinforce dressing; healthcare provider to change first dressing
☐ Cover with 4 x 4s and gauze wrap   ☐ Remove dressing
☐ Dakin solution   ☐ Remove staples/sutures per protocol
☐ Dressing change every :_ hour(s)   ☐ Semipermeable membrane dressing to skin tear
☐ Dressing change every shift   ☐ Staple removal tray to room
☐ Dressing change order :_   ☐ Suture removal tray to room
☐ Dressing location(s) :_   ☐ Use cloth tape only
☐ Elastic wrap to :_   ☐ Use paper tape only
☑ Incision line care per protocol   ☐ Wet-to-dry dressing using normal saline
☐ Irrigate wound with normal saline solution   ☐ Whirlpool every :_
☐ Keep dressing clean and dry   ☑ Wound care
☐ Physician change wound vacuum   ☐ Wound care consult :_
☐ Monitor wound drainage   ☐ Dressings/Wounds :_
☐ Nursing change wound vacuum

[Add Order]   [Clear Inputs]

Fig. 8.13 The provider's orders for the nursing team to perform wound care can be entered using a menu of check boxes. (From SimChart © 2021 Elsevier, Inc.)

Order Panels

Many facilities have created **order panels** to facilitate access to the most frequently ordered tests for certain complaints. Order panels aid in efficiency (not having to type in every test separately) and accuracy (not forgetting a test that should be ordered for a specific condition or complaint). Panels are always just starting points and are generally modified on a case-by-case basis. They may be somewhat different from facility to facility, depending on convention. The following are examples of order panels that might be found in an emergency department.

- *Abdominal pain panel*—CBC, BMP, lipase, LFT, urinalysis. Imaging and pregnancy tests could be added depending on history and physical.
- *Chest pain panel*—CBC, BMP, troponin and repeat troponin after 120 minutes, EKG standard 12 lead, and portable chest x-ray. Medications and other tests often need to be added.
- *Eye exam panel*—Fluorescein ophthalmic strip, alcaine 0.5% ophthalmic solution, as well as slit lamp, woods lamp, and tono-pen to bedside.

- *Dyspnea panel*—CBC, BMP, portable chest x-ray, and respiratory care per protocol. May need to add specific treatments, BNP (if possible heart failure), or EKG.
- *ObGyn panel*—Urinalysis with reflex microscopy, POC urine pregnancy, wet prep exam, STD panel PCR, pelvic exam set-up and notification of physician.
- *Psych panel*—CBC, CMP, drugs of abuse urine, serum toxicology screen, urinalysis with reflex microscopy, ED contact order to crisis-care consultant.
- *Sepsis panel*—CBC, CMP, blood cultures, lactate/lactic acid, portable chest x-ray, urinalysis with reflex microscopy, urine culture. Fluids and antibiotics will likely be added.
- *Weak and dizzy panel*—EKG standard 12 lead, CBC, BMP, urinalysis with reflex microscopy, NPO nursing communication, bedside glucose, LFT, TSH with reflex free T4.
- *Stroke non-hyperacute* (over 3-4 hours post symptom onset) *panel*—CBC, BMP, bedside glucose, EKG standard 12 lead, CT head W/O contrast, NPO nursing communication, vital signs every 15 minutes, nursing swallow assessment, protime-INR.
- *Stroke hyperacute* (under 3-4 hours post symptom onset) *panel*—Activate stroke alert team, CBC, BMP, bedside glucose, EKG standard 12 lead, CT head W/O contrast stroke hyperacute, NPO nursing communication, take vital signs every 15 minutes, nursing swallow assessment, protime-INR, NIH stroke scale, partial thomboplastin (PTT).
- *Trauma panel*—EKG standard 12 lead, CBC, BMP, amylase, protime-INR, partial thromboplastin time, platelet function test-EPI, ethanol, drugs of abuse urine, urinalysis with reflex microscopy, bedside glucose, lipase, troponin and repeat troponin after 120 minutes, type and screen, portable chest x-ray.

Dispositions

Transition of care is a term to describe patient flow from one aspect of care to another. This could include transitioning from the doctor's office to the emergency department, from the emergency department to inpatient, from inpatient to a specialist's office, from a specialist's office back to the family doctor.

It is important that communication is intact as a patient goes from one area to the next, so that the follow-on provider does not have to repeat testing and the patient obtains the best medical outcome. The scribe obviously has an important function as the one responsible for documenting the information that will travel with the patient from one area of care to the next.

Transition of care may look something like this:

Scenario 1: Patient comes to the emergency department because they have a perceived emergency and are admitted to the hospital. They are cared for by the hospitalist (inpatient) or another specialist (inpatient). The admitting physician may consult others from different specialties (inpatient). All of these providers will coordinate the patient's care. The patient will eventually be sent for outpatient follow-up with their primary care provider, another specialist, skilled nursing facility, or long-term acute care facility (outpatient).

Scenario 2: Patient comes to the emergency department because they have a perceived emergency and are discharged with instructions to see their outpatient primary care provider (outpatient). They may also need to follow-up with a specialist (outpatient). Will eventually return to their primary care for routine follow-up (outpatient).

Let's begin our detailed discussion about transition of care in the emergency department because this is where our fictional patient began.

Disposition is the status change at the end of the patient's visit in the emergency department or an inpatient facility. Patients cannot stay in the hospital forever and transition of care must take place. Patients will be transferred to another care setting, admitted as an inpatient, discharged to their homes, or they may leave against medical advice (AMA). Death is also a type of disposition.

Admission or **transfer** is the transition of a patient from the emergency department to a bed in the hospital or another facility. An admission requires a physician's order to admit, and this results in inpatient status. Although some admissions are planned (such as before surgery or at the order of the patient's primary care physician), most patients are admitted to the hospital through the ED. The emergency medicine provider will decide to admit the patient when he or she feels that the patient is not safe to go home and would benefit from additional medical evaluation and treatment in the hospital. As an alternative to inpatient admission, some hospitals have **observation** status, which is a shorter stay meant for brief work-ups, or to "observe" the patient a while longer (usually less than 24 hours). Otherwise, patients are considered to be *full admissions*, which implies that they will stay in the hospital until deemed stable enough to be discharged for outpatient follow-up (usually the anticipated stay is longer than 24 hours).

Patients may be admitted to different parts of the hospital. **Intensive care unit (ICU)** admissions are reserved for patients needing critical care. Hospital admissions may be placed in **telemetry** (a monitored bed) or a regular bed. The patient may go to a hospitalist (general medical physician) or to a specialist such as a surgeon. Other types of specialized physicians may consult on patients during their hospital stay, even if the specialist did not accept the admission themselves. This entails seeing the patient and giving their specialty advice to the admitting physician.

Discharge is the process of sending the patient to another setting. The patient may return home, or go to a more permanent facility like an extended care facility (ECF), nursing home, or skilled nursing facility (SNF), pronounced "sniff." Discharge occurs when the medical provider has cleared the patient, and the patient is deemed safe from any acute medical issues.

Although it is ideal for the patient to remain in the emergency department until a decision is made regarding the most appropriate disposition, sometimes a patient may decide to leave before their evaluation is complete. This is called leaving **against medical advice (AMA)** and happens for a variety of reasons. If the patient leaves AMA, the provider will give the patient discharge instructions with the safest plan of care (given the circumstances) and also discuss possible consequences of leaving before their evaluation is complete. **Eloping** is when the patient leaves before their evaluation is complete but they do not stay for the circumstantial discharge instructions.

A patient may also **leave without being seen (LWBS)**. This is a different situation in which a patient may check into an emergency department at triage (the front desk), but leave before being brought to a room or otherwise seen by the physician or other provider. In this case, the provider is not given the opportunity to evaluate the patient.

Outpatient facilities function a little differently than what has been described above. Because they are typically only open during normal business hours, patients are almost always sent home at the end of the appointment with a new appointment date and time for their next follow-up visit. Sometimes very ill patients are sent from the office to the emergency department for emergent care, or for **direct admission** into the hospital.

A scribe may complete disposition or follow-up paperwork for their provider, so long as they complete the paperwork as it is instructed by the provider. Because the outpatient paperwork is much more simple as compared to the emergency department or inpatient, here we will discuss the latter in much more detail.

DISPOSITION

Documentation of disposition is required for all discharges. In the EHR, this appears as an option to select admit, transfer, discharge, leaving against medical advice or eloping. Making this selection will officially change the patient's status. From the inpatient perspective, Table 8.2 lists selected discharge dispositions and the codes used by the Centers for Medicare and Medicaid Services and other payers to record the disposition.

TABLE 8.2 ■ **Discharge Disposition Codes**

Code	Discharge Status
01	Discharged to home or self-care
02	Discharged/transferred to another short-term general hospital for inpatient care
03	Discharged/transferred to a skilled nursing facility (SNF) with Medicare certification in anticipation of covered skilled care
04	Discharged/transferred to a facility that provides custodial or supportive care
05	Discharged/transferred to a designated cancer center or children's hospital
06	Discharged/transferred to home under care of organized home health service organization in anticipation of covered skilled care
21	Discharged/transferred to court/law enforcement
43	Discharged/transferred to a federal health care facility
50	Discharged/transferred to hospice—home (inpatient only)
51	Discharged/transferred to hospice—medical facility (inpatient only)
61	Discharged/transferred within this institution to a hospital-based Medicare-approved swing bed
62	Discharged/transferred to an inpatient rehabilitation facility, including distinct part units of a hospital
63	Discharged/transferred to a long-term care hospital (LTCH)
64	Discharged/transferred to a nursing facility certified under Medicaid but not certified under Medicare
65	Discharged/transferred to a psychiatric hospital or psychiatric distinct-part unit of a hospital
66	Discharged/transferred to a critical access hospital (CAH)
70	Discharged/transferred to another type of health care institution not defined elsewhere in the code list

A *swing bed* hospital is a hospital or critical access hospital (CAH) participating in Medicare that has CMS approval to provide post-hospital SNF care and meets certain requirements. A swing bed is an acute bed used by such a hospital to provide this service. http://www.cms.gov/Medicare/Medicare-Fee-for-Service-Payment/SNFPPS/SwingBed.html.
A long-term care hospital (LTCH) is defined by Medicare as a hospital having an average length of stay over 25 days. http://www.cms.gov/Outreach-and-Education/Medicare-Learning-Network-MLN/MLNProducts/downloads/LTCH-News.pdf.
A critical access hospital (CAH) is a special designation to hospitals that provide necessary care in remote locations. http://www.cms.gov/Outreach-and-Education/Medicare-Learning-Network-MLN/MLNProducts/downloads/CritAccessHospfctsht.pdf.
From Davis N: *Foundations of health information management*, ed 5, St. Louis, 2020, Elsevier.

CONDITION

Discharge paperwork also includes the patient's medical condition at time of disposition. This is required for all dispositions.

Examples: *good, fair, stable, serious, poor, or critical.*

FOLLOW-UP INSTRUCTIONS

The provider will make recommendations for outpatient follow-up after leaving the hospital. Follow-up could include the following:

1. Follow up with their primary care physician within "x" amount of days
2. Return to the emergency department if symptoms worsen
3. Follow up with additional specialists for further evaluation

Generally, including the first two in the discharge paperwork is recommended.

WORK/SCHOOL EXCUSE

The discharge "paperwork" may include a written excuse for work or school or elsewhere stating that the patient was in the hospital, and giving any specific instructions for limitations. This can be given to patients who are being discharged, but is not required. These should generally be signed by the provider prior to being given to the patient.

DISCHARGE INSTRUCTIONS

Discharge instructions may be added from a template or free texted, and given to a patient prior to discharge. They typically describe the diagnosis and how the patient can care for themselves at home.

ORDERS

The orders component includes any orders the provider requires for this disposition. This can be used for any disposition, but is not required. For patients who will be admitted to inpatient status, this could include medications or treatment that the patient will need prior to entering the hospital. An **ED contact order** may need to be ordered. This order often goes under another name such as consult order. This is a request for the receptionist to page the hospitalist or another specialist so the emergency medicine provider can discuss the patient's case and confirm the status change. For discharged patients or patients who leave AMA, orders could include medications or treatment that the patient needs prior to discharge, or prescriptions for them to take with them.

PROBLEM LIST

A **problem list** contains all current medical problems that a patient is known to have. This may include any combination of diagnoses, symptoms and signs, or clinical impressions. Every patient is different and may have multiple problems in their problem list.

All types of problems are documented using ICD-10-CM codes. There are tens of thousands of choices. Ultimately, there must be a code associated with each encounter in order to bill for that encounter. To bill at the highest level, it is always best to use the most specific code possible. For example, instead of using "nonspecific abdominal pain," try using specifics such as quadrant or chronicity pattern.

Clinical Impression

A **clinical impression** is typically ascertained after a rapid work-up in the emergency department. It is an assessment of the patient's condition based upon their symptoms and results, but may or may not be a diagnosis. A definitive diagnosis could be dependent upon additional testing deemed safe to be done after discharge the emergency department. Clinical impressions are required for all dispositions from an emergency department. New clinical impressions, especially if they are diagnoses, will often be included in the patient's problem list, in order to keep it up to date.

Diagnosis

A **diagnosis** is a more definitive description of a disease or condition than a clinical impression. If a definitive diagnosis has not yet been made, signs and symptoms codes are used until a diagnosis is found that explains the patient's presentation. After this point the signs and symptoms codes should be removed from the problem list and the diagnosis should be added in their place.

This month, Roz Yoder marked the second year of her battle against metastatic breast cancer. She has been through two courses of chemotherapy, and tried alternative therapies such as acupuncture and mindfulness meditation. Although Roz and her oncologist have celebrated several wins in the course of her treatment, Mrs. Yoder no longer has an appetite and is losing weight rapidly. Leaving bed is a difficult task, and she tires very quickly. She can no longer drive a car and it takes all the strength she can muster to leave the house for medical appointments and labs.

On Wednesday afternoon, Roz was gasping for breath. Her breathing was rapid and shallow, so her worried husband called the oncologist's office, who told him to take her to the ED immediately. The ED physician ordered a dyspnea panel and she received oxygen.

The lab results showed severe thrombocytopenia, a very low platelet count. Roz would need a platelet transfusion, but this did not explain her shortness of breath. She was admitted that evening.

The attending physician, Dr. Kishore, ordered the platelets. She also ordered Valium to help Roz relax, and breathing exercises, which the nursing staff would administer. Her respiratory rate slowly improved. Dr. Kishore monitored her condition the next day, and discharged her home the following morning in stable condition with instructions to see her oncologist within 14 days. Because she could not determine a cause for Mrs. Yoder's shortness of breath, Dr. Kishore suspected the patient was understandably anxious. She prescribed 5 mg diazepam (Valium) prn.

QUESTIONS

1. What type of imaging did Roz have in the ED?
2. What lab testing revealed the patient's thrombocytopenia?
3. What is the generic name of the drug Dr. Kishore prescribed?
4. What type of order did Dr. Kishore write so that Mrs. Yoder would do breathing exercises?
5. According to the Sig, when should Roz take the prescription?

Practice Questions

1. Complete the prescriptions template using the following information: A 36-year-old female patient presents with muscle spasm. Give her Flexeril 10 mg. Dispense 20 tablets. Take one tablet by mouth twice a day for 10 days. Take with or without food.

Name: _____

Dose: _____

Formulation: _____

Route: _____

Frequency: _____

Duration: _____

Patient Sig: _____

2. Complete the prescriptions template using the following information: A 42-year-old male patient presents with nausea. Give him Phenergan 25 mg rectal suppositories. Dispense 12. Use every 4 hours as needed.

Name: _____

Dose: _____

Formulation: _____

Route: _____

Frequency: _____

Duration: _____

Patient Sig: _____

Dispense: _____

Write the name for the diagnostic order that matches the description.

3. Blood cell count, type, & viscosity: _____

4. Electrolytes, glucose, renal function: _____

5. Radiographic images spliced together for a 3D image: _____

6. Hepatic function: _____

7. Contrast dye used on radiographic imaging of blood vessels:_____

8. Screening for toxins in the blood: _____

9. Examines pulmonary air and blood flow: _____

10. Electrical activity of the brain: _____

11. A patient presents to the emergency department with chest pain and the attending physician wants to order a test to measure heart enzymes. What is the name of this test?
    a. d-dimer
    b. sedimentation rate
    c. troponin
    d. ANA (antinuclear antibodies)

12. A patient is being seen by a family physician for pleuritic chest pain, shortness of breath, and tachycardia. The physician wants to order a test to screen for a blood clot. What is the name of this test?
    a. d-dimer
    b. sedimentation rate
    c. troponin
    d. ANA (antinuclear antibodies)

13. A pregnant patient is being seen by her obstetrician for a follow-up on the baby's health. What imaging study is the obstetrician going to use to assess fetal health?
    a. x-rays
    b. computed tomography (CT)
    c. magnetic resonance imaging (MRI)
    d. ultrasound

Match the situation on the left with the term on the right.

_____	**14.** Patient leaves before being brought to a room	A. Elope
_____	**15.** Patient is brought into the hospital for work-up	B. AMA
_____	**16.** Patient leaves before their work-up is complete but is not able to receive instructions	C. Transfer
_____	**17.** Patient is sent home from the ED	D. LWBS
_____	**18.** Patient is transported to another hospital	E. Admission
_____	**19.** Patient leaves before their work-up is complete but is able to receive instructions	F. Discharge

There are a variety of things that may be included on the patient's problem list. For each of the patient's problem list below, indicate whether it is a diagnosis, sign, symptom, or clinical impression.

20. Abdominal pain _____

21. Cirrhosis _____

22. Fever _____

23. Ascites _____

24. Hyperbilirubinemia (found in the ED) _____

Medical Terminology and Abbreviations

- Build and define medical terms using word parts.
- Explain the use of abbreviations in medicine.

Acronym	Prefix
Combining form	Suffix
Eponym	

Medical Terminology

Medicine uses an entire vocabulary unique to its profession. Entire books and courses are devoted to the instruction of medical terminology, and this chapter does not intend to replace those resources. However, because the medical scribe is working at the intersection of medical practice and documentation, a brief introduction to the workings of medical language is appropriate.

Medical terminology is based in a large part on ancient Greek and Latin, owing to the long period of history when those languages were well known by people of advanced learning. Because Greek and Latin were understood by physicians all over Europe—regardless of their country of origin or native tongue—they served as a universally understood means to communicate ideas and treatments.

The value of standardized communication is no less important today. Using medical terminology, healthcare professionals reduce confusion related to language changes and regional terms. This standardized language improves patient care, increases efficiency, and reduces potentially fatal errors.

WORD PARTS

Many medical terms based on Greek and Latin roots are easily constructed by assembling a standard set of word parts. The meaning of the word can be deciphered by understanding the meaning of the parts. Medical professionals can utilize the same parts in different combinations to build and decode a distinct vocabulary to refer to human anatomy and physiology, diseases, and procedures.

Combining Forms

The basis of the medical term is the **combining form**, which is a word root with a vowel. (The combining vowel allows the root to be joined to other word parts that begin with a consonant.) A selection of combining forms and their meanings are listed in Table 9.1. To the combining form can be added prefixes and suffixes. Combining forms can also be added to other combining forms. In addition to those shown in Table 9.1, each chapter in Part III of this book, Body Systems for the Medical Scribe, lists and defines combining forms relevant to the vocabulary in that chapter.

Prefixes

A **prefix** is a word part that appears at the beginning of a word. Prefixes alter the meaning of the root to indicate the absence of something (using *a-* or *an-* to mean *without*), define its location (such as adding *epi-* meaning *above*, or *sub-* meaning *below*), to indicate number or quantity (such as *bi-* meaning *two*), or to give the root a characteristic (such as *dys-* meaning *difficult*, or *brady-* meaning *slow*). Selected prefixes are shown in Table 9.2.

Suffixes

A **suffix** is a word part that appears at the end of the term. Usually, a suffix indicates a type of anatomy, a type of pathology (disease or disorder), or a type of procedure. Common suffixes are listed in Table 9.3. Sometimes, a term can be built from only a prefix and suffix (no combining form needed).

BUILDING AND DEFINING TERMS

Let's build a few words for practice, using the parts listed in Tables 9.1, 9.2, and 9.3.

The physician asks the patient about her surgical history, and she remarks that she had a "nose job" a few years ago. The combining form for nose is **rhin/o**, and the suffix for surgical formation is **-plasty**.

$$\text{rhin/o} + \text{-plasty} = \text{rhinoplasty}$$

What kind of instrument is used to view (-**scope**) the eye (**ophthalm/o**)?

$$\text{ophthalm/o} + \text{-scope} = \text{ophthalmoscope}$$

One of the most common pathological findings is inflammation, denoted by the suffix **-itis**. What term would you use to describe inflammation of the gums?

$$\text{gingiv/o} + \text{-itis} = \text{gingivitis}$$

Note that in the case of gingivitis, the combining vowel was not needed. This is because the suffix already begins with a vowel.

What about when your patient has inflammation of the both the stomach and the small intestine? Here, we need two combining forms: one for the stomach (**gastr/o**) and one for the small bowel (**enter/o**):

$$\text{gastr/o} + \text{enter/o} + \text{-itis} = \text{gastroenteritis}$$

Now let's try adding a prefix. We want to talk about something pertaining to (-**ic**) above (**epi-**) the stomach (**gastr/o**). How are these word parts combined?

$$\text{epi-} + \text{gastr/o} + \text{-ic} = \text{epigastric}$$

Finally, let's try using only a prefix and suffix to denote difficult breathing:

$$\text{dys-} + \text{-pnea} = \text{dyspnea}$$

TABLE 9.1 ■ **Selected Combining Forms**

Combining Form	Definition	Combining Form	Definition
aden/o	gland	leuk/o	white
adip/o	fat	lip/o	fat
angi/o	blood vessel	lith/o	stone
ankyl/o	stiff	mast/o	breast
anter/o	front	medi/o	middle
arter/o	artery	morph/o	shape
arthr/o	joint	my/o	muscle
articul/o	joint	necr/o	death
ather/o	fatty plaque	nephr/o	kidney
aur/o	ear	neur/o	nerve
axill/o	armpit	olig/o	scanty
bi/o	life	onych/o	nail
blephar/o	eyelid	oophor/o	ovary
bucc/o	cheek	ophthalm/o	eye
carcin/o	cancerous	orch/o	testis
cardi/o	heart	orth/o	straight
cephal/o	head	oste/o	bone
colp/o	vagina	ot/o	ear
crani/o	skull	path/o	disease
cutane/o	skin	phleb/o	vein
cyan/o	blue	proxim/o	near
cyst/o	urinary bladder	prurit/o	itching
cyt/o	cell	pseud/o	false
dipl/o	double	psych/o	mind
dors/o	back	py/o	pus
encephal/o	brain	pyel/o	renal pelvis
enter/o	small intestine	pyr/o	fever
erythem/o	flushed, red	ren/o	kidney
gastr/o	stomach	somat/o	body
gingiv/o	gums	splen/o	spleen
gloss/o	tongue	stomat/o	mouth
gluc/o	sugar, glucose	thorac/o	chest
hem/o	blood	thromb/o	clot
hepat/o	liver	tox/o	poison
hist/o	tissue	ur/o	urine
hydr/o	water	varic/o	varicose veins
hyster/o	uterus	vascul/o	vascular
jaund/o	yellow	ventr/o	front
kines/o	movement	vesic/o	bladder
lact/o	milk	viscer/o	internal organs
later/o	side	vit/o	life

TABLE 9.2 ■ **Selected Prefixes**

Prefix	Definition	Prefix	Definition
a- an-	without	macro-	large
ante-	before	mal-	bad
anti-	against	mega-	large
auto-	self	neo-	new
bi-	two	pan-	all
brady-	slow	para-	near, beside
contra-	against	per-	through
dys-	painful, abnormal, difficult	peri-	surrounding
endo-	within	poly-	many, much
epi-	above	post-	after
eu-	good; normal	pre-	before
exo-	outside	quadri-	four
hemi-	half	rhin/o	nose
hyper-	above; excessive	semi-	half
hypo-	deficient	sub-	under
infra-	below	supra-	above
inter-	between	tachy-	fast
intra-	within	trans-	across; through
		tri-	three

OTHER TERMS

Of course, not all medical terms are neatly made from a finite list of word parts. Sometimes, a medical term has origins in Greek or Latin, but the literal meaning of the root is not helpful for understanding the word. For example, the endocrine disorder *diabetes* comes from the Greek meaning "siphon"; *cataracts*, the clouding of the lenses of the eye, is another Greek word meaning "a high waterfall." The meanings of these terms and many like them cannot be decoded and must be memorized.

As medicine advances and new technologies are invented, the healthcare industry has had to adopt new words and means of describing things. Sometimes, we use **eponyms**, named after a person who studied a disease or anatomic region. *Parkinson disease* and *Down syndrome* are examples of eponyms, and there are many more.

Still other terms are **acronyms**—words formed from the initial letters of other words. Acronyms are especially prominent in medicine when there is a need to refer to a new technology or procedure. For example:

- CABG, pronounced "cabbage," which means **c**oronary **a**rtery **b**ypass **g**raft.
- LASIK, which is easier to say than **l**aser-**a**ssisted **i**n **s**itu **k**eratomileusis.
- DEXA, a bone scan, short for **d**ual **e**nergy **x**-ray **a**bsorptioimetry.

Abbreviations

There are medical abbreviations in the EHR written by many different types of medical professionals. There are different and sometimes conflicting opinions regarding their use and place

TABLE 9.3 ■ Selected Suffixes

Suffix	Definition	Suffix	Definition
-ac -al	pertaining to	-oma	tumor, mass
-algesia	sensitivity to pain	-osis	abnormal condition
-algia	pain	-penia	deficiency
-cardia	heart condition	-pepsia	digestion
-cele	hernia	-pexy	fixation
-centesis	surgical puncture	-phagia	eating
-derma	skin	-phasia	speech
-dynia	pain	-plasty	surgical forming
-ectasia	dilation, stretching	-plegia	paralysis
-ectomy	excision	-pnea	breathing
-emesis	vomiting	-poiesis	formation
-emia	blood condition	-prandial	meal
-esis	condition	-ptosis	drooping; sagging
-genesis	forming	-rrhage	bursting forth
-globin	protein	-rraphy	suturing
-gram	a recording	-rrhea	flow
-graphy	process of recording	-sclerosis	hardening
-iasis	abnormal condition	-scope	instrument to visualize
-ic	pertaining to	-scopy	process of viewing
-lapse	to sag	-stasis	to stop
-lithiasis	condition of stones	-stenosis	narrowing
-logy	study of	-stomy	new opening
-lysis	to break down	-tomy	cutting
-malacia	softening	-tresia	opening
-megaly	enlargement	-tripsy	to crush
		-uria	urinary disorder

within the health record. The guidelines in this text regarding the use of medical abbreviations are written in consideration of the following: a medical scribe's primary function is to document a patient encounter within the medical record. As such, pride should be taken in one's work and it is best to take the time to spell most things out.

Thus as a general rule, abbreviations are to be avoided. Some abbreviations can mean many different things. For example, "MS" can mean mental status, multiple sclerosis, morphine sulfate, or magnesium sulfate. The Joint Commission (TJC) maintains an official "Do Not Use" list for abbreviations, which applies to all orders, and all medication-related documentation that is handwritten (including free-text computer entry) or on pre-printed forms (Table 9.4). Abbreviations may however be used for those terms which are frequently used within a provider's area of practice, and which are known to be universally accepted and already in use by others.

TABLE 9.4 ■ **The Joint Commission's Official "Do Not Use" List**

Do Not Use	Potential Problem	Use Instead
U, u (unit)	Mistaken for "0" (zero), the number "4" (four) or "cc"	Write "unit"
IU (International Unit)	Mistaken for IV (intravenous) or the number 10 (ten)	Write "International Unit"
Q.D., QD, q.d., qd (daily)	Mistaken for each other and period mistaken for an "I"	Write "daily"
Q.O.D., QOD, q.o.d, qod (every other day)	Mistaken for each other and period after the Q mistaken for "I" and the "O" mistaken for "I"	Write "every other day"
Trailing zero (X.0 mg)†	Decimal point is missed	Write X mg
Lack of leading zero (.X mg)	Decimal point is missed	Write 0.X mg
MS	Can mean morphine sulfate or magnesium sulfate	Write "morphine sulfate" or write "magnesium sulfate"
MSO_4 and $MgSO_4$	Confused for one another	Write "morphine sulfate" or write "magnesium sulfate"

† Exception: A "trailing zero" may be used only where required to demonstrate the level of precision of the value being reported, such as for laboratory results, imaging studies that report size of lesions, or catheter/tube sizes. It may not be used in medication orders or other medication-related documentation.
From The Joint Commission: The Joint Commission Fact Sheet: Official Do Not Use List. Available at https://www.jointcommission.org/-/media/tjc/documents/resources/patient-safety-topics/do_not_use_list_6_28_19.pdf. Accessed March 4, 2021.

Keep in mind that other members of the healthcare team (such as nurses) do not always spell things out, and therefore the scribe should become familiar with abbreviations and their meanings to facilitate communication and understanding.

SYMPTOMS

All symptoms should be spelled out. These are generally not accepted as abbreviations, as some share acronyms with diagnoses. For example, using "CP" for chest pain can easily be confused with the diagnosis *cerebral palsy* if no context is provided.

MEDICAL DIAGNOSES, LAB TESTS AND IMAGING, PROCEDURES

These are frequently abbreviated, as many have long spellings and for the most part are unanimously accepted as abbreviations.

SIGNS

It is commonplace for physical exam findings to be abbreviated and this use is often acceptable because of their ubiquitous use by many providers. In any case, it would be beneficial for a scribe to know physical examination abbreviations because often the provider will use these while dictating physical exam findings to the scribe.

MISCELLANEOUS OTHERS

These include acronyms for phrases generally used in the notes of medical assistants, nurses, and other medical or laboratory technicians. A common example is "ADLs," which stands for "activities of daily living." The meaning of these acronyms is generally known; however the scribe should spell these out unless there is a compelling reason to abbreviate.

As previously noted, these conventions may vary based on location and the practicing provider. There will be times when shortcuts are needed in order to be efficient and abbreviations may be required. A scribe must learn what is acceptable, and when in doubt spell it out!

CASE STUDY 9.1

The physician sees Maggie MacPherson, a 33-year-old female who is 4 months postpartum. Maggie is visiting because she is experiencing urinary incontinence, having to wear pads all day and night, while at the same time not being able to urinate very much when she sits on the toilet. The physician ordered an intravenous pyelogram (IVP) and performed a cystoscopy. The diagnostics revealed multiple vesicovaginal fistulae, abnormal connections. In this case the physician suspects they were incurred during Maggie's recent childbirth. She is admitted for repair, and the surgeon will perform endoscopic surgery using a transvaginal approach.

QUESTIONS

1. What is the meaning of the prefix post- in the term postpartum?
2. What term would describe Maggie's symptom of abnormal, scanty urine output?
3. What is a pyelogram?
4. What structure was viewed during the cystoscopy?
5. Where are the fistulae found?

Practice Questions

1. What term would mean abnormal condition of the mind?
   a. Craniotomy
   b. Psychosis
   c. Psychiatric
   d. Encephalogy

2. What term means pertaining to the chest?
   a. Thoracic
   b. Cardialgia
   c. Epidermis
   d. Ventral

3. How would you define the term rhinorrhea?

4. How would you translate osteomalacia?

5. What kind of a term is Cushing disease?

PART III

Body Systems for the Medical Scribe

Constitutional

1. Use medical terminology to document the provider's observations of the patient's general appearance and wellbeing.
2. Describe locations on the body using directional terms.
3. Document constitutional symptoms related during a review of systems.
4. Document signs related by the provider during a physical exam of the patient's appearance and wellbeing.

Afebrile	Fatigue	Pyrexia
Anatomic position	Febrile	Rectal
Anorexia	Habitus	Somnolence
Anterior	Inferior	Superficial
Asthenic	Ipsilateral	Superior
Aural	Latera	Syncope
Axillary	Laterality	Systemic
Bilateral	Lethargy	Temporal
Cachectic	Malaise	Toxic appearance
Caudad	Medial	Tympanic
Cephalad	Oral	Unilateral
Constitutional	Polydipsia	Ventral
Contralateral	Polyphagia	Vertigo
Distal	Posterior	Vital signs
Dorsal	Proximal	

Anatomy and Physiology

Although "**constitutional**" is not a classic body system, it is considered as a body system for billing in both review of systems and physical exam. It is used to describe a person's **systemic** (overall) health or appearance. It also includes recording of the patient's **vital signs** in the physical exam portion of the chart (Fig. 10.1).

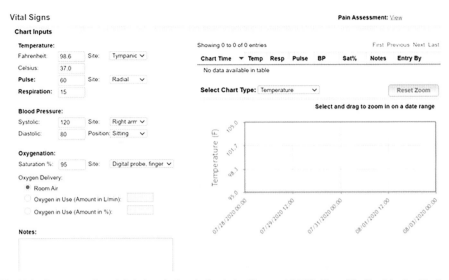

Fig. 10.1 Documentation of vital signs in the electronic health record (EHR). (From SimChart for the Medical Office, © Elsevier, Inc.)

VITAL SIGNS

Typically, the recorded vital signs are temperature, blood pressure, pulse (heart rate), and respiratory rate. In addition, some would add blood oxygenation ("pulse ox") and others might also include a pain scale rating along with the traditional vital signs. The pain scale rating is not measured of course, but is subjective and is reported by the patient.

Body temperature is usually measured on the Fahrenheit scale, with a normal range for adults between 97 °F and 99 °F. The patient's temperature can be taken at various sites, which is documented in the heath record along with the measurement:

- **Axillary** – the armpit
- **Oral** – the mouth
- **Temporal** – the forehead
- **Rectal** – the rectum
- **Tympanic/aural** – the ear

A fever, sometimes called **pyrexia**, is defined as a body temperature higher than 100.4 °F (38°C). The provider may describe a patient with a fever as **febrile**, while a patient without a fever is said to be **afebrile**. Fig. 10.2 illustrates terms used to describe temperature ranges in the adult patient.

Pulses are the result of arterial expansion as the beating heart forces blood through these vessels, which are detected as light taps. Thus, heart rate can be measured when the clinician counts the number of taps (per minute). The major pulse sites are depicted in Fig. 10.3.

Directional terms are used to designate the position of something on the body in relation to other bodily structures. All directional terms are paired as opposites, as follows and in Fig. 10.4:

Superior - closest to the top of the head
Inferior - closest to the bottom of the feet
Anterior (ventral) - front of the body
Posterior (dorsal) - back of the body
Proximal - closest to the center of the body
Distal - further from the center of the body
Lateral - away from the midline (Box 10.1)
Medial - towards the midline

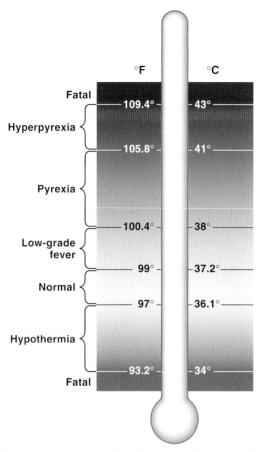

Fig. 10.2   Adult oral body temperature ranges and associated terminology. (From Bonewit-West K, Hunt SA: Today's medical assistant: clinical & administrative procedures, ed 4, St. Louis, 2021, Elsevier.)

Superficial - more externally located
Deep - more internally located
Cephalad – toward the head
Caudad – toward the tail

As shown in Fig. 10.4, when using directional terms, the observer's point of view should be from **anatomic position**, which is defined as the patient facing the examiner with arms at their side and the palms of both hands facing forward (also toward the examiner). Anatomic position is important to use because the changing point of view of the observer would otherwise change the meaning of directional terminology.

Review of Systems

As discussed in Chapter 5, the note for the review of systems is a listing of all subjective symptoms a patient denies or affirms, organized by system. Patients often describe what they are feeling in a manner which makes the most sense to them. It is the duty of the scribe to translate the patient's interpretation of their symptoms into medical terms. For example, if a patient says they have been really tired and not feeling well, the scribe should document "fatigue and malaise."

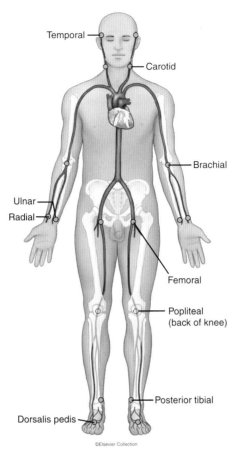

Fig. 10.3   Major pulse sites. (© Elsevier Collection.)

MEDICAL TERMINOLOGY WORD PARTS FOR THE CONSTITUTIONAL/PATIENT'S GENERAL APPEARANCE

Combining Forms

anter/o	front	somn/o	sleep
ventr/o	belly	phag/o	eat, swallow
poster/o dors/o	back	**Prefixes**	
		an-	without
super/o	upward	mal-	bad
infer/o	downward	poly-	much, many
later/o	side	**Suffixes**	
proxim/o	near	-al -ior	pertaining to
dist/o	far		
cephal/o	head	-ia	condition of
caud/o	tail	-dipsia	condition of thirst
orex/o	appetite	-thenic	condition of strength

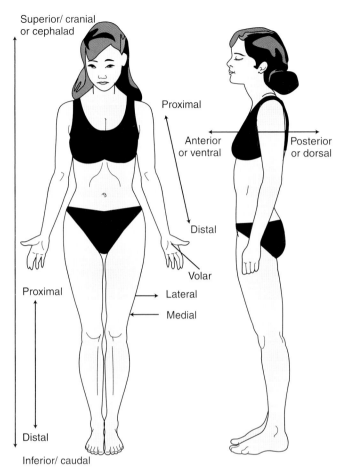

Fig. 10.4 Directional terminology shown on the body in anatomic position. (From Fritz S, Fritz L: *Mosby's essential sciences for therapeutic massage*, ed 6, St. Louis, 2021, Mosby Elsevier.)

BOX 10.1 ■ Laterality

The provider may describe a condition or problem as **unilateral**, meaning it pertains only to one side of the patient's body (the right side or the left side), or as **bilateral**, meaning that it occurs on both sides. Something that is **ipsilateral** pertains to the same side, and **contralateral** means that it pertains to the opposite side.

Laterality is important not only for patient care and safety, but also for proper coding and billing. Many ICD-10-CM diagnoses have three unique codes: one to specify that a condition occurs on the right, a separate code for a condition that occurs on the left lateral, and a third code to be used when the condition is bilateral.

Constitutional symptoms that can be placed in multiple systems have been designated below in italics. Remember to always maximize the number of <u>systems</u> that are included in the review of systems so that the chart can be billed at higher levels (if desired). For example: if a patient is having fatigue and malaise, it would be best to include fatigue in "*endocrine*" and malaise in "*constitutional*" (two billable systems), as opposed to including fatigue and malaise in "*constitutional*" (one billable system).

A patient reported fever is considered to be subjective history, just as the rest of the review of systems is considered to be subjective. However, the patient may report that they actually took their temperature and will give you a home temperature reading that you can record. If they only report feeling as if they had a fever, then that is recorded as a "subjective fever."

Anorexia (*digestive, endocrine, psychiatric*) - loss of appetite

Chills - involuntary shivering

Dizziness (*cardiovascular, neurologic*) - sensation that the room is spinning (**vertigo**), imbalance (**disequilibrium**) or feeling of blacking out (**near syncope**) (*note: placed here if uncertain cause*)

Falls - mechanical (falls that are due to slipping or tripping) or due to dizziness, palpitations, chest pain, etc.

Fatigue (*endocrine*) - feeling excessively tired

Fever (pyrexia) (*immunologic/allergic*) - temperature greater than 100.4°F (38°C)

Hot flash (*endocrine, genitourinary*) - feeling warm and sweaty

Lethargy - excessive fatigue and inactivity; suggests difficulty arousing and inability to be alert

Malaise - feeling unwell

Polydipsia (*digestive, endocrine*) - excessive thirst

Polyphagia (*digestive, endocrine*) - excessive hunger

Recent illnesses (*immunologic/allergic*) - any recent illnesses

Somnolence - sleepiness

Subjective fever - feeling warm without having taken a temperature (presumed fever, or feeling feverish)

CASE STUDY 1.1

Accompanied by the scribe, the emergency department physician sees Raul Lopez, a 21-year-old male who fell from a horse onto a steel fencepost. Mr. Lopez believes he lost consciousness briefly but appears alert and in no acute distress. His primary complaints are head pain, a sensation that the room is spinning, and tenderness at the anterior face of the distal right humerus, where there is a superficial laceration. He denies fatigue, lethargy, or malaise. In triage the nurse recorded a body temperature of 101.6°F (tympanic), a heart rate of 85, and an oxygen saturation of 95%.

QUESTIONS

1. How does the scribe record Mr. Lopez's sensation that the room is spinning?
2. At what site did the nurse take the patient's temperature?
3. Is the location of Mr. Lopez's laceration closer to the elbow, or closer to the shoulder?
4. The provider describes the patient's cut as superficial, meaning it is what?
5. The _____ are the problems Mr. Lopez denies having, including fatigue, lethargy, and malaise.

Physical Exam

The results of the physical exam are a listing of the provider's objective findings (signs), organized by system. The scribe will never be expected to interpret these findings, but rather must be diligent in recording exactly what the provider tells them to. The objective observations of the provider often are meant to convey the patient's general condition in terms of nutrition, body **habitus** (physique), and attention to self-care. This constitutional description should paint a picture for the next caregiver of the patient's general condition as judged by outward appearance at the time of the exam. Long-standing poor nutrition, whether due to chronic illness or inability to care for oneself could be reflected here. Poor grooming, state of dress, and even odors sometimes appear in this description and help to understand the patient's general condition. Of course normal body habitus and grooming are important to note here as well.

Physical findings may at times be appropriately placed in a different body system than what is listed, but less often than in the review of systems.

Asthenic - appearing weak

Cachectic - generalized bodily wasting

Disheveled - appearing not well put together

Toxic appearance - appearing severely ill; as opposed to an atoxic or nontoxic appearance, meaning that the patient does not appear sick

Well developed well nourished (WDWN) - appearing in good state of health and nutrition

Appearing older than stated age - a patient who looks to be older than their documented age

Practice Questions

1. The nose is _____, compared to the ear which is _____.

2. The nose is _____, compared to the mouth which is _____.

3. The chest is _____, compared to the back which is _____.

4. A 38-year-old male patient presents to his family doctor's office for evaluation of a new fever (with a high of 102 °F) that has been ongoing for a few days. He states that he has not been feeling well since developing the fever, and has been more tired than his normal. How should this be documented in the review of systems?

5. The family doctor examines this patient and notes that he is a well-developed and well-nourished male who appears his stated age. How should this be documented in the physical exam?

Integumentary System

1. Use medical terminology to document medical issues involving the integumentary system.
2. Describe the anatomy and physiology of the integumentary system.
3. Document integumentary system symptoms related during a review of systems.
4. Document signs related by the provider during a physical exam of the integumentary system.
5. Document operations and procedures for the integumentary system.
6. Document the integumentary system clinical impressions, diagnoses, and signs and symptoms commonly found in a problem list.

Abscess	Erythema	Pruritis
Avascular	Hair	Sebaceous gland
Avulsion	Hypodermis	Sebum
Biopsy	Impetigo	Stratified squamous epithelium
Candidiasis	Keratin	
Carbuncle	Lesion	Subcutaneous tissue
Connective tissue	Melanin	Tinea corporis
Contusion	Melanoma	Thrush
Cyanosis	Nail	Turgor
Dermis	Nail bed	Urticaria
Diaphoresis	Pallor	Vasoconstriction
Eczema	Paronychia	Vasodilation
Epidermis	Petechia	Vitiligo

Anatomy and Physiology

The skin is the largest organ of the body and is composed of many layers and types of cells. The skin serves many functions, including protection of internal bodily structures, temperature regulation, vitamin D absorption, and the sensation of touch.

The **epidermis** is the outermost layer of skin (Fig. 11.1). It mainly functions as a waterproof barrier against pathogens or extreme environmental conditions. The epidermis is composed of **stratified squamous epithelium**, a flat cell that makes the skin protective, and is often layered for extra protection. This explains why the thickness of skin varies in different areas of the body.

In regions where the skin experiences more abrasion or trauma, like the palms of the hands and soles of the feet, elbows, and mouth, there are more layers of epithelium for added protection. Skin is thinner over areas that have less exposure to such stress, such as over the back.

There are many types of epithelial cells, but there are two very important ones that reside in the epidermis. *Keratinocyte*s are cells that produce **keratin**, a protein that is responsible for the skin's protective function. Keratin also makes the skin waterproof. **Melanocytes** are highly specialized cells that produce melanin, a pigment that protects the skin from harmful ultraviolet (UV) radiation. The degree of melanin production varies between individuals, and impacts vitamin D absorption from the sun: less **melanin** is conducive to higher rates of vitamin D absorption.

Melanin is also responsible for producing variation in skin color: more melanin causes skin to appear darker (more protective against UV radiation, less conducive to vitamin D absorption), and less melanin makes skin lighter (less protective against UV radiation, but more conducive to vitamin D absorption). This explains the observed clinical variation in skin color. At the earth's equator the sun is the most intense, and thus it is more beneficial to have darker skin (more melanin). Further away from the equator where there is less sun exposure it is more beneficial to have lighter skin (less melanin).

The **dermis** is located below the epidermis and contains many structures, including nerves, vessels, and glands (Fig. 11.2). *Capillaries* and *lymph vessels* provide vascular supply to the skin and associated structures. Capillaries participate in temperature regulation. If the body's temperature is too high, capillaries will **vasodilate** (get larger), and heat will dissipate through the skin into the surrounding environment. If the body's temperature is too low, capillaries will **vasoconstrict** (get smaller), and heat will be preserved for the body's centrally located vital organs. It should be noted that some regions like cartilaginous structures (such as the nose and ears) are **avascular** and do not contain blood or lymph vessels. These structures take a longer time to progress through wound healing for this reason.

There are also several types of glands that can be found in the dermis. **Sebaceous glands** are one type of gland that produces **sebum** (a lubricant), which is secreted into *hair follicles* (containing

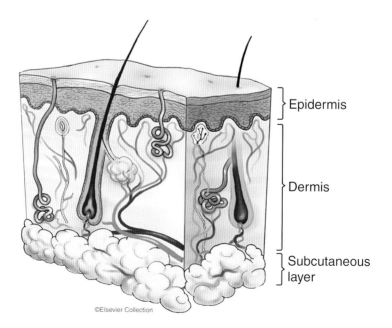

©Elsevier Collection

Fig. 11.1   Layers of the skin. (© Elsevier Collection)

hair, a sensory organ that can detect touch or movement) (Fig. 11.3). *Sweat glands* produce sweat, which plays a role in temperature regulation. When the body's temperature increases sweat is produced, and as it evaporates from the skin the body's temperature is cooled.

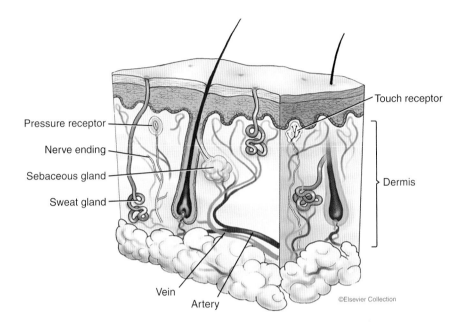

Fig. 11.2   The dermis. (© Elsevier Collection)

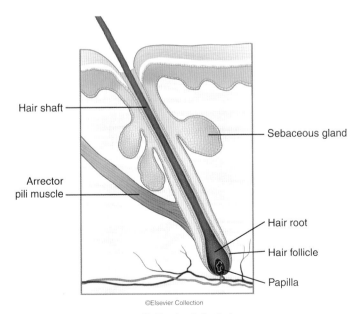

©Elsevier Collection

Fig. 11.3   Hair follicle and related structures. (© Elsevier Collection)

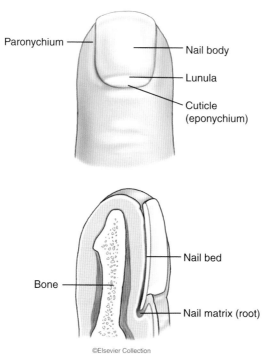

©Elsevier Collection

Fig. 11.4   Structures of the nails. (© Elsevier Collection)

Deep to the dermis is the **subcutaneous tissue** (**hypodermis**). This is primarily comprised of fat and connective tissue. Fat is a collection of *adipocytes*, or adipose cells, which store fat molecules. The fat in adipocytes is used for energy in times of famine and starvation, but accumulates when food intake is greater than energy output. Fat also contributes to temperature regulation, keeping the body warm through insulation and preservation of body temperature. **Connective tissue** is a type of tissue that separates groups of adipose cells and can also be found in the hypodermis.

Nails are considered to be an appendage of the skin and are visible above the epidermis. They participate in defining fine touch, and also protect the sensitive skin of the **nail bed**, which lies underneath the nail (Fig. 11.4).

Review of Systems

When documenting the review of systems for the integumentary system, be aware that the patient may use lay terms that are familiar to them such as "itchy rash" or "small blister." When there is a corresponding appropriate medical term that can be used, the scribe should 'translate' the patient's terminology into medical terms. For the examples above, the scribe may record "pruritic rash" and "vesicle."

Symptoms that can be placed in multiple systems have been designated as such in italics. Remember to always maximize the number of systems that are included in the review of systems so that the chart can be billed at higher levels (if desired). For example: if a patient is having a pruritic rash, it would be best to include pruritus in "*immune/allergy*" and rash in "*integumentary*" (two billable systems), as opposed to including pruritus and rash in "*integumentary*" (one billable system).

Blister - pocket of fluid in the upper layers of skin

Bruising (*hematologic/lymphatic*) - blue, purple, yellow, or green discoloration, usually from trauma

Medical Terminology Word Parts for the Integumentary System

Combining Forms	
derm/o dermat/o cut/o cutane/o	skin
trich/o pil/o	hair
onych/o ungu/o	nail
seb/o sebac/o	oil (sebum)
hidr/o sudor/i	sweat
adip/o lip/o	fat
squam/o	scaly
hemat/o	blood
melan/o	black
cyan/o	blue
erythr/o	red
purpur/o	purple
prur/o	itching
kerat/o	hard or horny

Combining Forms	
vesicul/o	blister
macul/o	spot
papul/o	pimple
corpor/o	body
crur/o	leg
ped/o	foot
cis/o	cut

Prefixes	
sub-	under, below
hypo-	under, below
dia-	through, across
epi-	above, upon

Suffixes	
-cyte	cell
-oma	mass
-itis	inflammation
-osis	abnormal condition
-phoresis	migration

Diaphoresis (*cardiovascular, endocrine*) – sweating
Drainage – fluid of any color or smell exuded by the skin
Dry skin (*endocrine*)
Erythema – redness
Insect bites or stings
Pruritus (*immunologic/allergic*) – sensation of itchiness
Rash (*immunologic/allergic*) – any abnormal change in the skin

Physical Exam

The physical exam is a listing of the provider's objective findings (signs), organized by system. The scribe will never be expected to interpret these findings, but rather must be diligent in recording the provider's exact findings.

Physical findings may at times be appropriately placed in a different body system than what is listed, but less often than in the review of systems.

Some unique aspects of documentation of the integumentary system are worth noting. The exam will likely record skin color, documenting whether there is pallor or flushing, or any findings of cyanosis or jaundice. The skin's **turgor** or elasticity is indicative of the patient's hydration status, assessed by pinching the skin and observing the speed at which it returns to its normal state; poor turgor is part of the clinical assessment for *dehydration*, or fluid loss. **Lesions** are alterations in body tissue caused by illness or injury and may require documentation of size and shape. Various lesions are listed below and illustrated in Fig. 11.5.

Burns are described in terms of their depth (first through fourth degree) and total body surface area covered (TBSA), which is expressed as a percentage. Scars, ecchymoses, and rashes will all be described. The following list illustrates some of the main findings that you may have to document.

Abrasion - superficial scrape of the epidermis

Abscess - collection of pus in body tissues

Avulsion - body structure or skin is forcibly detached

Blister - pocket of fluid in the upper layers of skin

Capillary refill - time it takes color (blood flow) to return to skin after pressure is applied (indicator of vascular health)

Contusion - bruise

Cyanosis - bluish discoloration due to hypoxia

Discharge - any fluid exuded from the skin described as purulent (pus-like), sanguinous (bloody), clear, or serosanguinous (blood + clear)

Ecchymosis - skin discoloration from bruising or bleeding internally

Erythema (rubor) - redness

Excoriation - abrasions due to mechanical irritation (like scratching)

Fissure – a cleft or groove (see Fig. 11.5)

Hematoma - collection of blood within the skin, usually due to trauma that ruptures blood vessels

Jaundice - yellow coloration of the skin/mucous membranes due to bilirubin excess from poor liver function

Laceration - a tear or cut wound in the skin

Lipoma - benign tumor of adipose tissue

Macule - skin change that appears as a change in surface color without a change in surface elevation (see Fig. 11.5)

Nodule - a small mass of tissue (see Fig. 11.5)

Pallor - pale skin

Paronychia - bacterial or fungal infection where the nail and skin meet, causing redness, swelling, and pain

Papule - skin change that appears as a raised area of skin often associated with a rash (see Fig. 11.5)

Petechiae - pinpoint erythematous rash often caused by superficial capillaries under the skin that rupture and bleed

Plaque - thick, red, and scaly patch of skin seen in psoriasis (commonly seen over the elbows and scalp)

Purpura - itchy purplish rash often caused by superficial blood vessels under the skin that rupture and bleed

Pustule - pus-filled elevation of skin (see Fig. 11.5)

Rash - many types often described by characteristics, such as macular (flat), papular (raised), maculopapular (flat + raised), urticarial (hive or welt-like), blanching and so on

Sebaceous cyst - a pocket containing fluid originating from sebaceous glands and containing sebum

Tenderness (dolor) - pain caused by touching an area

Ulcer - hollow area due to loss of the epidermis, dermis, and/or subcutaneous fat (commonly from poorly controlled diabetes)

Urticaria (hives) - welt-like rash notable for red, raised, pruritic bumps that is often due to an allergen

Vesicle - small blister (see Fig. 11.5)

Warmth (calor) - feeling hot to the touch

Wheal – a localized, raised, reddened, often pruritic lesion (see Fig. 11.5)

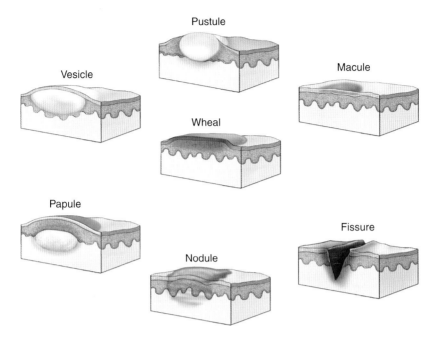

Fig. 11.5 Selected types of lesions. (© Elsevier Collection)

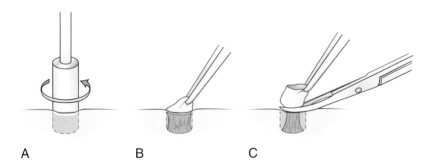

A   B   C

Fig. 11.6 Punch biopsy. (From Dehn R, Asprey D: *Essential clinical procedures*, ed 4, Philadelphia, 2021, Elsevier.)

Operations/Procedures

Any prior surgical history may be discussed during the patient interview. The scribe may record these procedures with the appropriate medical term if the patient uses a lay term. An integumentary example might be "lancing an abscess" which could be recorded as an I&D or "incision and drainage."

    Excisional biopsy - removal of a lesion or tumor with a scalpel for pathologic analysis

    Incision and drainage (I&D) - lancing an abscess to drain it; the fluid may be collected for analysis and the abscess cavity packed

    Phototherapy - exposure to wavelengths of light to treat skin disorders

    Punch biopsy - cylindrical core of tissue taken for analysis (Fig. 11.6)

Suturing (**stitches**) - pulling the sides of a laceration together with sutures to aid in the healing process

---

CASE STUDY 11.1

Eva is a medical scribe at Diamond Dermatology, a physician-owned practice. This morning she is assisting Dr. Bruccoleri, whose patient is a 26-year-old female presenting with an itchy rash on the abdomen, in the armpits, on the genitals, arms, and legs, and between the fingers. The patient states that it began about a week ago and has been getting worse, but is not painful. She claims the rash becomes unbearable at night. The patient is otherwise healthy and without SOB, fever, chills, nausea, vomiting, diarrhea, or urinary or other systemic symptoms. She lives with her sister, who does not have the same rash. She has tried taking Benadryl, and applying calamine lotion to the rash with little relief. During the physical examination, Dr. Bruccoleri notes normal lips and tongue and clear lungs. He describes a diffuse papular rash and takes skin scrapings for microscopic examination.

QUESTIONS
1. Who is the historian?
2. What term does Eva use to record the patient's itchiness?
3. The patient states that she noticed the rash about a week ago. Which descriptor (billable element) is this?
4. How might Eva record the timing of the chief complaint?
5. Should the scribe report that the patient's sister does not have the rash?

Problem List

Remember that the scribe will likely be asked to assist the provider with keeping the Problem List up to date and relevant.

A simple integumentary example might be the patient presenting with "pruritic rash." That symptom might be added into the problem list if a diagnosis is unknown. Once there is a specific diagnosis such as "contact dermatitis," the symptom or "clinical impression" would be removed from the list in favor of the final diagnosis, "contact dermatitis." A more complex example might be a patient who presents with both fever and an unexplained rash. These could both be entered into the problem list but would both need to be removed and replaced if a final diagnosis of "cellulitis" is made explaining both the fever and the rash.

Patients often do not know the name of a specific diagnosis, but will instead describe it to their provider. It is the scribe's duty to translate the lay terms into medical terminology. For example, if the patient says they have a history of athlete's foot, the scribe should document "tinea pedis."

Acne - blockage of sebaceous glands resulting in a variety of lesions (some can also be painful or pus-filled)

Basal cell carcinoma - skin cancer of the cells in the basal layer

Carbuncle - a large pustular lesion

Cellulitis - an infection of the skin that causes warmth, erythema, and tenderness; can progress and become an abscess

Contact dermatitis - erythematous and sometimes pruritic rash caused by a skin sensitivity (allergy)

Eczema (**dermatitis**) - skin inflammation with a variety of causes

Folliculitis - inflammation of hair follicles

Herpes simplex - oral or genital vesicular lesions (small fluid filled skin lesions) caused by the herpes simplex virus (Fig. 11.7)

Impetigo - contagious bacterial skin infection common in small children that usually localizes on the face, particularly around the mouth (Fig. 11.8)

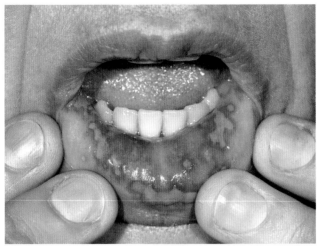

Fig. 11.7 Herpes simplex of the oral cavity. (From Dinulos JGH: *Habif's clinical dermatology*, ed 7, Philadelphia, 2021, Elsevier.)

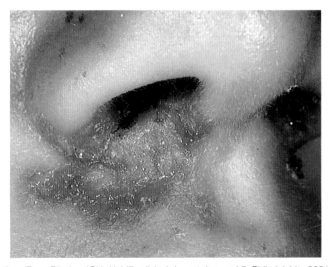

Fig. 11.8 Impetigo. (From Dinulos JGH: *Habif's clinical dermatology*, ed 7, Philadelphia, 2021, Elsevier.)

Melanoma - skin cancer of melanocytes (pigment containing cells)

Onychomycosis - fungal infection of the nail that causes the nail to appear yellow and thickened (Fig. 11.9)

Psoriasis - autoimmune disease characterized by patches of psoriatic plaques (scaly skin lesions), characteristically over the elbows, scalp, and behind the ears

Rosacea - a condition that causes facial redness and swelling

Squamous cell carcinoma - cancer of the epidermal squamous cells

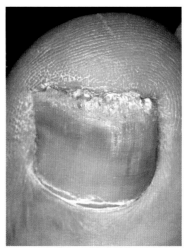

Fig. 11.9   Onychomycosis. (From Dinulos JGH: *Habif's clinical dermatology*, ed 7, Philadelphia, 2021, Elsevier.)

Thrush (candidiasis) - fungal infection of the mouth due to yeast
Tinea corporis (ringworm) - superficial fungal infection
Tinea pedis (athlete's foot) - fungal infection of the foot
Vitiligo - autoimmune destruction of melanocytes (pigment producing cells of the skin), causing the skin to lose its color

Practice Questions

1. _____ produce melanin and are protective against UV radiation.

2. _____ produce sebum into hair follicles.

3. _____ are the cell type in the hypodermis that store fat.

4. List the layers of the skin, superficial to deep.

5. A 19-year-old female patient presents to her dermatologist for evaluation of an itchy and red welt-like rash that develops randomly. She denies any residual bruising after the lesions resolve, nor recent illnesses. How should this be documented in the review of systems?

6. The dermatologist examines this patient and notes faint urticarial lesions over both arms and the upper chest. There is also some residual stippling and bruising near older lesions. She is well developed and well nourished. How should this be documented in the physical exam?

7. The patient's dermatologist would like to rule-out an urticarial vasculitis. He uses a scalpel to remove a lesion to send to pathology for analysis. What procedure should the scribe document?

8. Because the results of the biopsy are pending and a diagnosis has not yet been confirmed, what should be documented in the problem list?
   a. Urticaria
   b. Allergic dermatitis
   c. Urticarial vasculitis
   d. Contact dermatitis

Musculoskeletal System

1. Use medical terminology to document medical issues involving the musculoskeletal system.
2. Describe the anatomy and physiology of the musculoskeletal system.
3. Document musculoskeletal system symptoms related during a review of systems.
4. Document signs related by the provider during a physical exam of the musculoskeletal system.
5. Document operations and procedures for the musculoskeletal system.
6. Document the musculoskeletal system clinical impressions, diagnoses, and signs and symptoms commonly found in a problem list.
7. Document relevant drug classes and medications for the treatment of problems associated with the musculoskeletal system.

KEY TERMS

Abduction
Acromion process
Adduction
Analgesic
Ankylosing spondylitis (AS)
Antipyretic
Appendicular skeleton
Articulation
Atlas
Atrophy
Axial skeleton
Axis
Calcaneus
Carpal
Cauda equina syndrome
Cervical spine (c-spine)
Clavicle
Coccyx
Compartment syndrome
Cranial vault

Crepitus
Denervation
Depression
Dislocation
Dorsiflexion
Elevation
Eversion
Extension
Femur
Fibromyalgia
Fibula
Flexion
Fracture
Gout
Humerus
Hypertonic
Ilium
Innominate bone
Insertion
Inversion
Ischium pubis

Joint laxity (hypermobility)
Kyphosis
Lateral (external) rotation
Ligament
Lordosis
Lumbar spine
Malleolus
Mandible
Maxilla
Medial (internal) rotation
Meniscus
Metacarpal
Metatarsal
Origin
Osteoarthritis
Osteopenia
Osteoporosis
Patella
Pelvic girdle
Phalanx
Plantarflexion

Continued

Pressure ulcer (decubitus ulcer)	Scaphoid (navicular)	Tarsal
Pronation	Scapula	Temporomandibular joint (TMJ)
Protraction	Scoliosis	Tendon
Pubic symphysis	Sesamoid	Tibia
Radius	Spinal stenosis	Thoracic spine
Range of motion	Sprain	Ulna
Reflex	Sternum	Vertebral column
Retraction	Supination	Vertebral disc
Rheumatoid arthritis	Suture	Vertebral foramen
Ribs	Synovial fluid	
Sacrum	Systemic lupus erythematosus (SLE)	

Anatomy and Physiology

Joints are a point of connection between two bones that allows our bodies to move fluidly. Joints have varying limits of **range of motion**, which is the plane or degree of normal movement without joint injury. ***Ball and socket joints***, such as the shoulder or hip joints, are able to move in a 360° plane. ***Hinge joints***, such as the elbow or knee joints, are only able to move in a 180° plane. ***Pivot joints***, such as those between vertebrae, only allow rotation around a single axis. Movement outside of a joint's normal range of motion can result in joint injury or dislocation.

There are several types of joints, including synovial, fibrous, and cartilaginous. *Synovial joints* are the most common joint type, and contain **synovial fluid** within a *joint capsule*, which nourishes the joint and provides lubrication. Synovial joints have a large range of motion. Shoulder and knee joints are two examples.

Fibrous joints are sturdy and hold two bones together with minimal movement. The joints between the flat bones of the skull (**sutures**) are fibrous joints.

Cartilaginous joints are flexible, but are not as mobile as synovial joints. An example would be the pubic symphysis, which joins the two pubic bones. This is important in childbirth, where the pelvis needs to widen to allow the passage of a baby through the birth canal.

Although the types of joints differ in anatomy and function, ultimately all joints share a similar function of joining two bones together in an **articulation**.

Terms of movement describe the movement of a body part, typically across one or more joints (*range of motion*). These terms are often paired by oppositional actions. For example: flexion and extension both change the angle of a joint, but in opposite directions. Pairs of terms are listed together in Table 12.1.

The skeleton is divided into two categories: the axial skeleton and the appendicular skeleton. The **axial skeleton** comprises the centralized components, including the skull, vertebral column, sternum and ribs. The **appendicular skeleton** comprises the appendages of the skeleton, which includes everything that is not classified as axial. In Fig. 12.1, the portion of the skeleton in yellow is the axial skeleton, while the blue denotes the appendicular skeleton. Use these images as a reference for the anatomy in this chapter.

TABLE 12.1 ■ Terms of Movement

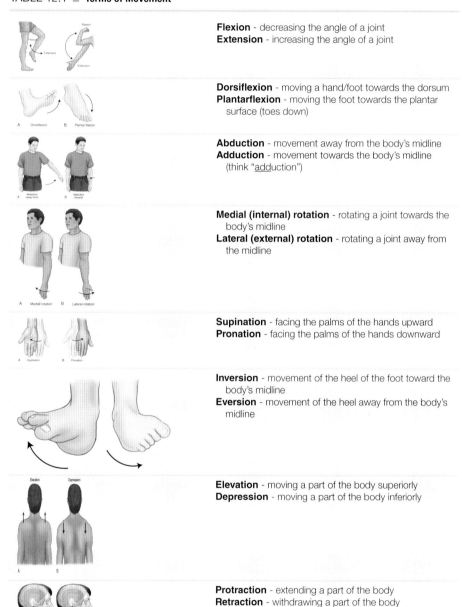

Flexion - decreasing the angle of a joint
Extension - increasing the angle of a joint

Dorsiflexion - moving a hand/foot towards the dorsum
Plantarflexion - moving the foot towards the plantar surface (toes down)

Abduction - movement away from the body's midline
Adduction - movement towards the body's midline (think "adduction")

Medial (internal) rotation - rotating a joint towards the body's midline
Lateral (external) rotation - rotating a joint away from the midline

Supination - facing the palms of the hands upward
Pronation - facing the palms of the hands downward

Inversion - movement of the heel of the foot toward the body's midline
Eversion - movement of the heel away from the body's midline

Elevation - moving a part of the body superiorly
Depression - moving a part of the body inferiorly

Protraction - extending a part of the body
Retraction - withdrawing a part of the body

Images from Kendrick LE, Lampignano JP: Bontrager's *textbook of radiographic positioning and related anatomy*, ed 10, St. Louis, 2021, Elsevier.

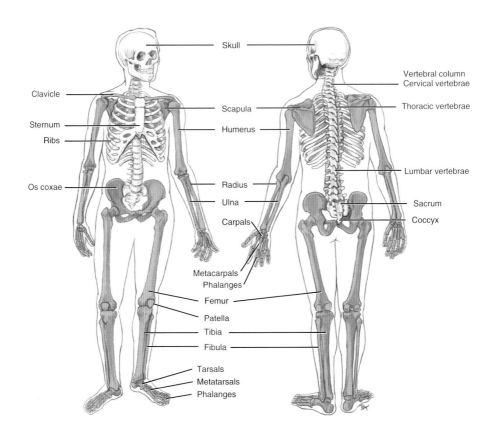

Fig. 12.1   Divisions of the skeleton with major bones identified. Yellow, axial skeleton. Blue, appendicular skeleton. (From Applegate E: *The anatomy and physiology learning system*, ed 4, St Louis, 2011, Saunders.)

AXIAL SKELETON

The **cranial vault** is the dome-like structure of the skull which is composed of four bones (Fig. 12.2). The *frontal bone* is most anterior and encompasses what is colloquially known as the "forehead." The paired *parietal bone*s are two symmetric bones that comprise the superior and lateral portion of the cranium. The *temporal bones* sit in the area known as the "temples" just posteriorly to the orbits. The *occipital bone* (or *occiput*) is the posterior portion of the skull, just superior to the nape of the neck. All of these bones are connected by cranial sutures (a fibrous joint). The function of the cranial vault is to protect the brain.

There are many facial bones but there are very few that a scribe should know. The *nasal bone* is located behind the bridge of the nose, between both eyes. The *zygomatic bones* are known colloquially as the "cheek" bones. The jaw is comprised of two bones: the **maxilla** is the upper part, and the **mandible** is the lower portion. The **temporomandibular joint (TMJ)** is a synovial joint between the temporal bone and the mandible.

An anterior view of the skull is depicted in Fig. 12.2, *B*, and a lateral view of the skull is depicted in Figure 12.2, *C*.

The **vertebral column** (Fig. 12.3) protects the spinal cord and helps provide support to stand upright and walk bipedally (with two legs). The primary function of the vertebrae is to protect the

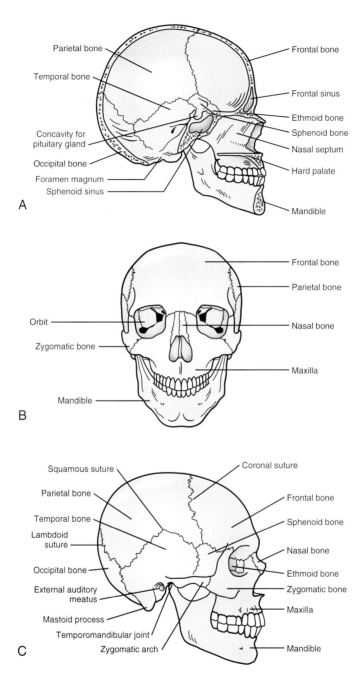

Fig. 12.2 Bones of the head and face. (A) Interior view. (B) Anterior view. (C) Lateral view. (From Magee DJ, Manske RC: *Orthopedic physical assessment*, ed 7, St. Louis, 2021, Elsevier. Redrawn from Jenkins DB: *Hollinshead's functional anatomy of the limbs and back*, Philadelphia, 1991, WB Saunders, pp 332–333.)

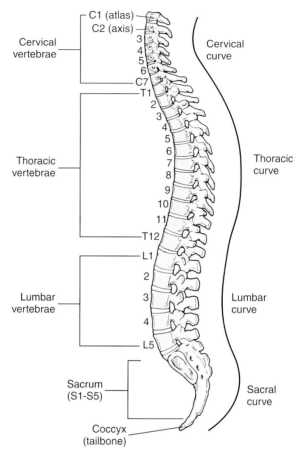

Fig. 12.3 Vertebral column. (From Koersterman JL: Buck's coding exam review 2021: the physician and facility certification step, St. Louis, 2021, Elsevier.)

spinal cord, which passes through the **vertebral foramen**, a large hole within the center of each vertebra. Vertebrae are connected pivot joints, which only allow rotational movement around a single axis.

The vertebral column is divided into four parts. The **cervical spine** *(c-spine)*, comprises the neck and consists of seven vertebrae (C1-C7: "C" for cervical, and numbered from superior to inferior). The cervical vertebrae articulate with the base of the skull superiorly and the thoracic vertebrae inferiorly. Sometimes, the first and second cervical vertebrae (C1 and C2) are referred to as the **atlas** and the **axis**, respectively.

The **thoracic spine** *(t-spine)* comprises the upper back and consists of twelve vertebrae (T1-T12: "T" for thoracic, and numbered from superior to inferior). The thoracic vertebrae articulate with the 7th cervical vertebra (C7) superiorly and the lumbar vertebrae inferiorly.

The **lumbar spine** *(l-spine)* comprises the lower back and consists of five vertebrae (L1-L5, same nomenclature as above). The lumbar vertebrae articulate with T12 superiorly and the sacral spine inferiorly.

The *sacrococcygeal spine* consists of a few vertebrae that have fused together, and is divided into two parts: the **sacrum** *(s-spine)* and the **coccyx**. The sacrum is the superior portion and articulates with the fifth lumbar vertebra superiorly, and the coccyx inferiorly. The sacrum is also part of the **pelvic girdle**. The coccygeal portion is known in lay terms as the "tailbone."

Between vertebrae are **vertebral discs**, which are cartilaginous discs that reduce the transmission of force between vertebrae and protect the bony structures of the vertebral column.

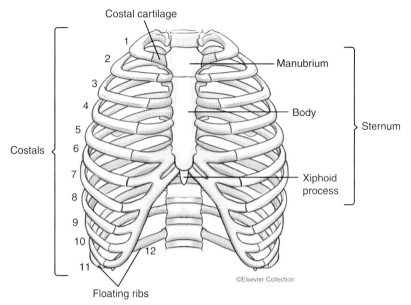

Costal cartilage

1

2

3

4

5

Costals

6

7

8

9

10

11

12

Floating ribs

Manubrium

Body

Sternum

Xiphoid process

©Elsevier Collection

Fig. 12.4 The thoracic cage. (© Elsevier Collection)

The thoracic cage is composed of the **sternum**, which is the flat bone in the center of the anterior chest, and twelve pairs of long and curved **ribs**, which articulate with the thoracic spine and curve around the body anteriorly to form the *thoracic cage* (Fig. 12.4). Some of these ribs articulate with the sternum. The pairs of ribs most inferiorly are known as *floating ribs*, as they do not articulate with anything anteriorly.

> **NOTE**
>
> When *cardiopulmonary resuscitation (CPR)* is performed, the sternum is pushed inward causing compression of the intrathoracic space and the heart, thus pumping blood. Ribs articulating with the sternum are sometimes fractured during CPR, and make cracking or crunching noises. This may be documented as **crepitus** on exam.

APPENDICULAR SKELETON (UPPER EXTREMITY)

Scapulae (**scapula**, singular) are a pair of flat bones located over the posterior upper thorax. These are colloquially called "shoulder blades".

The scapula forms two articulations. The **acromion process** of the scapula (a bony process is a knob or a protuberance of bone) articulates with the distal clavicle, forming the *acromioclavicular (AC) joint* (a synovial joint). The *glenoid fossa* (a shallow cup in the scapula) articulates with the head of the humerus, forming the *glenohumeral joint* (also a synovial joint). The *shoulder girdle* is this point of connection between the arm and the thorax across these two joints (Fig. 12.5).

> **NOTE**
>
> A *shoulder dislocation* occurs when the humeral head is forced out of the glenoid fossa. This is a fairly common dislocation because the glenoid fossa is shallow, thus an innate cause of joint instability. After a shoulder dislocation there will often be residual **joint laxity**, also called **hypermobility**—the ability to extend the joint to a greater degree than normal—on exam.

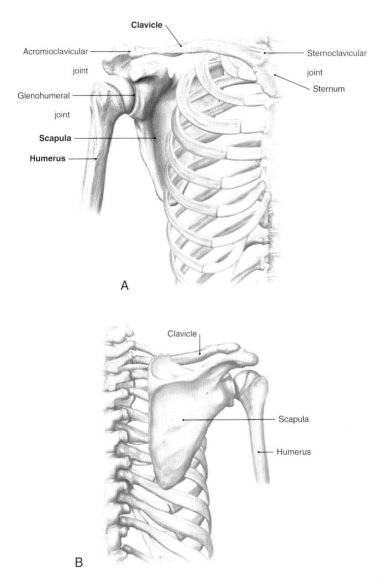

Fig. 12.5   The shoulder girdle. (a) Anterior. (b) Posterior. (From Hombach-Klonisch S, Klonisch T, Peeler J: *Sobotta: clinical atlas of human anatomy*, München, 2019, Elsevier/Urban & Fischer.)

Clavicles are a pair of thin narrow bones that cross over the anterior upper chest. These are also known as "collar bones" because they sit where a shirt collar would naturally lie. The clavicles articulate with the sternum proximally forming the ***sternoclavicular (SC) joint***, and the scapulae distally forming the ***acromioclavicular (AC) joint***. Both are synovial joints.

The **humerus** is the long bone of the arm. It is the attachment site of many muscles. The humerus articulates with the scapulae proximally, and the ulna and radius distally forming the elbow joint (synovial).

The elbow joint is a synovial hinge joint between the humerus (proximal) and ulna and radius (distal).

The **ulna** (medial) and **radius** (lateral) are the two bones of the forearm. Both articulate with the humerus proximally (elbow joint), and the small bones of the wrist (**carpals**) distally forming the wrist joint (synovial).

The wrist joint is a synovial joint consisting of many small bones (Fig. 12.6). The most notable of these bones is the **scaphoid (navicular)**. Located on the radial aspect of the wrist (thumb-side), this small bone is frequently fractured when someone falls with their arms outstretched.

The **metacarpals** are the bones of the hand (not including the fingers). In each hand there are five metacarpals, and they are numbered laterally to medially (thumb to pinky) as "1" to "5". The metacarpals articulate with the carpals proximally, forming *carpometacarpal (CMC) joints* (synovial joints).

The **phalanges** (**phalanx**, singular) are the most distal bones of the upper extremity and they comprise the fingers. The fingers are not numbered, but rather should be referred to as the following (medial to lateral): pinky, ring, middle, and index fingers and the thumb.

As aforementioned there are three sets of phalanges, designated as proximal, intermediate, and distal phalanges. The *proximal phalanges* articulate with the metacarpals proximally, forming *metacarpophalangeal (MCP) joints*, and intermediate phalanges distally, forming *proximal*

BONES AND JOINTS OF THE WRIST AND HAND

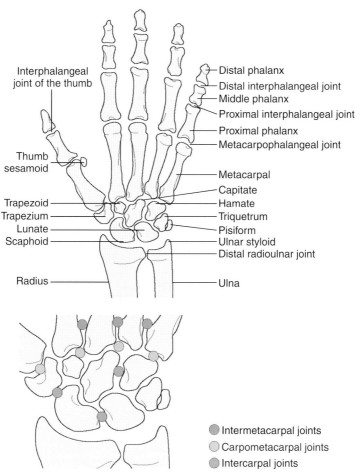

Fig. 12.6 Bones of the wrist and hand. (From Douglas MM, Thibodeau GA, Patton KT: *Essentials of anatomy and physiology*, St. Louis, 2012, Elsevier.)

interphalangeal (PIP) joints. The *intermediate phalanges* articulate with the distal phalanges distally, forming *distal interphalangeal (DIP) joints*. All finger joints are synovial joints.

A special mention of the thumb should be made, which only has two phalanges (proximal and distal). The articulation between the proximal and distal phalanx is the *interphalangeal (IP) joint*.

APPENDICULAR SKELETON (LOWER EXTREMITY)

Innominates (pelvic bones) are two bowl-shaped bones that together form the pelvis (Fig. 12.7). These consist of the fusion of three bones - the ilium, ischium, and the pubis. The **ilium** comprises the "wings" of the pelvis, and articulates with the sacrum forming the *sacroiliac joint* (a synovial and fibrous joint). This articulation forms the **pelvic girdle**. The **ischium** is the most inferior of the three pelvic bones, and is the bone that is sat upon. The **pubis** is a small portion of the pelvis that forms an articulation with the contralateral pubic bone, forming the **pubic symphysis** (a cartilaginous joint) of the anterior pelvis.

The ilium, ischium, and pubis join together to form the *hip joint*, which articulates with the head of the femur. This is a synovial ball and socket joint, but unlike the shoulder the hip joint is deeper and more stable, therefore harder to dislocate.

The **femur** is the long bone of the lower extremity. It is the attachment site of many muscles. It articulates proximally with the pelvis (hip joint), and distally with the tibia and fibula to form the knee joint.

The *knee joint* (synovial, hinge) is the articulation between the femur and tibia and fibula (Fig. 12.8). **Menisci** (**meniscus**, singular) are cartilages between these bones that absorb impact and reduce force exerted on the tibia. **Ligaments** are connective tissue that connect two bones together, typically across a joint. Their primary function is to provide stability to the joint. Many ligaments contribute to the stability of the knee joint. These include the *lateral* and *medial collateral ligaments* (located laterally and medially, respectively), and *anterior* and *posterior cruciate ligaments* (located anteriorly and posteriorly, respectively).

The **patellae** (**patella**, singular) is a **sesamoid** bone, a bone that grows in a tendon that runs over a bony prominence). The patella lies atop the knee joint and is the attachment point of the *quadriceps tendon* superiorly. The *patellar tendon* originates from the patella inferiorly and inserts onto the tibia. The patella is also known as the "kneecap".

The **tibia** (medial) and **fibula** (lateral) are the two bones of the shin. Both articulate with the femur proximally (knee joint) and calcaneus distally to form the ankle joint. The tibia is the weight bearing bone of the body.

The *ankle joint* is a synovial hinge joint consisting of articulations between the tibia and fibula superiorly, and the calcaneus and talus inferiorly (Fig. 12.9). Be aware that there are many ligaments

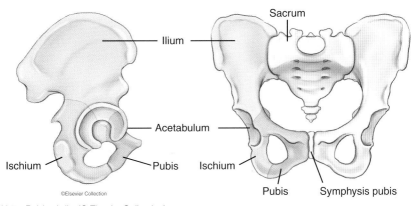

Fig. 12.7 Pelvic girdle. (© Elsevier Collection)

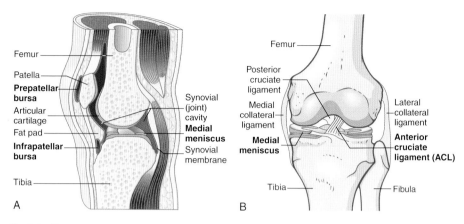

Fig. 12.8 The knee joint. (A) lateral view. (B) frontal section. (From Chabner D. *The language of medicine*, ed 12, St. Louis, 2021, Elsevier.)

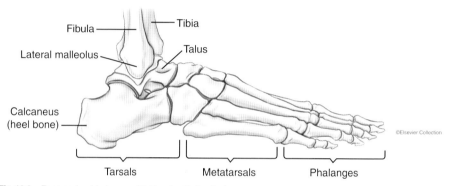

Fig. 12.9 Foot and ankle bones. (© Elsevier Collection)

of the ankle joint and sprains are very common. The ankle has three **malleoli** (**malleolus**, singular), which are bony prominences. These include the lateral, medial and posterior malleoli.

There are many small bones that comprise the foot and ankle (**tarsals**), but be familiar with the calcaneus and talus. The **calcaneus** is the heel of the foot. The **talus** is the major weight bearing bone of the ankle and the primary articulation of the ankle joint.

The **metatarsals** are the bones of the foot (not including the toes). In each foot there are five metatarsals, and they are numbered medially to laterally (big toe to little toe) as "1" to "5". The metatarsals articulate with the tarsals proximally, forming *tarsometatarsal (TMT) joints* (synovial joints).

The anatomy of the toes (*phalanges*) is very similar to that of the fingers. The only difference is that the toes are numbered from medially to laterally (1 to 5), as opposed to being named like the fingers. Please refer to the discussion of phalanges above for additional details.

MUSCLES

Muscles are the contractile force behind movement. Muscles attach to bones via **tendons** (or may just directly attach to the bone) (Fig. 12.10). The **origin** is the attachment site where the muscle begins. The attachment at the origin is immobile. The **insertion** is the attachment site where the muscle ends. The attachment at the insertion is mobile. All muscles have at least one (many have more) origin and insertion.

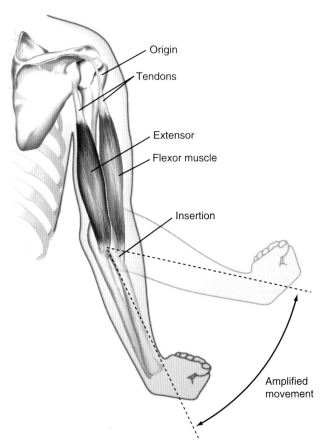

Fig. 12.10   The origin and insertion of a skeletal muscle. (From Koeppen BM, Stanton BA: *Berne & Levy physiology*, ed 6, Philadelphia, 2010, Mosby.)

Many of the bony enlargements and prominences on bones are the sites of tendinous or muscular attachment (origins or insertions). When muscles are frequently used and enlarge, bone compensates by growing at these attachment sites.

All muscles are innervated by a nerve. Nerves essentially act as a two way highway of information flow: from the brain to muscle, and vice versa. Without a nerve supply (**denervation**), the muscle would not be usable and would **atrophy** (shrink). Nerves will be discussed further in the chapter over the nervous system.

Every muscle has an *action*, which is the movement that the muscle elicits. Many muscles have primary, secondary, and sometimes even tertiary actions. ***Primary actions*** are the main movement that the muscle creates. As intuited, ***secondary*** and ***tertiary actions*** are other movements of the muscle that are less important than the primary action.

During contraction, a muscle becomes shorter and moves one or more of the bones that it is attached to. During relaxation, the muscle elongates and no bony movement occurs. Muscles often work in pairs to create opposing movements across a joint. These are termed ***agonist-antagonist muscles***. For this to happen, when one muscle is contracting the other has to be relaxed. For example, the biceps muscle flexes the elbow, whereas the triceps muscle extends it. Both muscles are often activated simultaneously. This allows controlled movements to occur. It should also be noted that not all muscles are paired in such a way.

There are three primary types of muscles. ***Skeletal muscle*** is the muscle type we have been discussing here, as it moves bone to create body movement. Skeletal muscle is under voluntary control.

This means that aside from some exceptions (such as reflexes), a conscious decision is made to move a skeletal muscle before it is moved. Fig. 12.11 shows anterior and posterior views of the skeletal muscles.

For completeness, mention will be made of the other two muscle types.

Cardiac muscle is a type of muscle that is found only in the heart. It has special properties which allow the heart to function properly. Cardiac muscle is involuntary, meaning that the muscle cycles through contraction and relaxation without the conscious decision to do so.

Smooth muscle is found in the walls of many body organs and the vasculature. Smooth muscle is also involuntary, and is responsible for body functions such as peristalsis (movement of food through the GI tract), and dilation and constriction of arteries.

It is not important for a scribe to know all of the origin and insertion sites of muscles. However, knowing the general location and the primary action is recommended. Table 12.2 lists the major muscles of the thorax, abdomen, and extremities, and each muscle's primary action.

Medical Terminology Word Parts for the Musculoskeletal System

synovi/o	synovial	cox/o	hip
articul/o arthr/o	joint	pub/o	pubis
		femor/o	femur/thigh bone
oste/o osse/o oss/i	bone	menisc/o	meniscus
		ligament/o syndesm/o	ligament
crani/o	skull, cranium	chondr/o	cartilage
mandibul/o	mandible/lower jaw bone	patell/o	patella/knee cap
maxill/o	maxilla/upper jaw bone	tendin/o ten/o tend/o	tendon
vertebr/o spondyl/o	vertebra	tibi/o	tibia
cervic/o	neck	fibul/o	fibula/smaller lower leg bone
thorac/o	chest, thoracic	tars/o	tarsus/foot bone
lumb/o	lumbar	calcane/o	calcaneus/heel
sacr/o	sacral	tal/o	talus
coccyg/o	tailbone/coccyx	muscul/o my/o myos/o	muscle
disc/o	disc	rhabdomy/o	skeletal muscle
pelv/o	pelvis	leiomy/o	smooth muscle
stern/o	sternum	myocardi/o	heart muscle
cost/o	rib	ankyl/o	stiff joint
scapul/o	scapula	burs/o	bursa/fluid filled joint sac
acromi/o	acromion process	condyl/o	condyle
clavicul/o	collar bone/clavicle	lamin/o	lamina
humer/o	humerus/upper arm bone	**Prefixes**	
uln/o	ulna	ab-	away from
radi/o	radius	ad-	toward
carp/o	wrist	circum-	around
phalang/o	phalanges, fingers or toes		
ili/o	ilium/a pelvic bone		
ischi/o	ischium/another pelvic bone		

Continued

Medical Terminology Word Parts for the Musculoskeletal System—Cont'd

ex-	out		-algia	pain
in-	in		-osis	abnormal condition
inter-	between		-itis	inflammation
intra-	within		-pathy	disease
peri-	around, surrounding		-trophy	growth
epi-	above, upon		-oma	tumor, mass
hyper-	excessive		-tomy	cutting
post-	after		-plasty	surgical formation
Suffixes			-ectomy	removal
-oid	resembling, like			
-ar	pertaining to			

Review of Systems

Remember that the patient will give their symptoms in their own language and the scribe will have to record in medical language whenever possible. If the patient complains of achy joints, for example, the scribe will record arthralgias. Other common colloquialisms are listed below. Note that some of the complaints that are part of the musculoskeletal system can be recorded in other body systems and these are listed in italics.

Remember to always maximize the number of systems that are included in the review of systems so that the chart can be billed at higher levels (if desired). For example: if a patient is having back pain with radicular symptoms, it would be best to include back pain in "*musculoskeletal*" and radicular symptoms in "*neurologic*" (two billable systems), as opposed to including back pain and radicular symptoms in "*musculoskeletal*" (one billable system).

Arthralgia - joint pain

Joint swelling - any swelling involving one or more joints

Joint stiffness - the sensation that a joint has become more difficult to move, often after periods of inactivity or certain times of the day

Low back pain (**lumbago** - less commonly used)

Myalgia - muscle pain

Neck pain (**cervicalgia** - less commonly used)

Pleuritic chest pain (*respiratory*) - chest pain with inspiration

Posttussive chest pain (*respiratory*) - chest pain after coughing

Radicular symptoms (*neurologic*) - radiating pain down an extremity due to injury or irritation of a nerve

Physical Exam

The physical exam is a listing of the provider's objective findings (signs), organized by system. The provider will convey to the scribe any abnormal physical findings on the musculoskeletal exam. Some common exam findings are listed below along with some of the more common maneuvers used in the exam to elicit disease specific findings.

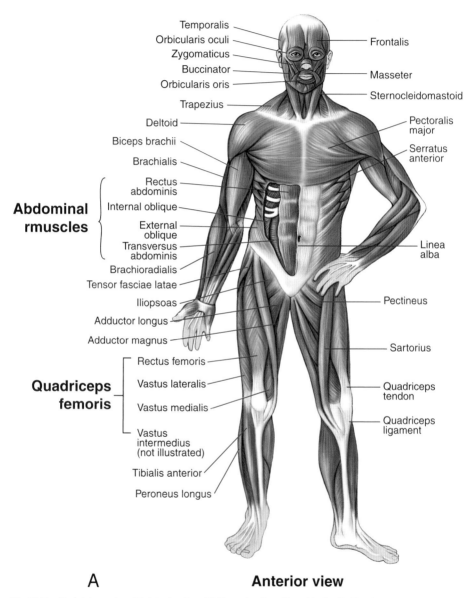

Temporalis
Orbicularis oculi
Zygomaticus
Buccinator
Orbicularis oris
Trapezius
Deltoid
Biceps brachii
Brachialis
Rectus abdominis
Internal oblique
External oblique
Transversus abdominis
Brachioradialis
Tensor fasciae latae
Iliopsoas
Adductor longus
Adductor magnus
Rectus femoris
Vastus lateralis
Vastus medialis
Vastus intermedius (not illustrated)
Tibialis anterior
Peroneus longus

Frontalis
Masseter
Sternocleidomastoid
Pectoralis major
Serratus anterior
Linea alba
Pectineus
Sartorius
Quadriceps tendon
Quadriceps ligament

Abdominal rmuscles

Quadriceps femoris

A

Anterior view

Fig. 12.11   Skeletal muscles. (A) Anterior view. (B) Posterior view. (From Herlihy B: *The human body in health and illness*, ed 6, St Louis, 2018, Elsevier.)

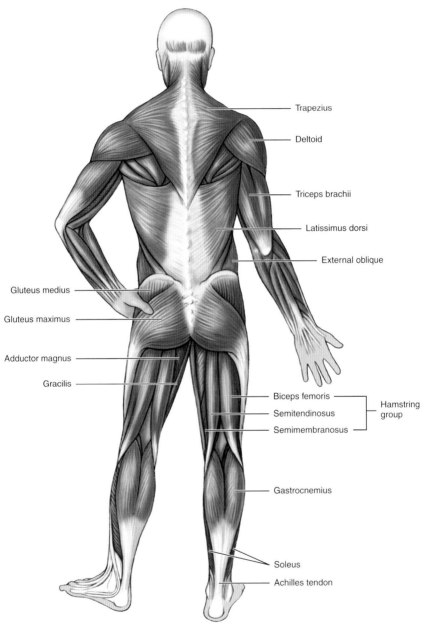

Trapezius

Deltoid

Triceps brachii

Latissimus dorsi

External oblique

Gluteus medius

Gluteus maximus

Adductor magnus

Gracilis

Biceps femoris

Semitendinosus

Semimembranosus

Hamstring group

Gastrocnemius

Soleus

Achilles tendon

B

Posterior View

TABLE 12.2 ■ Muscles of the Thorax, Abdomen, and Extremities, and Primary Actions

Muscle(s)	Location	Primary Action
Anterior Thorax (Chest and Abdomen)		
Pectoralis major m.	Located in the anterior thorax over the breast region	Arm adduction and medial rotation
Rectus abdominis m.	Most superficial abdominal muscle	Low back flexion
Posterior Thorax (Back)		
Trapezius m.	Triangular muscle located in the upper back, extending from the occiput to the thoracic vertebrae and both scapulae	Movement of the scapula
Deltoid m.	Pair of muscles that sit atop either shoulder	Abduction of the arms
Latissimus dorsi m.	Fan-like muscle in the mid-back	Adduction of the arms
Rhomboid m.	Rhomboid shaped muscle located in the upper back between the thoracic spine and the scapulae	Retraction of the scapulae
Upper Extremity		
Biceps brachii m.	Located in the volar region of the upper arm	Forearm supination and elbow flexion
Triceps brachii m.	Located in the dorsal region of the upper arm	Elbow extension
Brachioradialis m.	Crosses the elbow joint from the lateral humerus to the lateral wrist (radial)	Forearm supination
Forearm flexors (anterior compartment)	Group of muscles in the volar forearm	Wrist flexion
Forearm extensors (posterior compartment)	Group of muscles in the dorsal forearm	Wrist extension
Lower Extremity		
Gluteus maximus m.	Largest muscle in the gluteal region	Hip external rotation and extension
Tensor fascia latae m. (TFL)	Muscle of the hip that continues to the lateral knee as the *iliotibial tract* (tendon)	Hip external rotation and extension
Adductor group	Group of muscles in the inner thigh	Hip adduction
Abductor group	Deep group of muscles in the gluteal region	Hip abduction
Quadriceps group	Group of muscles in the anterior thigh	Knee extension
Hamstring group	Group of three muscles in the posterior thigh	Knee flexion
Gastrocnemius	Two muscles in the calf that terminate as the calcaneal tendon (*Achilles tendon*) on the calcaneus	Plantar flexion
Posterior compartment	Group of muscles in the calf	Plantar flexion
Anterior compartment	Group of muscles in the anterior shin	Dorsiflexion
Lateral compartment	Group of muscles in the lateral shin	Ankle eversion

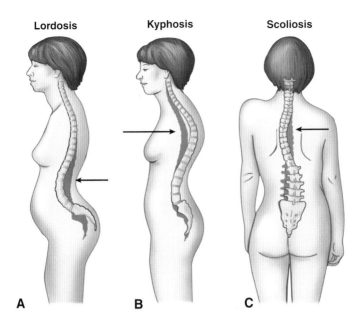

Fig. 12.12   Kyphosis (A) lordosis (B) and scoliosis (C) in relation to normal spinal curvature. (From Thibodeau GA, Patton KT: *The human body in health & disease*, ed 7,m St. Louis, Mosby.)

Physical findings may at times be appropriately placed in a different body system than what is listed, but less often than in the review of systems.

Compartment syndrome – when there is increased pressure within a muscle region (compartment) causing decreased blood flow and death of muscle tissue *(see detail below)*

Dislocation - a joint that has been removed from normal articulation *(see detail below)*

Drawer sign - anterior or posterior cruciate ligament testing *(see detail below)*

Effusion - excessive and abnormal fluid within a joint

Hammertoe deformity - the toes become permanently bent at the PIP joints (usually due to wearing poorly fitting footwear or heels)

Kyphosis - excessive convex curvature of the thoracic spine (Fig. 12.12, A)

Lordosis - excessive concave curvature of the lumbar/cervical spine (Fig. 12.12, B)

McMurray's test - knee meniscal (cartilage) testing

Muscle spasm - involuntary muscle contraction

Pressure (decubitus) ulcer – an erosion of the skin, sometimes called a bedsore, that results from prolonged pressure to an area *(see detail below)*

Scoliosis - abnormal lateral curvature of the spine (Fig. 12.12, C)

Snuffbox (anatomic) - a depressed area on the wrist overlying the scaphoid bone (one of the wrist bones/carpels) *(see detail below)*

Step-off deformity - apparent misalignment between two bones suggesting fracture or displacement.

Synovitis - joint swelling

Tendon reflex (sometimes called *deep tendon reflex* or *DTR*) – the rapid contraction of a stretched muscle in response to sudden stimulus, classically when the provider strikes a tendon with his/her reflex hammer (knee jerk for example) *(see detail below)*

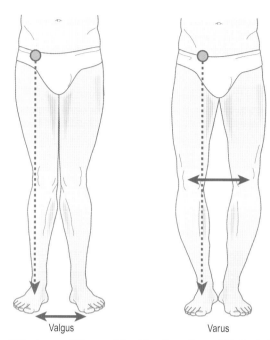

Valgus   Varus

Fig. 12.13 Illustration of (A) valgus and (B) varus deformities. (From Bowen WT, Cho L, Dennis M: *Mechanisms of clinical signs*, ed 3, Chatswood: New South Wales, 2020, Elsevier Australia.)

Thompson test - the examiner squeezes the patient's calf to test the integrity of the Achilles tendon (a positive test will not elicit plantar flexion, indicating that the Achilles tendon is not intact)

Tinel's sign - test to detect irritated or entrapped nerves that is conducted by lightly tapping the nerve (positive test will elicit pain)

Ulnar deviation - the fingers of a hand deviate (or drift) towards the ulna (pinky side) - usually due to inflammatory joint degeneration

Valgus – at a joint where the distal segment bends outward, or laterally (Fig. 12.13, *A*)

Varus – at a joint where the distal portion is bent inward, or medially (Fig. 12.13, *B*)

The following explanations give some additional information about some of the common physical findings mentioned.

When a bone is displaced from its position within a joint, this is a **dislocation**. Often there will be a visible deformity at the site of the dislocation. Range of motion will also be severely limited, and the area will be diffusely tender.

The *anatomic snuffbox* is the divot formed on the dorsum of the hand when the thumb is hyperextended (the hitchhiking thumb). The scaphoid lies just under this region, so when the snuff box is examined for tenderness the scaphoid is actually being examined for possible fracture. Sometimes scaphoid fracture cannot be seen on x-rays. This is termed an **occult** (hidden) **fracture**. If there is snuffbox tenderness the injury will be treated as a fracture until further evaluation is possible.

Pressure ulcers (decubitus ulcers) are common among elderly or disabled patients who are unable to move much on their own. They often develop over bony prominences that can become pressure points such as the ischium, which is a major pressure point when one is seated.

Ligaments and menisci are often torn when the knee is forced past the limits of its normal range of motion. *Anterior and posterior drawer testing* assesses the stability of the anterior and posterior cruciate ligaments, respectively. ***Varus and valgus stress testing*** assesses the stability of the lateral and medial collateral ligaments, respectively.

The ***patellar reflex*** (knee jerk test**)** assesses the reflex arc beginning at the patellar tendon. **Reflexes** are an involuntary response to a stimulus. In this case, the shortening of the patellar tendon results in contraction (shortening) of the quadriceps muscle to prevent injury, and extension of the leg. Reflexes can range from ***absent*** to ***normal*** to **hypertonic**.

Muscles enlarge by **hypertrophy**. When muscles shrink (from disuse or denervation, the loss of a supplying nerve), this is **atrophy**. Both of these findings can be observed during a physical exam, and have different implications depending on the clinical scenario.

The legs and arms are divided into compartments, which are separated by fascia (connective tissue). When there is swelling or fluid accumulation in a compartment, there can be ***muscle ischemia*** (lack of blood flow) leading to ***necrosis*** (death). This is a **compartment syndrome**. During exam, the compartments will feel hard and the patient will have a great deal of pain with little movement. A surgeon must make an incision over the affected compartment to relieve the pressure.

Operations / Procedures

Any of the patient's prior surgical history (including major operations or minor procedures) may be discussed in the context of a patient's medical history. Patients often do not know the name of the operation and will describe their understanding of the procedure in lay terms. It is the scribe's duty to translate the patient's procedural description into the equivalent medical term. For example, if a patient says they had fluid drained from a joint, the scribe should document "arthrocentesis."

Above the knee amputation (AKA) - amputation of a leg above the knee, often due to ulcerations and gangrene from diabetes

Arthrocentesis - a needle is inserted into a joint to drain excess fluid

Below the knee amputation (BKA) - amputation of a leg below the knee, often due to ulcerations and gangrene from diabetes

Hip replacement - replacing a partial or whole hip joint

Knee replacement - replacement of a partial or whole knee joint (TKR = total knee replacement)

Kyphoplasty - use of a balloon to reexpand a collapsed vertebra and then inject cement into that space to stabilize the vertebra and relieve pain

Laminectomy - removal of the vertebral lamina often for decompression of the spinal cord

Vertebroplasty - use of pressure to inject cement into a fractured vertebra to relieve pain

Problem List

Patients often do not know the name of a specific diagnosis, but will instead describe it to their provider. It is the scribe's duty to translate the lay terms into medical terminology. For example, if the patient says they have a history of wear and tear arthritis, the scribe should document "osteoarthritis."

Ankylosing spondylitis (AS) - inflammatory back disease that forms bony syndesmoses around the vertebrae, resulting in loss of flexibility and back stiffness

Bursitis - inflammation of bursae (sacs of synovial fluid)

Cauda equina syndrome - a herniated disc compresses spinal roots causing neurologic deficits (this is a medical emergency!)

Degenerative disc disease (DDD) - intervertebral disc degeneration

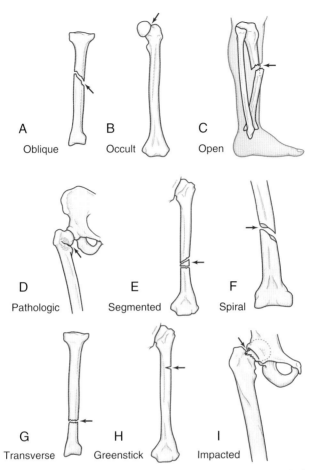

Fig. 12.14 Common types of fractures. (A) Oblique: fracture at oblique angle across both cortices. Cause: direct or indirect energy, with angulation and some compression. (B) Occult: fracture that is hidden or not readily discernible. Cause: minor force or energy. (C) Open: skin broken over fracture; possible soft tissue trauma. Cause: moderate to severe energy that is continuous and exceeds tissue tolerances. (D) Pathologic: transverse, oblique, or spiral fracture of bone weakened by tumor pressure or presence. Cause: minor energy or force, which may be direct or indirect. (E) Segmented: fracture with two or more pieces or segments. Cause: direct or indirect moderate to severe force. (F) Spiral: fracture that curves around cortices and may become displaced by twist. Cause: direct or indirect twisting energy or force with distal part held or unable to move. (G) Transverse: horizontal break through bone. Cause: direct or indirect energy toward bone. (H) Greenstick: break in only one cortex of bone. Cause: minor direct or indirect energy. (I) Impacted: fracture with one end wedged into opposite end of inside fractured fragment. Cause: compressive axial energy or force directly to distal fragment. (From Skidmore-Roth L, Richardson F. *Introduction to critical care nursing*, ed 8, St. Louis, 2021, Elsevier. In: Huether S, McCance K, eds. *Pathophysiology: the biologic basis for disease in adults and children*, ed 8, St. Louis, 2019, Elsevier.)

Degenerative joint disease (DJD) - degenerative changes to the joints

Fibromyalgia - hypersensitivity to pain accompanied by excessive fatigue without another explainable cause

Fracture - break in a bone (Fig. 12.14)

Gout - uric acid deposits in joints that cause pain, swelling, and redness

Herniated disc - tear in fibrous ring around a vertebral disc allowing the central portion to bulge, often against the spinal cord causing back pain and radiating pain down a limb

Lateral epicondylitis (tennis elbow) - inflammation of tendons in the lateral elbow that is usually caused by repetitive movement of the elbow such as when one plays tennis

Medial epicondylitis (golfer's elbow) - inflammation of tendons in the medial elbow that is usually caused by repetitive movement of the elbow such as when one plays golf

Myopathy - muscle disease

Osteoarthritis (OA) - degenerative joint disease ("wear and tear") that causes joint pain and deformity

Osteopenia - low bone mineral density, not to the point of osteoporosis but still increases risk of fracture

Osteoporosis (OP) - decreased bone mineral density that significantly increases risk of fracture

Psoriatic arthritis - inflammatory joint disease with concomitant manifestation of psoriatic plaques (scaly skin lesions)

Rheumatoid arthritis (RA) - inflammatory autoimmune disease resulting in joint destruction manifested as joint pain, swelling, and deformity that typically affects smaller synovial joints

Septic joint - infection within a joint capsule

Spinal stenosis - narrowing of the vertebral foramen that may cause nerve compression

Sprain - ligaments are over extended and partially or completely tear

Systemic lupus erythematosus (SLE) - inflammatory autoimmune disease affecting multiple organ systems, including the joints which manifests as joint pain, stiffness, and swelling

Tendinitis - tendon inflammation

Tendinosis - tendon degeneration

Tenosynovitis - inflammation of the synovium (fluid filled sheath) around a tendon

---

CASE STUDY 12.1

Bonnie Jurista is an 89-year-old woman whose daughter has brought her to the emergency department after a fall at home. Bonnie is conscious but confused and does not answer the questions asked by the triage nurses or the physician. Her daughter Lynette tells the ED physician that around 6:45 AM, about 2 hours ago, she fell in her bathroom, hitting her head on the bathtub. Lynette further relates that her mother complained of lower back pain on the way here in the car.

Lynette tells the physician that her mother has "weak bones" and is taking calcium and vitamin D supplements. Plain x-ray images reveal compression fractures of T8-T10, along with kyphosis and a slight scoliosis. An examination of the occipital region of her head reveals a gash that requires stitches.

1. Who is the historian?
2. How would the scribe construct the first sentence of the HPI?
3. What do you think Lynette means when she describes her mother's "weak bones?"
4. In what region of the spine are Bonnie's fractures?
5. The gash is on the occipital side of Bonnie's head, meaning it is where?

Medications

A scribe should be able to diligently record the patient's medication list, which includes the drug name (generic or brand), dose, frequency, and indication (reason for taking the drug). Table 12.3 lists relevant drug classes and medications for the musculoskeletal system.

TABLE 12.3 ▪ Selected Musculoskeletal Medications

Drug Class and Uses	Generic Name (Brand Name)
Muscle relaxants • Reduce muscle spasm and induce relaxation	baclofen (Lioresal) carisoprodol (Soma) cyclobenzaprine (Flexeril) metaxalone (Skelaxin) methocarbamol (Robaxin) tizanidine (Zanaflex)
Neuromuscular blocking drugs (paralytics) • Antagonize transmission of signal at the neuromuscular junction (synapse) • Used to induce muscle paralysis (e.g. during surgery or procedures)	succinylcholine vecuronium
NSAIDs (non-steroidal anti-inflammatory drugs) • Inhibit the COX enzyme (**COX inhibitor**), reducing inflammatory molecules • Used to reduce inflammation, pain (**analgesic**), and fever (**antipyretic**)	aspirin/acetylsalicylic acid (Bayer) celecoxib (Celebrex) diclofenac (Voltaren) ibuprofen (Motrin) or (Advil) ketorolac (Toradol) meloxicam (Mobic) nabumetone (Relafen) naproxen (Aleve) or (Naprosyn)

Practice Questions

1. The joint between the humerus and scapula is the _____.
2. The joint type of the joint described above is the _____.
3. Movement away from the body's midline is _____.
4. What are the levels of the spine, from superior to inferior?
   a. _____
   b. _____
   c. _____
   d. _____
   e. _____
5. A 36-year-old female presents to a rheumatologist for evaluation of a 6-month history of joint pain, stiffness, and swelling, particularly in the small joints of her hands, both wrists, elbows, and toes. She has had intermittent rashes and fevers during this time but denies any other illnesses. How should this be documented in the review of systems?
6. During physical exam the rheumatologist notes synovitis diffusely in the MCP joints of both hands and the left wrist. There is ulnar deviation bilaterally. Hammertoe deformities are seen in both feet but there is no synovitis. Effusion is noted in the left knee with some loss in range of motion. Range of motion is otherwise intact throughout. No rashes were observed. The patient appears disheveled. How should this be documented in the physical exam?
7. The rheumatologist decides to insert a needle into the left knee to drain some of the excess fluid from the effusion. What is the name of this procedure?
8. The rheumatologist determines that the patient likely has a systemic autoimmune inflammatory disease affecting her joints. Lab work (including antibody assays) and x-rays of the

hands, feet, and knees are ordered to narrow down the differential. Which of the following is a systemic autoimmune inflammatory disease consistent with the patient's affected joint distribution?

   a. Ankylosing spondylitis

   b. Fibromyalgia

   c. Rheumatoid arthritis

   d. Osteoarthritis

9. The patient is discharged on an NSAID to reduce some of the inflammation until the pending lab work and x-rays return with results. Which of the following is an NSAID?

   a. baclofen

   b. methotrexate

   c. prednisone

   d. naproxen

CHAPTER 13

HEENT (Head, Eyes, Ears, Nose, Throat)

LEARNING OBJECTIVES

1. Use medical terminology to document medical issues involving the head, eyes, ears, nose, throat (HEENT).
2. Describe the anatomy and physiology of the HEENT.
3. Document HEENT symptoms related during a review of systems.
4. Document signs related by the provider during a physical exam of the HEENT.
5. Document operations and procedures for the HEENT.
6. Document the HEENT clinical impressions, diagnoses, and signs and symptoms commonly found in a problem list.
7. Document relevant drug classes and medications for the treatment of problems associated with the HEENT.

KEY TERMS

Age-related macular degeneration (ARMD)
Aphtha
Aqueous humor
Auricle
Benign paroxysmal peripheral vertigo (BPPV)
Caries
Cataract
Cerumen
Cochlea
Congestion
Conjunctiva (conjunctival membrane)
Conjunctivitis
Cornea
Diplopia
Edentulous
Epiglottis
Epistaxis

Eustachian tube (auditory tube)
Extraocular muscles
Exudates
Fundoscopy
Hard palate
HEENT (head, eyes, ears, nose, throat)
Iris
Laryngopharynx
Lavage
Lens
Macula lutea
Myringotomy
Naris
Nasal turbinate (concha)
Nasopharynx
Normocephaly
Nystagmus

Ophthalmoscope
Optic disc
Optic nerve
Oropharynx
Otalgia
Otitis media
Otoscope
PERRL (pupils are equal, round, and reactive to light)
Pharynx
Pinna
Pupil
Pupillary light reflex
Retina
Retinal subluxation
Rhinorrhea
Sclera
Scleral icterus

Continued

Anatomy and Physiology

HEENT (head, eyes, ears, nose, throat) is not a traditional body system, but rather a group of organs or body structures that are often organized together. Many of these organs are **special sensory** organs, meaning that they participate in collecting special sensory information such as sight (eyes), hearing and balance (ears), smell (nose), and taste (taste buds in the mouth and throat).

HEAD

Not much comment will be made about the head during history or physical exam. Mainly, trauma or **normocephaly** (having a normally developed head) will be noted.

EYE

The external eye can be examined grossly (Fig. 13.1). The **pupil** is an adjustable aperture through which light enters to project to the retina. It is located centrally in the **iris**, which is the colored portion of the eye. The iris is actually a muscle that adjusts the size of the pupil depending on levels of ambient light. In situations of high light, the normal pupil should become smaller (*constriction*), and in low light the normal pupil should enlarge (*dilation*). The **sclera** ("white" of the eye) surrounds the iris. The **cornea** is a transparent thickening of the sclera over the pupil and iris that refracts light as it enters the eye (Fig. 13.2). The **conjunctival membrane** (or **conjunctiva**) covers the external eye and the internal eyelids.

The **uvea** is a layer beneath the sclera, comprising the *choroid* (at the posterior), the iris, and the *ciliary body*. The *anterior chamber* is a space between the cornea (superficial) and iris (deep) that is filled with **aqueous humor**. Deep to the iris is the **lens**, which is responsible for *accommodation*—the ability to adjust between looking at near versus far objects. Posterior to the lens is the *vitreous chamber*, filled with **vitreous humor**. The **retina** is the most posterior structure of the eye, and contains *rods* and *cones*—the cells that are responsible for *phototransduction*, the conversion of light into electrical signal.

The **optic disc** is the point at which the **optic nerve (CN II)** enters the eye. The **macula lutea** is the area of highest visual acuity of the retina.

There are six **extraocular muscles** that work together to move the eye in various directions. These muscles are innervated by three cranial nerves.

EAR

The *external ear* can be examined grossly. The **pinna** (or **auricle**) is the oval-like cartilaginous tissue that most recognize as the ear (Fig. 13.3). The pinna's shape funnels sound into the *ear* *canal (auditory canal)*. The auditory canal terminates at the **tympanic membrane (TM)**, which separates the external ear from the middle ear. The *tragus* is a flap of tissue on the side of the canal opposite the pinna.

The *middle ear* is an air-filled cavity behind the tympanic membrane. The **auditory tube** or **eustachian tube** is located in the middle ear, and connects the middle ear to the nasal cavity. It

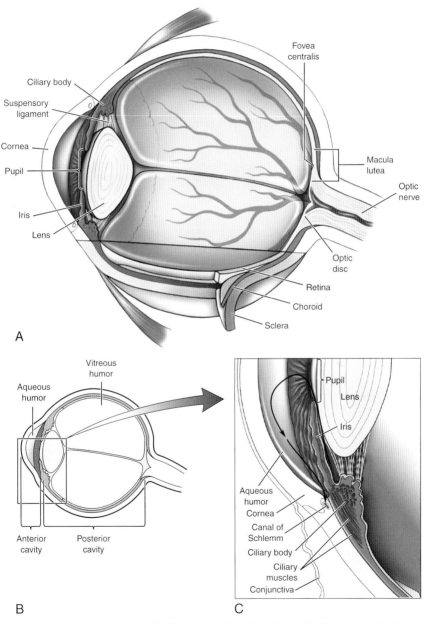

Fig. 13.1 Anatomy of the external eye. (LaFleur Brooks M, LaFleur Brooks D: *Exploring medical language*, ed 11, St. Louis, 2021, Elsevier.)

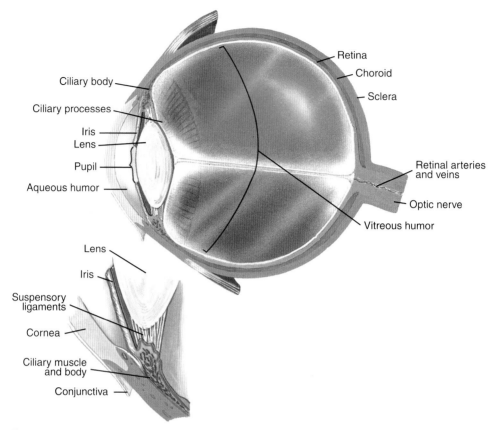

Fig. 13.2 (A) Structure of the eyeball. (B) Cavities and fluids. (C) Flow of aqueous humor from the ciliary body to the canal of Schlemm (arrow), Cross-section of the eye. (LaFleur Brooks M, LaFleur Brooks D: *Exploring medical language*, ed 11, St. Louis, 2021, Elsevier.)

equalizes pressure between these two air-filled compartments. Also in the middle ear are three small bones (*malleus, incus, stapes*) that function in sound transmission.

When sound contacts the tympanic membrane, vibrations are generated. The vibrations are transferred via the small bones of the middle ear to the *oval window*, which separates the middle ear from the fluid-filled inner ear. Within the *inner ear* are the hearing and balance organs - the **cochlea** and **semicircular canals**, respectively. These are both innervated by **CN VIII**, the **vestibulocochlear nerve**.

NOSE

The nose is primarily comprised of cartilage, although the two *nasal bones* also contribute to its structure. The nose opens externally through the two **nares** (singular **naris**) (Fig. 13.4).

The *nasal septum* is the wall of cartilage that divides the left and right nares. *Kiesselbach's plexus* is a highly vascularized portion of the anterior inferior septum. These arteries are the most prone to bleed.

Nasal turbinates (conchae [plural] or **concha** [singular]), are bony structures located on the lateral walls of the *nasal cavity* that direct airflow into the **nasopharynx**.

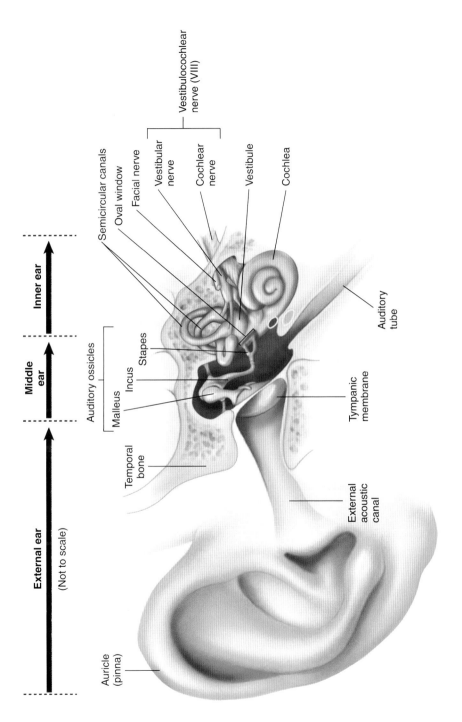

Fig. 13.3 Structures of the external, middle, and inner ear. (Patton KT, Thibodeau GA: *Human body in health & disease*, ed 7, St. Louis, 2018, Elsevier.)

Medical Terminology Word Parts for the HEENT

Head Combining Forms

norm/o	normal
ceph/o	head

Eyes Combining Forms

opt/o optic/o ophthalm/o	vision
conjunctiv/o	conjunctiva
ocul/o ophthalm/o	eye
blephar/o palpebr/o	eyelid
corne/o kerat/o	cornea
uve/o	uvea
irid/o ir/o	iris
pupil/o core/o cor/o	pupil
retin/o	retina
scler/o	sclera
choroid/o	choroid
vitre/o	vitreous humor
macul/o	macula
phak/o phac/o	lens
canth/o	corner (of eye)
dipl/o	double
fund/o	the base, or part farthest from the opening
angi/o	vessel

Ears Combining Forms

acous/o audi/o aur/o	hearing
ot/o	ear
tympan/o myring/o	tympanic membrane/ eardrum
vestibul/o	vestibule
cochle/o	cochlea

Nose Combining Forms

nas/o rhin/o	nose
turbin/o	nasal turbinate
sept/o	septum

Throat and Mouth Combining Forms

stomat/o or/o	mouth
bucc/o	cheek
gloss/o lingu/o	tongue
gingiv/o	gums
dent/i odont/o	teeth
palat/o	palate
mandibul/o	mandible (lower jawbone)
adenoid/o	adenoid
tonsil/o	tonsils
uvul/o	uvuvla
pharyng/o	throat, pharynx
laryng/o	larynx
aphth/o	ulceration
sial/o	saliva
lith/o	stone

Prefixes

extra-	outside
sub-	under
par-	near
peri-	surrounding
epi-	above, upon
hyper-	excessive

Suffixes

-y	condition, process of
-ar -id	pertaining to
-acusis -cusis	hearing
-rrhea	discharge, flow
-algia	pain
-itis	inflammation
-trophy	growth
-oma	tumor, mass
-tomy	cutting
-plasty	surgical formation
-ectomy	removal

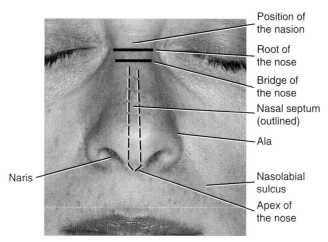

Fig. 13.4   Landmarks of the nasal region. (From Fehrenbach M, Herring S: *Illustrated anatomy of the head and neck*, ed 4, St. Louis, 2012, Elsevier.)

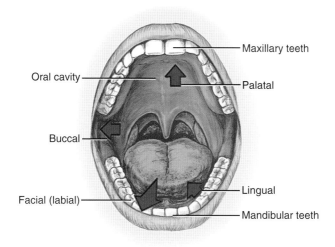

Fig. 13.5   Regions of the oral cavity. (From Fehrenbach M, Herring S: *Illustrated anatomy of the head and neck*, ed 4, St. Louis, 2012, Elsevier.)

THROAT

The ***oral cavity*** (mouth) is comprised of several distinct regions (Fig. 13.5). Laterally is the *buccal region*, which is the cheek area. Inferiorly is the *lingual region*, which consists of the tongue and the floor of the oral cavity. The *tongue* is a large muscle that functions to move food into the pharynx. It also plays a role in speech. *Taste buds* are located on the surface of the tongue, and they function to convert chemical to electrical signals, creating taste. The tongue has a complex innervation, but taste is primarily a function of the ***facial nerve (CN VII)*** and the ***glossopharyngeal nerve (CN IX)***.

BOX 13.1 ■ Counting Teeth

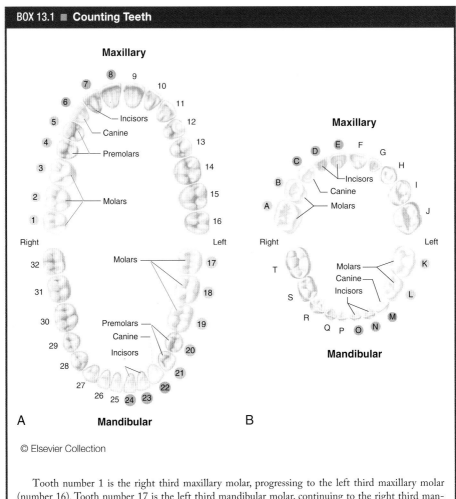

© Elsevier Collection

Tooth number 1 is the right third maxillary molar, progressing to the left third maxillary molar (number 16). Tooth number 17 is the left third mandibular molar, continuing to the right third mandibular molar (number 32).

Superiorly, the **hard palate** (anterior) and **soft palate** (posterior) compose the roof of the mouth. The **uvula** is a muscular tissue that dangles from the soft palate and plays a role in the gag reflex.

Within the oral cavity are *salivary glands* that function to secrete saliva, which aids in digestion and lubricates the mouth. The three pairs of salivary glands are the *parotid*, *submandibular*, and *sublingual glands*. The *teeth* (32 in an anatomically normal adult individual) are used to break-up food for digestion (Box 13.1).

Tonsils are immune tissues in the oral cavity. The *lingual tonsils* are located on the root of the tongue. The *palatine tonsils* are located on the roof of the posterior oral cavity.

The **pharynx** (throat) is subdivided into various regions (Fig. 13.6). Most superiorly, the nasopharynx is the region posterior to the nasal cavity. Below this is the **oropharynx**, which is posterior to the oral cavity. The most inferior region is the **laryngopharynx**, which contains the vocal cords. The **vocal cords** (or **vocal folds**) participate in the generation of sound and voice. They also separate

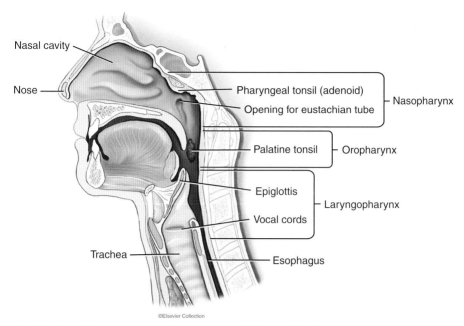

Fig. 13.6 Parts of the pharynx and adjacent anatomy. (© Elsevier Collection)

the pharynx from the trachea (part of the pulmonary tree) and the esophagus (part of the gastrointestinal tract). The trachea is located anteriorly to the esophagus. The main structure preventing food or foreign objects from entering the trachea is the **epiglottis**. This cartilaginous structure covers the opening of the trachea while swallowing, thus routing everything into the esophagus.

Review of Systems

Patients often describe what they are feeling in a manner which makes the most sense to them. It is the duty of the scribe to translate the patient's interpretation of their symptoms into medical lingo. For example, if a patient says they have been having "double vision," the scribe should document **diplopia**. A "stuffy nose" is properly recorded as **nasal congestion**, the result of the tissues surrounding the turbinates swelling during allergies or illness.

Symptoms that can be placed in multiple systems have been designated as such in italics. Remember to always maximize the number of <u>systems</u> that are included in the review of systems so that the chart can be billed at higher levels (if desired). For example: if a patient is having blurred vision and otalgia, it would be best to include blurred vision in "*neurologic*" and otalgia in "*HEENT*" (two billable systems), as opposed to including blurred vision and otalgia in "*HEENT*" (one billable system).

Blurred vision (*neurologic*)—loss of visual clarity

Congestion *(immunologic/allergic)*—swelling and/or irritation of the nasal tissues that causes the sensation of not being able to inhale through the nasal cavity

Deafness (*neurologic*)—complete or partial hearing loss

Dentalgia/odontalgia—tooth pain

Diplopia (*neurologic*)—seeing double

Epistaxis (*hematologic/lymphatic*)—nose bleed

Eye problems—redness, pain, swelling, itching, drainage, etc.

Head injury/pain—any trauma or pain to the face or skull

Otalgia—ear pain

Post nasal drainage *(immunologic/allergic)*—mucus drainage down the throat that causes voice clearing, a sore throat, and hoarseness

Rhinorrhea *(immunologic/allergic)*—runny nose

Sinus pain/pressure *(immunologic/allergic)*—facial pain or pressure

Tinnitus *(neurologic)*—hearing sound (e.g. ringing) when none is present

Voice hoarseness *(neurologic)*—changes in the sound of voice

Physical Exam

The result of the physical exam is a listing of signs, organized by system. Physical findings may at times be appropriately placed in a different body system than what is listed, but less often than in the review of systems. The scribe will never be expected to interpret these findings, but rather must be diligent in recording the provider's exact objective findings as related by the provider.

FINDINGS

In a patient with nasal congestion, *turbinate swelling* is notable during exam. *Secretions* (mucus) may also be observed.

Sometimes tonsils can become infected with *streptococcus bacteria* (strep throat). The patient will often present with a sore throat, fever, and malaise. On examination, findings may include *pharyngeal erythema* (redness), *tonsillar edema* (swelling), and *tonsillar* exudates (pus). *Uvular deviation* (deviation of the uvula from midline) is a more ominous sign, possibly indicative of *peritonsillar abscess*.

TESTS

The provider may utilize several tests during the physical examination. For the eyes, the *pupillary light reflex* is used to test the integrity of the optic nerve (CN II, containing only *afferent* nerve fibers for input) and the oculomotor nerve (CN III, containing only *efferent* nerves for output). A light is shone into one eye and pupillary constriction should be observed in both eyes (consensual constriction). This is often documented as **pupils are equal, round, and reactive to light (PERRL)** if the response is normal. Sometimes accommodation, the ability of the eyes to adjust between near and far sightedness, will also be tested, and is therefore documented as *PERRLA*.

Extraocular movement (EOM) testing evaluates the integrity of the muscles that move the eyes (and the three cranial nerves that innervate them). Often this is done by drawing an "H" in the air and asking the patient to follow the examiner's finger.

Vertigo (dizziness) can be caused by disease that affects the balance organs of the inner ear. A common cause of vertigo is **benign paroxysmal peripheral vertigo (BPPV)**, in which *otoconia* (small stones) become loose in the balance organs of the inner ear. The Dix-Hallpike maneuver (Fig. 13.7) is a test that can be done to confirm a peripheral cause of vertigo (such as BPPV) as opposed to a central cause (like a brain tumor). The Epley maneuver can be performed in attempt to move the otoconia back into proper position.

INSTRUMENTATION

The internal components of the eye can be viewed with the aid of an **ophthalmoscope**, which is a handheld device equipped with a light and magnification. The examination of the internal

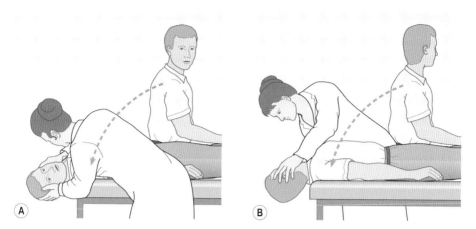

Fig. 13.7　The Dix Hallpike maneuver. (From Dari Boon NA, Colledge NR, Walker BR: *Davidson's principles & practice of medicine*, ed 20, Edinburgh, 2006, Churchill Livingstone.)

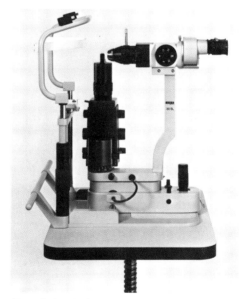

Fig. 13.8　Zeiss slit lamp. (From Stein HA, Stein RM, Freeman MI: *The ophthalmic assistant: a guide for ophthalmic and medical personnel*, ed 10, Edinburgh, 2018, Elsevier.)

eye structures with an ophthalmoscope is a **fundoscopic exam**. A **slit lamp** (Fig. 13.8) is frequently used to magnify and examine both the external eye and the anterior portion of the internal eye.

　　Some internally located structures of the external ear (namely the auditory canal and tympanic membrane) are examined with the aid of an **otoscope**, a handheld device with a light and magnifying glass. The interior structures of the nose can also be visualized with the aid of an otoscope through the nares. The middle ear cannot be visualized with an otoscope.

　　Aphthae (aphtha, singular)—oral or aphthous ulcers

　　Caries (cavities)—tooth decay

Cataract—clouding of the lens in the eye that causes visual loss

Cerumen—ear wax

Cobblestoning—post nasal drainage in the oropharynx gives the throat a bumpy or cobble-stone appearance

Conjunctival injection—eye redness

Dix-Hallpike—a test in which the head is rapidly moved to determine a peripheral versus central cause of vertigo (a positive test in which nystagmus is produced indicates a peripheral cause) (see Fig. 13.7).

Edentulous—toothlessness

EOMI (extraocular muscles intact)—the muscles that move the eyes are tested to evaluate function of the muscles and the cranial nerves that innervate them (often done by drawing an "H" in the air and asking the patient to follow with their eyes)

Epley maneuver—a maneuver in attempt to move otoconia (small stones in the inner ear) back into proper position and alleviate vertigo

Exudates—pustular patches typically found near the tonsils that can indicate infection by streptococcus bacteria

Fundoscopy—using an ophthalmoscope to examine the fundus of the eye and other internal structures

Hard of hearing—difficulties hearing

Hemotympanum—blood in the middle ear (behind the tympanic membrane) that can indicate basilar skull fracture

Mallampati score—assessment of the oropharynx to predict difficulty of intubation (a higher score indicates a narrower pharyngeal opening)

Nystagmus—involuntary rapid eye movement with a variety of causes

Ocular angioedema—eye swelling

Oropharyngeal angioedema—lip or throat swelling

PERRLA (pupils equal, round, reactive to light and accommodation)—the pupil's response to light and accommodation is evaluated to determine functionality of some cranial nerves

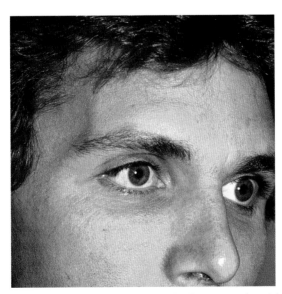

Fig. 13.9 Scleral icterus. (Kyle WL, High WA, Fitzpatrick JE: *Urgent care dermatology: symptom-based diagnosis*, Philadelphia, 2018, Elsevier.)

Scleral icterus—yellow discoloration of the conjunctiva that is caused by jaundice (accumulation of bilirubin often due to liver failure) (Fig. 13.9)

Septal deviation—displacement of the nasal septum

Septal hematoma—blood in the septum usually from trauma

Strabismus ("lazy eye")—inability to direct both eyes towards the same point simultaneously

Tonsillar edema (hypertrophy)—swelling of the tonsils

Uvular deviation—uvula that has moved from the midline (can be due to peritonsillar abscess or allergic reaction, which is an emergency)

Uvular edema—swelling of the uvula

Operations/Procedures

Any of the patient's prior surgical history (including major operations or minor procedures) may be discussed in the context of a patient's medical history. Patients often do not know the name of the operation and will describe their understanding of the procedure in lay terms. It is the scribe's duty to translate the patient's procedural description into the equivalent medical term. For example, if a patient says they had their tonsils and adenoids removed, the scribe should record that the patient had an "tonsillectomy & adenoidectomy".

Dental extraction—removal of teeth

Lavage—washing out (or irrigation) of a body cavity, such as the ear canal or nose

Myringotomy—small incision in the tympanic membrane to relieve fluid accumulation that causes increased pressure

Septoplasty—surgically correcting the nasal septum

Tonsillectomy and adenoidectomy (T&A)—removal of the tonsils and adenoids usually because of recurrent infections

Turbinectomy—removal of the nasal turbinates

Tympanostomy (pressure equalizer [PE]) tubes—tubes placed in the tympanic membrane to prevent fluid accumulation (usually because of recurrent middle ear infections)

Problem List

Since the problem list is to be maintained as an up-to-date recording of all of the patient's current clinical impressions, diagnoses and signs and symptoms, it should be updated at each visit. Any new or resolved HEENT problems or symptoms should be added or removed as appropriate. Thus, if the patient had vertigo that has now resolved, it should be removed with the provider's instruction. And if the patient has presented with new symptoms such as recurring gum inflammation, these should be added either as the symptom or as the diagnosis if known; in this case the scribe should "translate" to the medical term "gingivitis."

Age-related macular degeneration (ARMD)—degeneration of the macula that causes vision loss (can be wet or dry)

Benign paroxysmal peripheral vertigo (BPPV)—stones in the inner ear (otoliths) become loose and move, causing vertigo

Blepharitis—inflammation of the eyelids and eyelashes

Conjunctivitis (pink eye)—conjunctival inflammation caused by chemical irritants or infectious agents such as bacteria, viruses, or fungi

Episcleritis—inflammation of the tissue superficial to the sclera

Gingivitis—gum inflammation

Glaucoma—elevated intraocular pressures

Iritis—uveal inflammation

Keratitis—corneal inflammation

Labyrinthitis—inflammation in the inner ear

Macular edema—swelling of the macula

Maculopathy—disease of the macula

Nasal polyps—benign tissue growths (polyps) within the nasal cavity

Otitis externa ("swimmer's ear")—inflammation of the outer ear and/or ear canal that causes itching and pain

Otitis media—inflammation in the middle ear

    Acute otitis media (AOM)—sudden onset infection in which fluid and mucus becomes trapped in the middle ear, presenting with swelling, redness, fever, and ear pain

    Serous otitis media/otitis media with effusion (OME)—Inflammation caused by **serous** (thin) fluid accumulation in the middle ear following an acute infection; commonly presents with hearing loss rather than pain

    Chronic suppurative otitis media (CSOM)—Persistent inflammation of the middle ear with a **suppurative** (pus-like) discharge, signifying a bacterial infection

Periodontitis—periodontal inflammation

Peritonsillar abscess—collection of pus around a tonsil

Pharyngitis—pharynx inflammation

Retinal subluxation (detachment)—retina separates from surrounding support tissues

Retinitis—retinal inflammation

Retinopathy—disease of the retina (often due to diabetes)

Sialolithiasis—salivary stones in a salivary gland

Streptococcal infection ("strep throat")—streptococcal bacterial infection of the tonsils that can cause a sore throat, fevers and malaise

Tonsillitis—tonsil inflammation

Tracheitis—tracheal inflammation

Uveitis—uveal (middle layer of the eye) inflammation

CASE STUDY 13.1

The patient today is a 40-year-old male who has had persistent right ear pain and a feeling of fullness for over a year. He says it began after he took a long soak in the bathtub. Since then he has tried clearing the liquid with Q-tips and an over-the-counter "ear dry" remedy, which he believes was alcohol-based. The patient had been to his family doctor two months ago about the problem, who ordered a lavage and prescribed antibiotic ear drops. He states that a "huge hunk of wax" came out while the nurse flushed his ear, and he had some temporary relief. But after finishing the antibiotic course, the patient says the ear pain and fullness has recurred.

QUESTIONS

1. What is the patient's chief complaint?
2. What is the medical term for earwax?
3. What is the duration of the chief complaint?
4. What instrument would the provider use to examine the patient's external ear?
5. How might the scribe document the treatment before arrival?

Medications

Many drugs are related to other drugs in both function and chemical composition. These drugs would be considered to be in the same drug class. This gives the provider options within a class to choose different drugs with slightly different profiles (actions and side-effects).

A scribe should be able to diligently record the patient's medication list, which includes the drug name (generic or brand), dose, frequency, and indication (reason for taking the drug). Table 13.1 lists relevant drug classes and medications for the HEENT.

TABLE 13.1 ■ **Selected HEENT Medications**

Drug Class and Uses	Generic Name (Brand Name)

Antihistamines
• Used to treat:
  • Motion sickness
  • Dizziness
  • Allergic reactions
	diphenhydramine (Benadryl)
	fexofenadine (Allegra)
	loratadine (Alavert) or (Claritin)
	meclizine (Antivert)

Decongestant • Not a class • Used to treat nasal/sinus congestion	guaifenesin (Mucinex) pseudoephedrine (Sudafed)
Steroidal anti-inflammatories • Reduce inflammation and histamine release	methylprednisolone (Medrol) prednisone (Deltasone)

Practice Questions

1. The _____ is the portion of the throat posterior to the oral cavity.

2. Tonsils are the _____ tissues of the oral cavity.

3. The _____ tonsils are located at the root of the tongue.

4. The muscular appendage of the soft palate is the _____.

5. A 20-year-old male patient presents to an urgent care center for evaluation of a two-day history of a sore throat associated with drainage at the back of his throat, and a stuffy and runny nose. He has been having fevers with a maximum temperature of 101 °F, chills, and he has not been feeling well. He denies blurred or double vision, muscle aches or joint pains, or rashes. How should this be documented in the review of systems?

6. On exam, conjunctiva are clear and pupils are equal, round, and reactive to light. Turbinates are swollen and there is scant clear rhinorrhea. Tonsillar enlargement, erythema, and exudates bilaterally but no uvular deviation. Tympanic membranes are pearly white with intact light reflexes. No rashes are noted. He has full range of motion in all major joints. The patient is otherwise atoxic and well developed and well nourished. How should this be documented in the physical exam?

7. As the physician is verbalizing the physical exam findings to you (the scribe), note is made of the patient's deviated septum as part of the nose exam. The patient mentions that he has had surgery in attempt to correct this in the past. How should this be documented in the surgical history?

8. At the end of the visit the patient shared that he has a history of recurrent strep throat infections since childhood, and once had to have surgery for a particularly nasty infection that he explained as a collection of pus around his tonsils. What diagnosis is the patient describing?

9. The patient is given a prescription for Amoxicillin to treat the bacterial infection, and prednisone to reduce some of the pharyngeal inflammation. He is also instructed to use which of the following medications for symptomatic treatment of the nasal congestion?
   a. azithromycin (Zithromax)
   b. Vitamin C
   c. dapsone (Aczone)
   d. pseudoephedrine (Sudafed)

Nervous System

1. Use medical terminology to document medical issues involving the nervous system.
2. Describe the anatomy and physiology of the nervous system.
3. Document nervous system symptoms related during a review of systems.
4. Document signs related by the provider during a physical exam of the nervous system.
5. Document operations and procedures for the nervous system.
6. Document the nervous system clinical impressions, diagnoses, and signs and symptoms commonly found in a problem list.
7. Document relevant drug classes and medications for the treatment of problems associated with the nervous system.

Affect
Afferent
Alzheimer's disease
Amnesia
Anorexia nervosa
Aphasia
Arachnoid mater
Asterixis
Ataxia
Brain
Brainstem
Cauda equina
Cauda equina syndrome
Central nervous system (CNS)
Cephalgia
Cerebellum
Cerebral cortex
Cerebrospinal fluid (CSF)
Cerebrovascular accident
Cerebrum
Concussion

Cranial nerves
Disequilibrium
Dura mater
Efferent
Electromyogram (EMG)
Epidural space
Epilepsy
Foramen magnum
Gait
Glasgow coma scale
Gyri
Hallucination
Lumbar puncture
Mania
Meninges
Meningismus
Meningitis
Motor neuron
Multiple sclerosis (MS)
Neuron
Neurotransmitters

Nuchal rigidity
Obsessive compulsive disorder (OCD)
Paranoia
Paresthesia
Parkinson disease
Peripheral nervous system (PNS)
Pia mater
Psychosis
Reflexes
Schizophrenia
Spinal cord
Subarachnoid space
Subdural space
Suicidal ideation
Sulci
Synapse
Ventricles
Ventriculoperitoneal (VP) shunting
Vertigo

Anatomy and Physiology

The nervous system has several divisions, all with varying functions (Fig. 14.1). The **central nervous system (CNS)** includes the brain and spinal cord. Most major neurological functions and decision making occurs somewhere in the central nervous system. The **peripheral nervous system (PNS)** includes any nervous tissue that is not part of the central nervous system. The peripheral nervous system is essentially a highway of bidirectional information flow. Input from the body is sent via the **afferent** neurons of the peripheral nervous system to the central nervous system for interpretation. Subsequently, output is generated by the central nervous system and is sent via the **efferent** neurons of the peripheral nervous system to elsewhere in the periphery (or elsewhere in the central nervous system).

> **NOTE**
>
> The exception to normal information flow in the nervous system are **reflexes**, in which the input (stimulus) is not sent to the brain for interpretation before an output (response) is generated. One way reflexes can be tested during physical exam is with a reflex hammer (e.g. *knee jerk reflex*). The stimulus is a sudden lengthening of a tendon or muscle that results in contraction of that muscle and subsequent shortening. This is a protective mechanism meant to prevent overstretching and injury.

The peripheral nervous system is further classified into two divisions (Fig. 14.2). The *somatic nervous system* consists of peripheral components that innervate skeletal muscle. This part of the nervous system is responsible for voluntary muscle movement. The *autonomic nervous system* consists of peripheral components that are responsible for the involuntary functions of the body. Some examples include sweating, production of glandular secretions, peristalsis in the GI tract, and heart rate.

The autonomic nervous system is also divided into two components. The *sympathetic nervous system* is responsible for the body's response to possible danger. Some effects of SNS activation include a racing heart, sweating, and feeling on edge. This is due to the generation of *catecholamines* (one that might be familiar is *epinephrine*). Contrarily, the *parasympathetic nervous system* is responsible for the body's normal homeostatic functions. Such functions include digestion and producing glandular secretions.

As mentioned above, the central nervous system consists of the brain and spinal cord. The **brain** is the most centralized organ of the nervous system, protected within the hard cranial vault of the skull. There are many components that comprise the brain, but the most relevant to the scribe are the cerebrum, brainstem, and cerebellum (Fig. 14.3).

The **cerebrum** is the largest part of the brain, and is responsible for higher level thought and decision making, interpretation of the senses, and execution of voluntary motor function (amongst many other functions). It contains the **cerebral cortex**—the outer layer of grey matter—as well as several other subcortical structures. The cortex is divided into four primary lobes, including the paired *parietal* and *temporal lobes*, and the single *frontal* and *occipital lobes* (Fig. 14.4). As the names imply, these are located in the same place as the similarly named bones of the skull. Each primary lobe is subdivided into smaller lobes, all of which serve a different function (the details of which are not pertinent for a scribe to know). The grooves of the cerebral cortex are called **sulci**, while the folds are termed **gyri**.

The **brainstem** (Fig. 14.5) is located on the ventral aspect of the cortex and is responsible for more life dependent functions, such as respiration and heart rate. It is comprised of three sections, the *midbrain*, *pons*, and *medulla*.

The **cerebellum** is located ventrally and posterior to the cortex (see Fig. 14.3). Its primary role is motor function, especially involving coordination and balance.

Within the brain there are several compartments, termed **ventricles. Cerebrospinal fluid (CSF)** is produced and contained within the ventricles, and functions to nourish and protect the entire central nervous system. In the spinal canal, CSF is located in the subarachnoid space (discussed below).

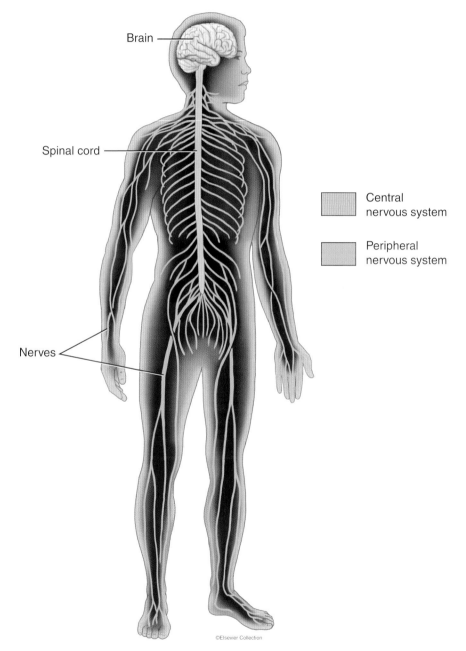

Brain

Spinal cord

Nerves

Central
nervous system

Peripheral
nervous system

©Elsevier Collection

Fig. 14.1   Components of the nervous system. (© Elsevier Collection)

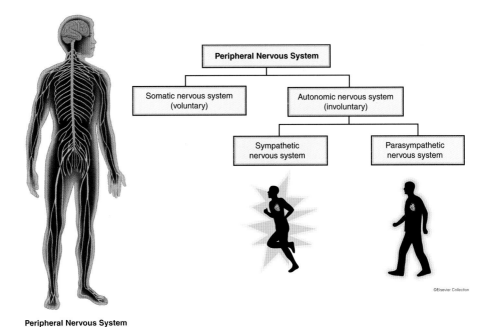

Peripheral Nervous System

Fig. 14.2　Functions of the peripheral nervous system. (© Elsevier Collection)

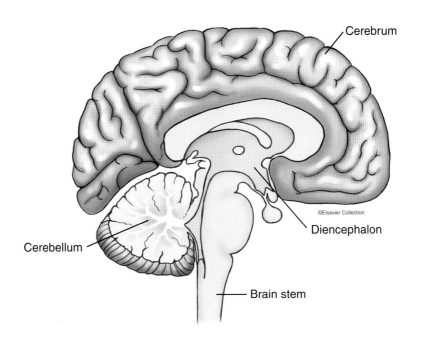

Fig. 14.3　Parts of the brain. (© Elsevier Collection)

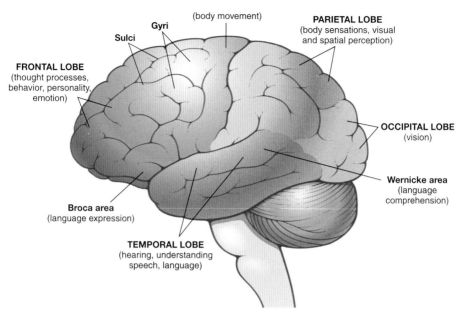

Fig. 14.4 Lobes of the cerebral cortex and their functions. (From Chabner, D. *Language of medicine*, 12th edition, St. Louis, 2021, Elsevier.)

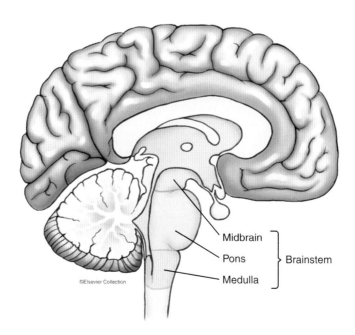

Fig. 14.5 Parts of the brainstem. (© Elsevier Collection)

The **spinal cord** is essentially a continuation of the CNS outside the skull. It is contained within the *spinal canal*, extending from the brain to the lumbar spine (Fig. 14.6). The spinal cord exits the skull via the **foramen magnum**, which is a large hole at the base of the skull. The spinal cord terminates as the **cauda equina** ("horse's tail")—a group of nerve roots located in the lumbar region.

Meninges are layers of connective tissue that form several compartments within the central nervous system (Fig. 14.7). They surround both the brain and spinal cord, and are continuous as they travel through the foramen magnum at the base of the skull to enter the *vertebral foramen*.

The **dura mater** is the most superficial meningeal layer. In the spinal canal, the **epidural space** is located between the dura mater and the vertebrae. In the spinal canal this is a normal anatomical space. In the head, however, the epidural space is known as a potential space. This is because it is not normally present, but can be created with a certain type of bleeding in the head (epidural hematoma).

NOTE

The epidural space is used for epidural injections, such as those given prior to childbirth or for pain management.

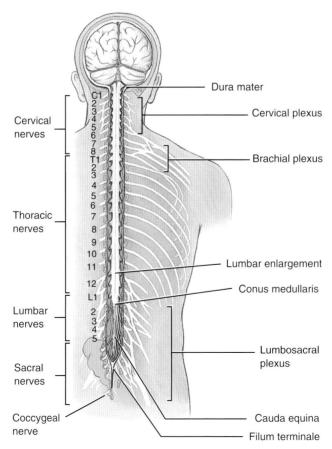

Fig. 14.6   Gross anatomy of the spinal cord. (From Shiland, BJ: *Medical terminology and anatomy for coding*, ed 4, St. Louis, 2021, Elsevier.)

Deep to the dura mater is the **arachnoid mater**. Between the dura mater and the arachnoid mater is the **subdural space**. Sometimes excessive fluid (such as blood) can accumulate in the subdural space and cause problems (subdural hematoma).

Deep to the arachnoid mater is the **subarachnoid space**. Cerebrospinal fluid circulates through the spinal canal in the subarachnoid space. The meningeal layer that lies deep to the arachnoid mater is the **pia mater**. The pia mater is directly adherent to the brain and spinal cord.

> **NOTE**
>
> The subarachnoid space is the compartment that is accessed during a **lumbar puncture** (spinal tap), in which CSF is collected for analysis. (Refer to Fig. 14.10 below.)

From the spinal cord, *dorsal* and *ventral spinal roots* arise and exit the vertebral canal via the *intervertebral foramen* (Fig. 14.8). A dorsal and ventral spinal root at the same level join to

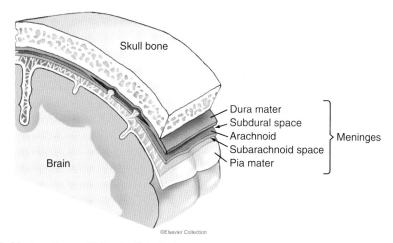

Fig. 14.7 Meningeal layers. (© Elsevier Collection)

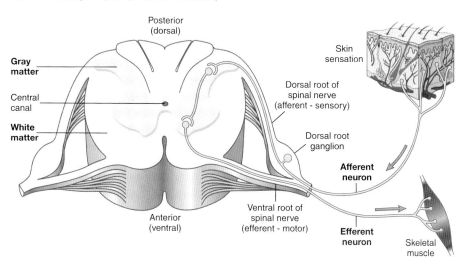

Fig. 14.8 Dorsal and ventral spinal roots forming the spinal nerves. (From Chabner, D. *Language of medicine*, 12th edition, St. Louis, 2021, Elsevier.)

form a *spinal nerve*. This is part of the peripheral nervous system: spinal nerves transmit sensory information from the body to the CNS (input, or *afferent*), and motor information from the CNS to the body (output, or *efferent*). Autonomic information from the parasympathetic and sympathetic nervous systems has bidirectional information flow.

In the head, an equivalent set of nerves to the spinal nerves are the **cranial nerves** that arise from the brain. Like spinal nerves, cranial nerves also transmit sensory information from the head and neck to the CNS (input), and motor information from the CNS to the head and neck (output). Cranial nerves also supply sensory organs in the head: eyes (sight), ears (hearing and balance), the nose (smell), and tongue (taste).

A **neuron** is a specialized cell found in the nervous system. A **motor neuron** is a neuron that innervates muscles and glands. Motor neurons have two components. An *upper motor neuron*

Medical Terminology Word Parts for the Nervous System

Combining Forms

neur/o	nerve
somat/o	body
cerebr/o	cerebrum
cortic/o	(cerebral) cortex
ventricul/o	ventricle
cerebell/o	cerebellum
spin/o	spinal
mening/o meningi/o	meninges
dur/o	dura mater
crani/o	skull
rhiz/o radicul/o	nerve root
phas/o	speech
tax/o	order, coordination
cord/o chord/o myel/o	spinal cord
nuch/o	neck
my/o	muscle
carp/o	wrist
dipl/o	double
schiz/o	split
phren/o psych/o	mind

Prefixes

a- an-	without

Prefixes

sub-	under
inter-	between
para-	near, beside, abnormal
par-	near
dys-	bad
epi-	above, upon
intra-	within

Suffixes

-al -ic	pertaining to
-esthesia	sensation
-phobia	fear
-sterixis	fixed position
-algia	pain
-sclerosis	abnormal condition of hardening
-itis	inflammation
-trophy	growth
-kinesis	movement
-oma	tumor, mass
-tomy	cutting
-ectomy	removal
-rrhage	bursting forth
-lepsy	seizure
-pathy	disease process
-osis	abnormal condition

begins in the brain or spinal cord and synapses with a *lower motor neuron*, which innervates the muscle or gland. A **synapse** is an electrochemical junction at which signal is transmitted between neurons, or between a neuron and its target. Often signal is transmitted with the aid of **neurotransmitters** (chemical messengers). Some that may be familiar are *dopamine, acetylcholine*, and *serotonin*.

Review of Systems

Patients often describe what they are feeling in a manner which makes the most sense to them. It is the duty of the scribe to translate the patient's interpretation of their nervous system symptoms into medical lingo. For example, if a patient says they have been having a "pins and needles" tingling sensation, the scribe should document "paresthesias."

Symptoms that can be placed in multiple systems have been designated as such in italics. Remember to always maximize the number of systems that are included in the review of systems so that the chart can be billed at higher levels (if desired). For example: if a patient is having weakness and urinary incontinence, it would be best to include weakness in "*neurologic*" and urinary incontinence in "*genitourinary*" (two billable systems), as opposed to including weakness and urinary incontinence in "*neurologic*" (one billable system).

The scribe should understand that *dizziness* is rather non-specific as a complaint, and could have *neurological* causes (**vertigo** or **disequilibrium**) or *cardiovascular/constitutional* causes (such as pre-syncope due to anemia, dehydration, or cardiac causes). Dizziness should be placed under "neurologic" if/when the symptoms are associated with a headache or seizure or if the cause is unclear.

Amnesia - memory loss

Anesthesias - numbness

Aphasia - inability to express speech

Blurred vision (*HEENT*) - loss of visual clarity

Deafness (*HEENT*) - complete or partial hearing loss

Diplopia (*HEENT*) - seeing double

Dizziness (*cardiovascular, constitutional*) - sensation that the room is spinning (**vertigo**) or balance is off (**disequilibrium**) or feeling like one is about to black out (**near syncope**)

Dysesthesias - abnormal and often painful sensation

Facial droop - unilateral facial weakness

Fecal incontinence (*digestive*) - involuntary bowel movement

Cephalgia – a headache; sensation of discomfort or pain in any region of the head

Paresthesias - tingling "pins and needles" sensation that is usually due to nerve injury

Radicular symptoms (*musculoskeletal*) - radiating pain down an extremity due to injury or irritation of a nerve

Saddle anesthesia - numbness of the groin region that can be indicative of *cauda equina syndrome* (a medical emergency, discussed below)

Scintillating scotoma (*HEENT*) - visual disturbances with light that typically precede a migraine

Tinnitus (*HEENT*) - hearing sound (e.g. ringing) when none is present

Unilateral weakness - weakness of one side

Urinary incontinence (*genitourinary*) - loss of urinary control

Voice hoarseness (*HEENT*) - changes in the sound of voice

Cauda equina syndrome occurs when there is compression of the terminal nerve roots of the spinal cord. This may cause low back pain with numbness in the groin (documented as **saddle anesthesias), leg weakness**, and **urinary** or **bowel incontinence** (loss of bladder or bowel control). This is a medical emergency and should be addressed right away.

PSYCHIATRIC SYMPTOMS

"*Psychiatric*" is classified and billed as an individual system in review of systems, however it has been included in this chapter because of the pathophysiology. The following symptoms should be documented in "*psychiatric*" for review of systems:

Anorexia (*constitutional, digestive, endocrine*) - loss of appetite

Anger outbursts - episodes of anger with little to no provocation

Anxiety - feeling uneasy

Auditory hallucinations - hearing things that are not really there

Germaphobia - having unrealistic fears of microbes

Homicidal ideation - thinking or planning to hurt or kill someone else

Nonrestorative sleep - waking up feeling unrefreshed

Sleep disturbances - any disruption in sleep

Suicidal ideation - thinking or planning on hurting or killing oneself

Visual hallucinations - seeing things that are not really there

Physical Exam

During the physical exam of the nervous system, provider's objective findings are often supported by several evaluations and tests. There are twelve pairs of cranial nerves (CN I-XII) that can be tested on physical exam (Fig. 14.9). CN I (olfaction) is often not tested unless by a specialist. CN II - XII are routinely tested in any setting if clinically warranted. If normal, **CN II-XII intact** should be documented.

The sobriety testing that law enforcement officers do is actually an evaluation of cerebellar function (since alcohol mainly affects the cerebellum). Many of these tests are also performed medically. These include **finger-to-nose** or **heel-to-shin testing**, and **tandem walking** (walking heel-to-toe). Abnormalities in any of these tests indicate **cerebellar ataxia.**

Meningitis is inflammation of the meninges. **Meningismus** describes symptoms that are caused by the meningeal inflammation, typically including fever, neck stiffness, and headache. Meningismus can be elicited on physical exam (**signs of meningismus**). These include **Kernig's** and **Brudzinski's signs**, and **nuchal rigidity** (inability to flex the neck). Absence of nuchal rigidity may also be documented as **neck is supple**, implying range of motion is intact.

Alertness - awake and awareness of time, person, and place (aka: oriented ×3)

Asterixis - tremor of the hand when the wrist is extended that indicates a problem with the motor systems in the brain

Ataxia - poorly coordinated muscle movements (finger to nose and heel to shin tests) that typically indicates a cerebellar problem

Battle's sign - bruising over the mastoid process of the skull that could indicate possible basilar skull fracture

Brudzinski's sign - touching chin to chest causes neck pain and the urge to draw knees up (sign of meningismus)

Cranial nerve II-XII tests - set of commands used to determine functionality of the cranial nerves

Dix-Hallpike - a test involving rotation of the patient's head that is used to determine if dizziness results from positional changes (positive test reproduces vertigo and nystagmus)

Dysdiadochokinesia - impaired ability to perform rapid alternating movement typically due to a cerebellar problem

Focal neurologic deficit - acute changes in neurologic function (especially unilateral) that affects specific areas of the body

Gait (normal, tandem, heel or toe walking) - observed and described in any of a number of ways depending on the clinical presentation (e.g. spastic gait, limping or other gait type)

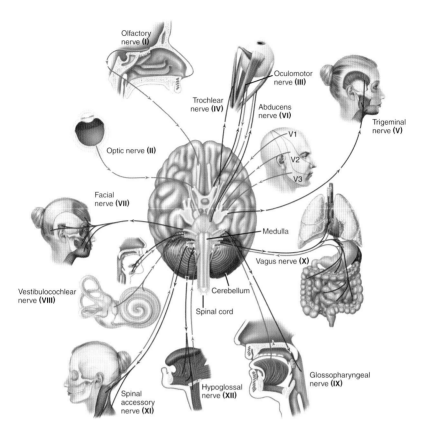

NERVE	TYPE	FUNCTION
(I) Olfactory	Sensory	Sense of smell
(II) Optic	Sensory	Sense of sight
(III) Oculomotor	Motor	Movement of eye muscles
(IV) Trochlear	Motor	Movement of eye muscles
(V) Trigeminal	Motor	Movement of muscles of mastication and other cranial muscles
	Sensory	General sensations for face, head, skin, teeth, oral cavity, and tongue
(VI) Abducens	Motor	Movement of eye muscles
(VII) Facial	Motor	Facial expression, functions of glands and muscles
	Sensory	Sense of taste on tongue
(VIII) Vestibulocochlear	Sensory	Senses of sound and balance
(IX) Glossopharyngeal	Motor	Functioning of parotid gland
	Sensory	General sensation of skin around ear
(X) Vagus	Motor	Moves muscles in soft palate, pharynx, and larynx
	Sensory	General sensation on skin around ear and sense of taste
(XI) Accessory	Motor	Movement of muscles of the neck, soft palate, and pharynx
(XII) Hypoglossal	Motor	Movement of muscles of the tongue

Fig. 14.9 Anatomy and function of the twelve pairs of cranial nerves. (© Elsevier Collection)

Glasgow Coma Scale (GCS) - score measuring a patient's conscious state that is used to predict morbidity/mortality from neurologic injury. Lower scores represent a more severe neurological problem (Table 14.1).

Kernig's sign - straightening the knee causes pain in the neck and/or back (sign of meningismus)

TABLE 14.1 ■ Glasgow Coma Scale

Response	Score	Significance
Eye Opening		
Spontaneously	4	Reticular activating system intact; patient may not be aware
To verbal command	3	Opens eyes when told to do so
To pain	2	Opens eyes in response to pain
No eye opening	1	Does not open eyes to any stimuli
Verbal Stimuli		
Oriented, converses	5	Relatively intact CNS, aware of self and environment
Disoriented, converses	4	Well-articulated, organized, but disoriented
Inappropriate words	3	Random exclamatory words
Incomprehensible	2	Moaning, no recognizable words
No verbal response	1	No response or intubated
Motor Response		
Obeys verbal commands	6	Readily moves limbs when told to
Localizes to painful stimuli	5	Moves limb in an effort to remove painful stimuli
Flexion withdrawal	4	Pulls away from pain in flexion
Abnormal flexion	3	Decorticate rigidity
Extension	2	Decerebrate rigidity
No motor response	1	Hypotonia, flaccid—suggests loss of medullary function or concomitant spinal cord injury

From Walls RM, Hockberger RS, Gaushe-Hill M: Rosen's emergency medicine: concepts and clinical practice, ed 9, Philadelphia, 2018, Elsevier.

Motor (strength) testing - muscle strength is evaluated and compared to the contralateral side to evaluate for possible nerve or muscle problem

National Institutes of Health (NIH) Stroke Scale - quantification of damage/disability caused by stroke

Pronator drift - test using both hands held pronated at shoulder level to evaluate upper motor neuron disease (hands drift in a positive test)

Raccoon eyes - bruising around both eyes (resembling a raccoon) that can indicate basilar skull fracture

Reflex testing - most commonly, muscular reflexes will be tested with a reflex hammer to evaluate damage to the reflex arc

Romberg's sign - testing **proprioception** (awareness of body position) by asking the patient to stand with both eyes closed (in a positive test the patient will sway and may even lose their balance)

Sensation testing - sensation to light touch, pain, pressure, vibration is tested to evaluate possible nerve injury

PSYCHIATRIC SIGNS

"*Psychiatric*" is classified and billed as an individual system in physical exam, however it has been included in this chapter because of the pathophysiology. The following signs should be documented in "*psychiatric*" for physical exam:

Affect - emotional tone

Compulsive behavior - having urges to do things in attempt to alleviate anxiety caused by obsessions

Depersonalization - when one distances themselves from reality

Insight - awareness of one's own situation

Judgement - a person's ability to appropriately assess a situation

Mania or hypomania - period of abnormally elevated mood and activity

Mood - emotional state (e.g. depressed, inappropriate, elated)

Obsessive - having intrusive, unwanted, or repeated thoughts or feelings

Paranoia - suspicion or mistrust that can be unrealistic or unwarranted

Pressured speech - speech pattern in which the individual seems rushed

Racing thoughts - when a person has a flight of ideas with poor flow or little connection between thoughts

Operations/Procedures

Any of the patient's prior surgical history (including major operations or minor procedures) may be discussed in the context of a patient's medical history. Patients often do not know the name of the operation and will describe their understanding of the procedure in lay terms. It is the scribe's duty to translate the patient's procedural description into the equivalent medical term. For example, if a patient says they had a shunt placed from their brain to their stomach, the scribe should record that the patient had "VP shunting".

Craniotomy - removal of a part of the skull to access the brain

Coiling - a coil is used in treating a brain aneurysm to prevent it from rupturing and bleeding

Deep brain stimulation (DBS) - electrical currents are delivered to the brain to help treat disease (such as Parkinson Disease)

Electroconvulsive therapy (ECT) - seizures are electrically induced to relieve psychiatric illness

Electromyogram (EMG) - nerve conduction testing

Lumbar puncture (LP) or **spinal tap** - Cerebral spinal fluid (CSF) is removed from the spinal canal by inserting a needle into the lumbar back and maneuvering it into the subarachnoid space (Fig. 14.10). Used to diagnose a variety of neurologic conditions and infections.

Ventriculoperitoneal (VP) shunting - a shunt (essentially a tube) is placed between the ventricles of the brain and abdominal cavity to drain excessive fluid in the brain (Fig. 14.11)

Problem List

The problem list should always be kept up to date and the practitioner may have the scribe assist in this process. Any new neurological or psychiatric diagnoses or signs and symptoms should be added while any resolved issues should be eliminated. Thus if the patient has developed recent onset of headaches these would be documented as "cephalgia" if the cause is still unknown, or perhaps "migraines" if that is the diagnosed cause of these new headaches. Sometimes the patient will call a bad headache a "migraine" but your provider will let you know if that is the correct term or not since "migraine" indicates a specific clinical condition and not any "bad headache."

Patients often do not know the name of a specific diagnosis, but will instead describe it to their provider. It is the scribe's duty to translate the lay terms into medical terminology. For example, if the patient says he or she had shingles last year, the scribe should document "herpes zoster."

Alzheimer's disease - neurodegenerative disease associated with plaques and tangles in the brain that cause memory loss and personality changes

Amyotrophic lateral sclerosis (ALS; Lou Gehrig's) - disorder of neuronal death in upper and lower motor neurons that causes loss of motor function and eventually death

Anorexia nervosa - eating disorder characterized by low weight, poor body image, and food restriction

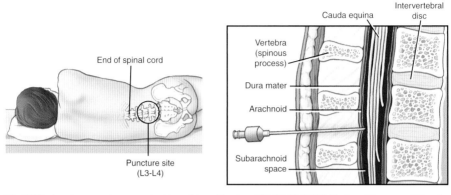

Fig. 14.10 Lumbar puncture or spinal tap. (From Elsevier: ICD-10-CM/PCS Coding: Theory and Practice: 2021/2022 Edition, St. Louis, 2021, Elsevier.)

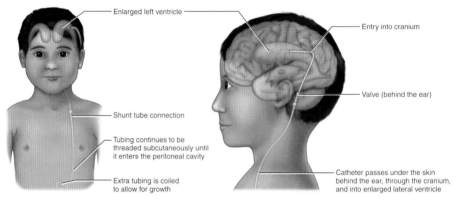

Fig. 14.11 A ventriculoperitoneal (VP) shunt in a child. (From Silvestri LA, Silvestri AE: *Saunders comprehensive review for the NCLEX-PN® examination*, ed 8, St. Louis, 2022, Elsevier.)

Anxiety disorder - excessive anxiety and fear

Attention deficit hyperactivity disorder (ADHD) - a condition that typically manifests in young children a combination of poor focus, excessive activity, and impulsivity

Bipolar disorder - disorder that can manifest as alternating periods of depression and mania or hypomania

Borderline personality disorder (BPD) - pattern of impulsivity and inconsistent relationships

Bulimia nervosa - eating disorder characterized by binge eating and purging by vomiting

Carpal tunnel syndrome - median nerve compression causing pain and sensation changes in the lateral hand

Cerebral contusion - brain bruise

Cerebral edema - brain swelling

Cerebral hemorrhage - intracranial hemorrhage within brain tissue

Cerebrovascular accident (CVA; stroke) - blood supply to a part of the brain is blocked, resulting in tissue injury or death

Concussion (mild traumatic brain injury) - a brain injury that temporarily affects brain function and may result in headaches and temporary short-term memory loss

Depression - having a low mood for a prolonged period of time

Epilepsy - seizure disorder

Herpes zoster (shingles) - reactivation of chickenpox virus along the distribution of a single nerve root

Intracranial hematoma - hemorrhage within the skull

Meningitis - inflammation of the meninges

Multiple sclerosis (MS) - demyelinating disease damaging the neuronal insulating covers and affecting the transmission of neuronal signal

Obsessive compulsive disorder (OCD) - obsessions associated with repeatedly doing things (compulsions) to alleviate the obsessions

Oppositional defiant disorder (ODD) - pattern of defiance in a child

Parkinson disease - degenerative brain disease that causes a dopamine deficiency manifested as muscle rigidity and tremor (Fig. 14.12)

Peripheral neuropathy - damage to peripheral nerves causing sensory changes or pain

Postpartum depression (PPD) - severe and sometimes prolonged depression after childbirth

Psychosis - having lost contact with reality

Radiculopathy - pain, weakness, or numbness radiating to any extremity from nerve dysfunction

Schizophrenia - disease characterized by episodes of psychosis

Sciatica - pain, weakness, or numbness radiating to a lower extremity from nerve dysfunction in the lower back

Seizure - episode of excessive neuronal activity that manifests in a variety of ways (e.g. jerking and relaxation (tonic-clonic), periods of 'absence' or blank staring)

Transient ischemic attack (TIA) - transient lack of blood flow to the brain causing tissue ischemia but not tissue death (not as severe as stroke)

Vertigo (dizziness) - sensation that the self or objects are moving when they are not (room is spinning)

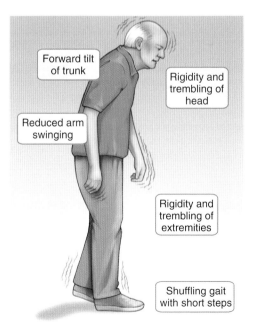

Fig. 14.12 The signs of Parkinson disease include (but are not limited to) rigidity and trembling of the head and extremities, a forward tilt of the trunk, and a shuffling gait with short steps and reduced arm swinging. (From Patton KT, Thibodeau: *The human body in health and disease*, ed 7, St. Louis, 2018, Elsevier.)

The police brought Mr. McCarthy, a 55-year-old male, to the emergency department (ED) because he has been combative and angry towards them. Visiting from out-of-state, Mr. McCarthy was on a hunting trip and had been playing darts this evening at a bar in town. He started a fight with three locals whom he accused of "messing" with his truck. Mr. McCarthy is hostile with the staff in the ED, is insisting the police investigate damage to his vehicle, and demands the nursing staff bring him a Mountain Dew.

Phil Dwyer, the medical scribe, accompanies the attending physician in the ED, Dr. Bloom, for Mr. McCarthy's H&P. The patient reports that he hasn't slept in three nights but that he feels great. "I'd be even better if someone here could get me a Mountain Dew," Mr. McCarthy says sarcastically. He tells Dr. Bloom that he has a bipolar diagnosis and that he stopped taking his medication about a week ago. He denies drinking alcohol but could not complete the finger-to-nose test administered by the physician.

QUESTIONS

1. What is Mr. McCarthy's chief complaint?
2. Dr. Bloom describes both the patient's mood and affect as "euphoric." Does Phil record this as part of the ROS or the PE?
3. Mr. McCarthy is worried that people have damaged his truck. What is the term for this state of suspicion or mistrust that can be unrealistic or unwarranted?
4. The sobriety test Dr. Bloom administered reveals an abnormal functioning in what part of Mr. McCarthy's brain?
5. In what part of the HPI would Phil document the patient's bipolar diagnosis?

Medications

A scribe should be able to diligently record the patient's medication list, which includes the drug name (generic or brand), dose, frequency, and indication (reason for taking the drug).

Although knowing the drug class mechanism of action isn't essential to become a great scribe, having familiarity with the mechanism can facilitate faster and more accurate documentation (Table 14.2). This is because within a class, the generic names tend to sound similar. This is usually a good way to identify a drug class from a generic name. For example, the serotonin agonists used to treat headache all end in "triptan."

You may hear terminology for different drug classes that is based on their general actions, like anti-psychotics, anti-depressants, mood stabilizers, **anxiolytic** (antianxiety) agents, or stimulants. You may also hear of classes of drugs that are based on their chemical formulation and so should be comfortable with terms like tricyclics, selective serotonin reuptake inhibitors (SSRIs) and monoamine oxidase inhibitors (MAOIs).

Psychiatric conditions are often the result of imbalances in **neurotransmitters** (chemical messengers) within the nervous system. Thus the most effective treatment for such conditions is to use drugs that correct these neurotransmitter imbalances.

TABLE 14.2 ■ **Selected Nervous System Medications**

Drug Class and Uses	Generic Name (Brand Name)
Antiepileptics (not a class) • Used to prevent and treat seizures	**Sodium channel antagonists** carbamazepine (Tegretol) lacosamide (Vimpat) lamotrigine (Lamictal) phenytoin (Dilantin) topiramate (Topamax) **Calcium channel antagonists** valproate (Depakote) **GABA/glutamate modifiers** levetiracetam (Keppra)

Continued

TABLE 14.2 ■ Selected Nervous System Medications—cont'd

Drug Class and Uses	Generic Name (Brand Name)
Serotonin agonists • Used to treat migraines and other headaches	eletriptan (Relpax) sumatriptan (Imitrex) zolmitriptan (Zomig)
Mood stabilizer • Not a class • Used to treat many mood disorders such as depression, bipolar disorder, and schizophrenia	Lithium (Eskalith, Lithobid)
Antidepressants • Not a classUsed to treat depression and some other mood disorders	**Selective serotonin reuptake inhibitors (SSRI)** citalopram (Celexa) escitalopram (Lexapro) fluoxetine (Prozac) paroxetine (Paxil) sertraline (Zoloft) **Serotonin norepinephrine reuptake inhibitors (SNRI)** duloxetine (Cymbalta) milnacipran (Savella) venlafaxine (Effexor) **Tricyclic antidepressants (TCA)** amitriptyline (Elavil) nortriptyline **Others** bupropion (Wellbutrin) pregabalin (Lyrica)
Sedative-hypnotics • Not a class • Anxiolytic (antianxiety) or for sleep induction	**Barbiturates** phenobarbital (Luminal) **Benzodiazepine** alprazolam (Xanax) clonazepam (Klonopin) diazepam (Valium) lorazepam (Ativan) temazepam (Restoril) **Others** zolpidem (Ambien)
Antipsychotics • Used to treat psychosis	aripiprazole (Abilify) clozapine (Clozaril) haloperidol (Haldol) quetiapine (Seroquel) risperidone (Risperdal) ziprasidone (Geodon)
CNS stimulants • From many classes) • Used to treat ADHD/ADD	amphetamine (Vyvanse) dextroamphetamine (Adderall) methylphenidate (Concerta) or (Ritalin)
Narcotics (opioid agonists) • Modify the pain-reward pathway to produce pleasure and reduce pain	hydrocodone (Vicodin) or (Norco) oxycodone (Percocet) morphine meperidine (Demerol) hydromorphone (Dilaudid) fentanyl (Duragesic) nalbuphine (Nubain) buprenorphine + naloxone (Suboxone) methadone (Dolophine) tramadol (Ultram)
Opioid antagonists • Reverse opioid overdose	naloxone (Narcan)

Practice Questions

1. The primary role of the part of the brain called the _____ is motor function, especially involving coordination and balance.
2. The _____ nervous system controls involuntary bodily functions.
3. The space between the dura and arachnoid mater is the _____ space.
4. The _____ nerves supply motor/sensory function to the head and neck.
5. A 42-year-old male patient presents to the emergency department for an evaluation of low back pain with shooting pains down his left leg, which has been ongoing for years now but have worsened in the last 72 hours. He is now having numbness in his groin region, weakness in both legs, and this morning awoke having urinated during the night without realizing it. He denies any recent falls or trauma to his back. No fevers. How should this be documented in the review of systems?
6. On exam the patient's motor strength is 5/5 in both arms but 3/5 in both legs. He has symmetric diminished sensation to light touch in the buttocks, inner thighs, and perineal region. Anal reflex is absent. Patellar and Achilles reflexes are diminished. There is diffuse low back tenderness in the paraspinal region but no vertebral step off or deformity. Range of motion is limited in flexion and extension of the low back. Skin exam is unremarkable. The patient appears to be in moderate distress. How should this be documented in the physical exam?
7. The patient reports a history of narrowing of the spinal canal that was diagnosed by his family doctor. What should be documented in the patient's medical history?
8. Given the patient's presentation and history of spinal stenosis the physician is concerned about cauda equina syndrome. She orders an emergent MRI of the patient's lumbosacral spine. If cauda equina syndrome is confirmed the patient will likely have decompression surgery to remove the lamina from the stenotic vertebrae. What is this operation called?
9. Cauda equina syndrome secondary to spinal stenosis is confirmed on the MRI and the patient is admitted for surgery. The emergency medicine physician gives the patient a narcotic pain medication until the surgery. Which medication is a narcotic?
   a. morphine
   b. naloxone (Narcan)
   c. amphetamine (Vyvanse)
   d. haloperidol (Haldol)

CHAPTER 15

Cardiovascular System

1. Use medical terminology to document medical issues involving the cardiovascular system.
2. Describe the anatomy and physiology of the cardiovascular system.
3. Document cardiovascular system symptoms related during a review of systems.
4. Document signs related by the provider during a physical exam of the cardiovascular system.
5. Document operations and procedures for the cardiovascular system.
6. Document the cardiovascular system clinical impressions, diagnoses, and signs and symptoms commonly found in a problem list.
7. Document relevant drug classes and medications for the treatment of problems associated with the cardiovascular system.

Aneurysm
Angina
Angiography
Aorta
Aortic coarctation
Aortic valve
Apex
Arrhythmia
Artery
Atherosclerosis
Atria (s. atrium)
Atrial fibrillation
Atrial flutter
Base (of the heart)
Bradycardia
Bruit
Capillary
Cardiovascular system
Cardioversion
Coronary artery bypass
  graft (CABG)

Deep vein thrombosis
  (DVT)
Diaphoresis
Dyspnea
Echocardiogram
Endocardium
Epicardium
Gallop
Heart
Holter monitor
Mitral (bicuspid) valve
Murmur
Myocardial infarction (MI)
Myocarditis
Myocardium
Palpitations
Pericardiocentesis
Pericardium (pericardial
  sac)
Pulmonary artery
Pulmonary embolism

Pulmonary hypertension
Pulmonary vein
Pulmonic (pulmonary)
  valve
Pulse
Regurgitation
Sick sinus syndrome (SSS)
Stenosis
Syncope
Tachycardia
Telangiectasia
Tricuspid valve
Varicose vein
Vasculature
Vein
Vena cava
Ventricle
Ventricular hypertrophy

Anatomy and Physiology

The **cardiovascular system** consists of the **heart**, a hollow muscular organ which is responsible for pumping blood throughout the **vasculature**, a network of arteries and veins (Fig. 15.1). Blood is the transportation system of our body. It is especially important in transporting oxygen from

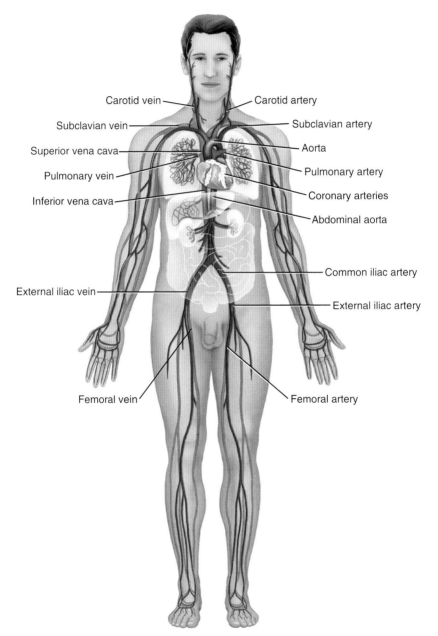

Fig. 15.1   The heart, arteries, and veins of the cardiovascular system. (From Leonard PC: *Quick & easy medical terminology*, ed 9, St. Louis, 2020, Elsevier.)

the lungs to the body's tissues for cellular respiration. Subsequently it transports carbon dioxide, a waste product from cellular respiration, back to the lungs for exhalation.

The heart is composed of four layers (Fig. 15.2). The innermost membranous layer is known as the **endocardium**. This layer makes contact with the blood that fills each of the chambers. The middle layer is the **myocardium**. This layer is composed of muscle cells that provide the force allowing the heart to contract. The superficial layers are the **epicardium**, which is the outermost layer of the heart, and the **pericardium (or pericardial sac)**, which is a fibrous sac that surrounds the entire heart. Together, these two layers form the *pericardial cavity*—a space between the epicardium and pericardium filled with *pericardial fluid* that reduces friction.

The heart's interior is sectioned into four chambers (Fig. 15.3). The superior two chambers are the left and right **atria** (**atrium**, singular). The two atria are separated by the *interatrial septum*. The atria receive blood from elsewhere in the body and direct it to the **ventricles**, which are the two chambers located inferiorly to the atria. The ventricles are separated by the *interventricular septum*. After receiving blood from the atria, the ventricles send it elsewhere in the body.

The chambers of the heart are separated from each other and from the great vessels by heart valves. The four heart valves ensure that blood flows unidirectionally. On the right side of the heart there are two valves. The **tricuspid valve** separates the right atrium and the right ventricle, and the **pulmonic (or pulmonary) valve** separates the right ventricle from the pulmonary artery, which directs blood to the lungs. On the left side of the heart there are also two valves. The **mitral (or bicuspid) valve** separates the left atrium from the left ventricle, and the **aortic valve** separates the left ventricle from the aorta, which directs blood to the rest of the body.

The circulatory system has three primary types of vessels. **Arteries** carry oxygenated blood away from the heart to the rest of the body (with the exception of the pulmonary artery, discussed below). **Veins** carry deoxygenated blood to the heart, so that it can be sent to the lungs for reoxygenation (with the exception of the pulmonary veins, also discussed below). **Capillaries** are tiny vessels that exchange gases, primarily oxygen and carbon dioxide, with the body's tissues. Capillaries connect the arterial (oxygenated) and venous (deoxygenated) systems (Fig. 15.4).

Pulses are the result of arterial expansion as blood is forced through these vessels. The major pulses are depicted in Fig. 10.3.

There are a few major veins and arteries that connect to the heart (Fig. 15.5). On the right side of the heart, the **superior** and **inferior vena cava** are major veins that direct deoxygenated blood from the body to the right atrium. The **pulmonary arteries**, which exit the right ventricle

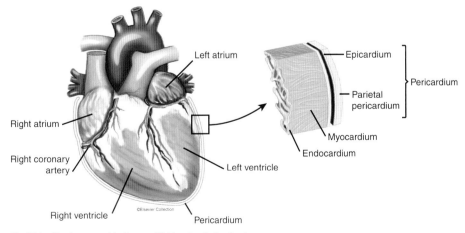

Fig. 15.2   The heart and its layers. (© Elsevier Collection.)

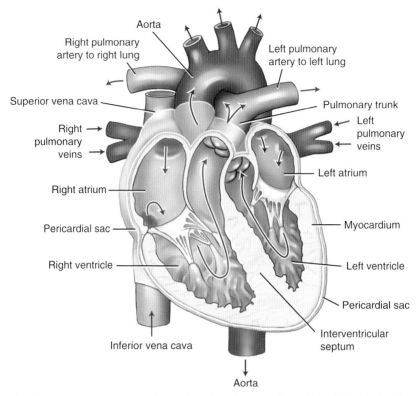

Fig. 15.3 Heart anatomy and the flow of blood through its chambers. (From Shiland, BJ: *Medical terminology and anatomy for coding*, ed 4, St. Louis, 2021, Elsevier.)

and transport blood to the lungs for reoxygenation, are the only arteries within the body that carry deoxygenated blood. On the left side of the heart are the **pulmonary veins**, which carry oxygenated blood from the lungs to the left atrium. These are the only veins in the body that carry oxygenated blood. The blood is sent from the left atrium to the left ventricle, and the **aorta** directs the oxygenated blood from the left ventricle to the body.

It is worth having a brief discussion about blood flow and how this relates to oxygen transport in particular. The circulatory system is actually divided into two separate systems—the deoxygenated system (the "right" sided system) and the oxygenated system (the corresponding "left" sided system). As intuited, the oxygenated system carries oxygen to the body's tissues. The deoxygenated system carries carbon dioxide (a waste product) to the lungs to be exhaled.

Let's first start with the deoxygenated system (the "right" side). Deoxygenated blood enters the right atrium of the heart via the superior and inferior vena cava. From here it enters the right ventricle, and is sent to the lungs via the pulmonary arterial trunk and the smaller pulmonary arteries (remember, this is the exception to the rule where arteries normally carry oxygenated blood). At the lungs the deoxygenated blood gets rid of the carbon dioxide it had been carrying (a waste product), and picks up oxygen instead. It is now oxygenated blood.

This brings us to the oxygenated system (the "left" side). Oxygenated blood leaves the lungs and enters the left atrium via the pulmonary veins (remember, this is the other exception to the rule where veins normally carry deoxygenated blood). From here it enters the left ventricle, and is sent throughout the body via the aorta and its various branches. At the body's tissues, the

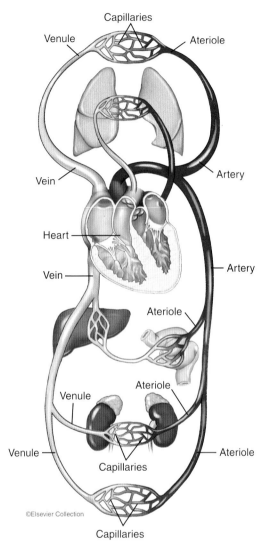

Fig. 15.4 Arteries, arterioles, and finally capillaries carry blood oxygenated by the lungs to the body's cells. Venules and veins return deoxygenated blood to the lungs where gases are again exchanged. (© Elsevier Collection.)

oxygenated blood gives up the oxygen it had been carrying (for cellular respiration), and instead picks up carbon dioxide (a waste product of cellular respiration). The now deoxygenated blood travels back to the right side of the heart for reoxygenation and the cycle begins anew.

Below is a diagram illustrating blood flow pertaining to gas exchange:

Deoxygenated (from body):

vena cava → right atrium → right ventricle → pulmonary artery → lungs

Oxygenated (from lungs):

pulmonary veins → left atrium → left ventricle → aorta → body tissues

Medical Terminology Word Parts for the Cardiovascular System

Combining Forms

cardi/o coron/o	heart
pulmon/o	lung
vascul/o angi/o vas/o	vessel
my/o	muscle
aort/o	aorta
atri/o	atrium, upper heart chamber
ventricul/o	ventricle, lower heart chamber
sept/o	septum
valvul/o, valv/o	valve
arter/o arteri/o	artery
ven/o ven/i phleb/o	vein
capillary/o	capillary
sphygm/o	pulse
ech/o	sound
cyan/o	blue
rhythm/o	rhythm
varic/o	dilated vein
thromb/o	clot
ather/o	yellowish plaque, fatty substance (Greek athere means porridge)
tens/o	stretching

Prefixes

peri-	surrounding
inter-	between
endo-	inner
epi-	above, on top of
a-	without
dia-	through
dys-	bad, difficult
intra-	within
peri-	around, surrounding
epi-	above, upon
hyper-	excessive
hypo-	below, deficient
brady-	slow
tachy-	fast

Suffixes

-oid	resembling, like
-ar -ary -ous	pertaining to
-algia	pain
-osis	abnormal condition
-sclerosis	abnormal condition of hardening
-itis	inflammation
-emia	blood condition
-pathy	disease
-cardia	heart condition
-trophy	growth
-pnea	breathing
-centesis	surgical puncture
-tomy	cutting
-plasty	surgical formation
-ectomy	removal

Review of Systems

Patients often describe their symptoms, or what they are feeling, in a manner which makes the most sense to them. It is the duty of the scribe to translate the patient's interpretation of their symptoms into medical lingo. For example, if a patient says they passed out or fainted, the scribe should document "syncope." Some common cardiovascular systems are listed below.

    Symptoms that can be placed in multiple systems have been designated as such in italics. Remember to always maximize the number of <u>systems</u> that are included in the review of systems so that the chart can be billed at higher levels (if desired). For example: if a patient is having chest pain and dyspnea, it would be best to include chest pain in "*cardiovascular*" and dyspnea in "*respiratory*" (two systems), as opposed to including chest pain and dyspnea in "*cardiovascular*" (one system).

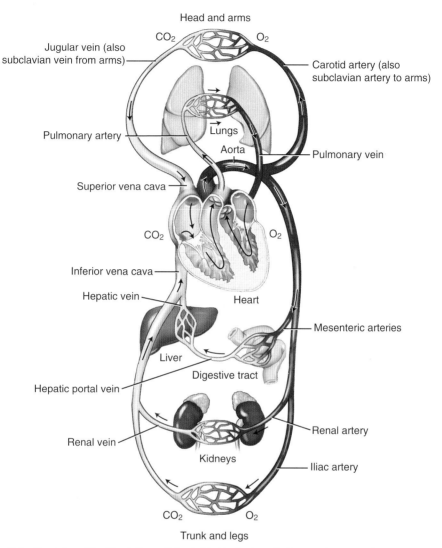

Fig. 15.5 Circulation of the blood. (From Shiland, BJ: *Medical terminology and anatomy for coding*, ed 4, St. Louis, 2021, Elsevier.)

Angina pectoris (Chest pain)—chest discomfort, pressure, heaviness, tightness, etc.

Diaphoresis (*endocrine, integumentary*)—sweating

Dizziness (*constitutional, neurologic*)—sensation that the room is spinning (***vertigo***) or balance is off (***disequilibrium***) or feeling that one is going to black out (near syncope) (*note: placed in the cardiovascular system if associated with chest pain*)

Dyspnea (*respiratory*)—shortness of breath

Dyspnea on exertion (DOE) (*respiratory*)—shortness of breath with exertion

Extremity swelling—collection of fluid in any extremity

High blood pressure—blood pressure above 130/90 for a prolonged period of time (*not the same as hypertension, a diagnosis*)

Orthopnea (*respiratory*)—shortness of breath that worsens lying supine

Palpitations (*endocrine*)—heart beats that are abnormal (such as beats that are irregular, hard, racing, fast, skipped, etc.)

Paroxysmal nocturnal dyspnea (PND) (*respiratory*)—sudden awakening at night with shortness of breath

Platypnea (*respiratory*)—shortness of breath that worsens sitting up

Syncope—brief loss of consciousness

Physical Exam

The heart is located in the thoracic cavity posterior to the sternum. The **apex**, or tip of the heart, is pointed towards the left arm and lies in the left *midclavicular line (MCL)*. (Think of an imaginary line extending from the middle of the clavicle to the inferior rib cage.) Much of the heart is actually located on the left side of the thorax because of this orientation (Fig. 15.6).

As the heart cycles through contraction and relaxation, the sound of the valves closing can be heard with a stethoscope. These are the normal heart sounds (*S1* and *S2*). **Heart murmurs** can be heard when a valve is not functioning properly and creates turbulent blood flow. **Regurgitation** occurs when the valve is unable to close properly and blood flows in the wrong direction. **Stenosis** occurs when the valve cannot completely open and blood is unable to flow freely in the correct direction.

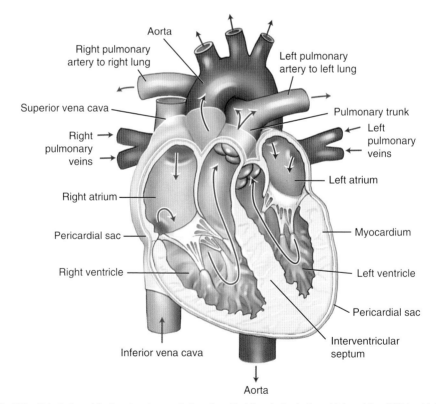

Fig. 15.6 Orientation of the heart and auscultation sites. Red lines indicate the midsternal line (MSL), midclavicular line (MCL) and anterior axillary line (AAL). *ICS*, Intercostal space; *PMI*, point of maximal impulse. (From Harding MM: *Lewis's medical-surgical nursing: assessment and management of clinical problems*, ed 11, St. Louis, 2020, Elsevier.)

The heart's orientation is very important when performing a physical exam. Heart valves are heard in different regions. The aortic valve is heard best at the ***right sternal border (RSB)***—just right of the upper sternum. The pulmonic valve is heard at the ***left sternal border (LSB)***—just left of the upper sternum. The tricuspid valve is best heard at the ***lower left sternal border (LLSB)***— just left of the lower sternum. The mitral valve is best heard at the apex in the MCL. See Fig. 15.6 for the sites where the heart sounds are best heard at during physical exam.

Bradycardia—slow heart rate (below 60 bpm)

Bruit—abnormal sound of arterial blood flow due to a partial blockage

Cyanosis—bluish discoloration often due to hypoxia

Edema—swelling of various parts of the body (most commonly the legs) due to water retention from a variety of causes (local injury, failure of the heart to pump adequately, fluid leakage from inside the blood vessels to the space in the tissues external to the blood vessels, and more). **Pitting edema** is a type of edema in which pressing on the area with edema leaves an indentation that returns to the former swollen state over seconds to minutes.

Gallop—extra heart sound (S3 or S4)

Hepatojugular reflux (HJR)—jugular vein distension elicited by applying pressure to the liver

Homan's sign—with the leg extended, the foot is forcefully dorsiflexed. A positive test will elicit pain in the calf or behind the knee and may be indicative of *deep vein thrombosis (DVT)*.

Jugular vein distention (JVD)—distention of the internal jugular vein on either side of the neck (Fig. 15.7)

Murmur—abnormal heart sound caused by turbulent blood flow through a heart valve

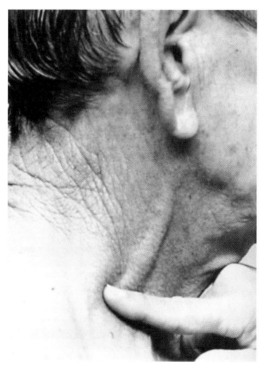

Fig. 15.7 Assessment of jugular vein distention (JVD). (From Urden LD, Stacy KM, Lough ME: *Priorities in critical care nursing,* ed 8, St. Louis, 2020, Elsevier.)

Pericardial friction rub—Velcro-like heart sound heard when there is excess fluid in the pericardial sac

Tachycardia—elevated heart rate (above 100 bpm)

Telangiectasia—small dilated blood vessels near the surface of the skin and mucous membranes (Fig. 15.8)

Varicose veins—veins that have become enlarged and tortuous (Fig. 15.9). The condition can increase susceptibility to **thrombophlebitis**, blood clots and inflammation in the veins.

Venous stasis—poor blood flow in veins that causes chronic discoloration/skin changes to the lower legs

Operations/Procedures

Any of the patient's prior surgical history (including major operations or minor procedures) may be discussed in the context of a patient's medical history. Patients often do not know the name of the operation and will describe their understanding of the procedure in lay terms. It is the scribe's duty to translate the patient's procedural description into the equivalent medical term. For example, if a patient says they had an ultrasound of their heart, the scribe should record that the patient had an "echocardiogram."

Ablation—termination of a faulty electrical pathway in the heart by chemical or electrical means

Angiography—dye and x-rays are used to visualize blood vessels and organs in "real time," often used during other procedures (Fig. 15.10)

Cardiac catheterization—inserting a catheter into the heart for diagnosis and/or intervention (e.g. stenting a coronary artery open during an MI)

Cardiac stents—hollow tubes placed into the coronary arteries to keep them open and prevent ischemia (Fig. 15.11)

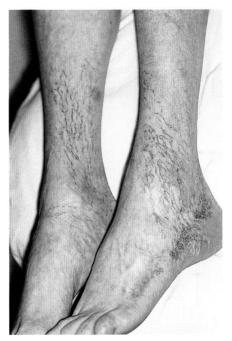

Fig. 15.8   Telangiectasia. (From James WD, Elston DM, Treat JR, Rosenbach MA, Neuhaus IM: *Andrews' diseases of the skin: clinical dermatology*, ed 13, Edinburgh, 2020, Elsevier.)

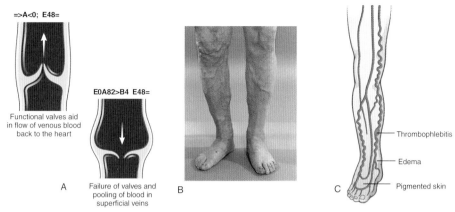

Fig. 15.9 (A) Valve function in normal vein and varicose vein. (B) Varicose veins. (C) The slow flow in veins increases susceptibility to thrombophlebitis (clot formation), edema, and pigmented skin (blood pools in the lower parts of the leg and fluid leaks from distended small capillaries). (From Chabner, DL: *The language of medicine*, ed 12, St. Louis, 2021, Elsevier.)

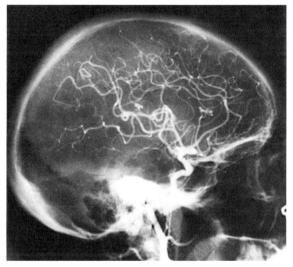

Fig. 15.10 Cerebral angiography. (From Ehrlich RA, Coakes DM: *Patient care in radiography*, ed 9, St. Louis, 2017, Elsevier.)

Cardioversion—using chemicals or electricity to convert an irregular rhythm into normal sinus rhythm

Coronary artery bypass graft (CABG)—the heart is put on bypass and a coronary artery graft is placed to restore blood flow (Fig. 15.12)

Echocardiogram—ultrasound of the heart

Electrophysiology (EP) study—testing the heart's electrical system

Endarterectomy—removal of plaques from the lining of an artery

Holter monitor—portable device that continuously monitors the electrical activity of the heart

Implantable cardiac defibrillator (ICD)—performs heart cardioversion, defibrillation, and pacing

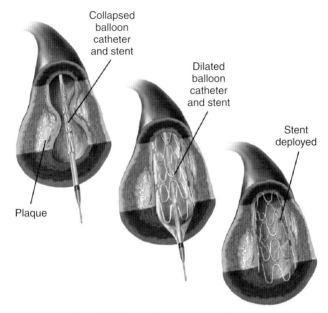

Fig. 15.11 Cardiac stent. (From Good VS, Kirkwood PL: *Advanced critical care nursing*, ed 2, St. Louis, 2018, Elsevier.)

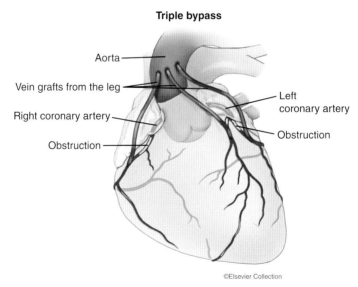

©Elsevier Collection

Fig. 15.12 Coronary artery bypass graft (CABG). (© Elsevier Collection.)

Pericardiocentesis—a long thin needle is advanced into the pericardial sac to drain excessive fluid

PICC line—tube in any of an extremity's larger veins for long-term antibiotic or other therapy

Sclerotherapy—injections into blood vessels to shrink them

Stress test—measures the heart's ability to respond to external stress (Fig. 15.13)

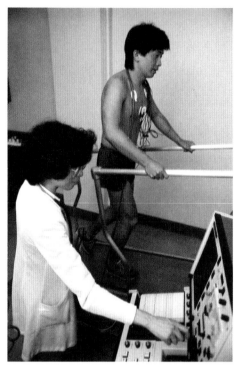

Fig. 15.13 During a stress test, the patient performs physical activity while heart function is monitored on an ECG. (From Pagana KD, Pagana TJ: *Mosby's manual of diagnostic and laboratory tests*, ed 3, St. Louis, 2006, Mosby.)

Transesophageal echocardiogram (TEE)—heart ultrasound that is done through the esophagus

Valvuloplasty—heart valve repair

Vena cava (Greenfield or IVC) filter—implanted in the inferior vena cava to trap emboli and prevent pulmonary embolism.

Problem List

The problem list contains current clinical impressions, diagnoses, and signs and symptoms. If a patient has specific signs or symptoms that are not yet explained by a specific diagnosis, they may be listed separately in the patient's problem list. Once these signs and symptoms are determined to be caused by a disease, the signs or symptoms are removed from the problem list and the diagnosis is added instead.

Patients often do not know the name of a specific diagnosis, but will instead describe it to their provider. It is the scribe's duty to translate the lay terms into medical terminology. For example, if the patient says they have a history of a bulging aorta in their stomach, the scribe should document "abdominal aortic aneurysm."

Abdominal aortic aneurysm (AAA)—localized enlargement of the abdominal aorta that is at risk to rupture and cause bleeding

Aortic coarctation—narrowing of the aorta that can cause cardiac hypertrophy and differences in blood pressure between the extremities; most often a congenital condition

Aneurysm—bulge in the wall of an artery that may rupture and bleed

Angina—chest pain with a cardiac etiology

Arrhythmia—irregular heartbeat

Atherosclerosis—arterial wall thickening due to plaque formation (Fig. 15.14)

Atrial fibrillation—arrhythmia of the atria, typically with a rapid and irregular heartbeat ("irregularly irregular" on physical exam); often designated as being with or without ***rapid ventricular response (RVR)***

Atrial flutter—arrhythmia of the atria that manifests as fluttering and is inefficient at pumping blood to the ventricles

Atrial septal defect—a hole in the atrium that allows blood to flow from one atrium to the other

Cardiac arrest—failure of the heart to contract (basically, death)

Cardiomyopathy—pathology of heart muscle from a variety of causes that usually results in heart failure and fluid retention

Congestive heart failure (CHF)—heart cannot effectively pump blood and causes accumulation of fluid ("congestion")

Coronary artery disease (CAD)—plaque accumulation in any of the arteries of the heart that may become blocked and cause a heart attack

Deep vein thrombosis (DVT)—venous blood clot, usually in the lower extremities that is known to cause unilateral leg pain and swelling and can embolize and cause **pulmonary embolism** (blood clot in the lungs; Fig. 15.15)

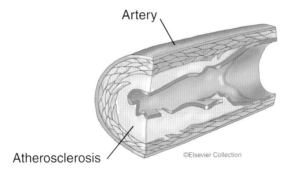

Artery

Atherosclerosis

©Elsevier Collection

Fig. 15.14	Atherosclerosis. (© Elsevier Collection.)

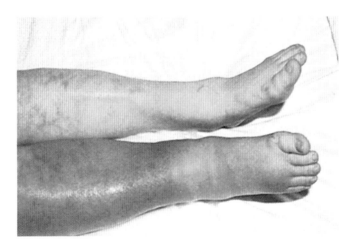

Fig. 15.15	Deep vein thrombosis. (From Lewis SM: *Medical-surgical nursing: assessment and management of clinical problems*, ed 8, St. Louis, 2011, Mosby.)

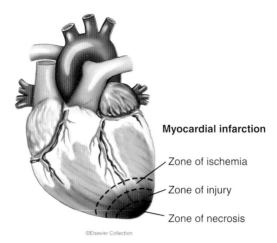

Myocardial infarction

Zone of ischemia

Zone of injury

Zone of necrosis

©Elsevier Collection

Fig. 15.16 Myocardial infarction (MI). (© Elsevier Collection.)

Dysrhythmia—irregular heartbeat

Endocarditis—inflammation or infection of the endocardium

Hyperlipidemia (HLD)—elevated blood cholesterol and/or triglycerides

Hypertension (HTN)—consistently elevated blood pressure (>130/90)

Hypotension—low blood pressure

Myocardial infarction (MI; heart attack)—blood is blocked from part of the heart, causing tissue ischemia (death) and necrosis (decomposition; Fig. 15.16)

Myocarditis—inflammation of heart muscle

Pericardial effusion—accumulation of fluid in the pericardial cavity

Pericarditis—inflammation of the pericardium

Peripheral artery disease (PAD)—narrowing of the extremity arteries that limits blood flow

Peripheral vascular disease (PVD)—narrowing of the extremity vasculature (arteries and veins) that limits blood flow

Pulmonary hypertension—elevated blood pressure in the pulmonary vasculature that increases resistance for the heart and may eventually lead to heart failure

Regurgitation—a heart valve is unable to completely close and blood flows (or leaks) in the wrong direction

Sick sinus syndrome (SSS)—arrhythmia caused by malfunction of the sinus node that results in a very slow heartbeat

Stenosis—a heart valve is unable to completely open and blood cannot flow freely in the correct direction

Supraventricular tachycardia (SVT)—improper electrical activity causing a rapid and dangerous arrhythmia

Valvular disease—disease of any heart valve

Vasculitis—inflammation of the blood vessels

Ventricular hypertrophy—enlargement of the ventricles

Ventricular septal defect—a hole in the ventricular septum that allows blood to flow from one ventricle to the other

Of note, **pericarditis** is inflammation of the pericardium. Patients with pericarditis will often complain of chest pain that worsens when they sit, and improves when lying supine. This is because when leaning forward, the heart contacts the inflamed pericardium and causes pain. When lying down, the heart is suspended in pericardial fluid and there is no pain.

Medications

A scribe should be able to diligently record the patient's medication list, which includes the drug name (generic or brand), dose, frequency, and indication (reason for taking the drug). Table 15.1 lists some of the drug classes useful in the treatment of cardiovascular problems.

Although knowing the drug class mechanism of action is not essential to become a great scribe, having familiarity with the mechanism can facilitate faster and more accurate documentation. This is because, within a class, the generic names tend to sound similar. This is usually a good way to identify a drug class from a generic name. For example, in the beta blocker class, all of the drug generic names end in "lol."

TABLE 15.1 ■ Selected cardiovascular system medications.

Drug Class and Uses	Generic Name (Brand Name)
Antiarrhythmics • Not a class • Prevent and treat arrhythmia	**Calcium channel blockers** amlodipine (Norvasc) diltiazem (Cardizem) nicardipine (Cardene) nifedipine (Procardia) verapamil (Calan) **Sodium channel blockers** flecainide (Tambocor) lidocaine (Xylocaine) procainamide (Pronestyl) **Potassium channel blocker** amiodarone (Pacerone) dofetilide (Tikosyn) sotalol (Betapace)
Digitalis • Treatment of arrythmia and CHF	digoxin (Lanoxin)
Nucleoside • Lowers heart rate	adenosine (Adenocard)
Beta Blockers • Reduce sympathetic tone (lowers heart rate, contractility, vasodilates) • Treat arrhythmia, hypertension • Reduce risk of subsequent MI after an initial heart attack	atenolol (Tenormin) carvedilol (Coreg) labetalol (Trandate) metoprolol (Lopressor) nadolol (Corgard) propranolol (Inderal)
Anticholinergics • Reduce parasympathetic tone (increases heart rate)	atropine
Alpha agonists • Increase sympathetic tone (increases heart rate, increases contractility, vasoconstricts)	clonidine (Catapres) dobutamine (Dobutrex) dopamine epinephrine (Adrenalin) norepinephrine
Diuretics • Increase water excretion to alleviate fluid retention • Treat CHF, pulmonary edema, kidney failure	bumetanide (Bumex) furosemide (Lasix) hydrochlorothiazide (HCTZ) (Hydrodiuril) spironolactone (Aldactone)
ACE (angiotensin converting enzyme) inhibitors • Vasodilate and increase water excretion • Treat hypertension and fluid overload	captopril (Capoten) enalapril (Vasotec) lisinopril (Zestril or Prinivil) ramipril (Altace)

Continued

TABLE 15.1 ■ Selected cardiovascular system medications. —Cont'd

Drug Class and Uses	Generic Name (Brand Name)
ARB (angiotensin II receptor blockers) • Vasodilate and increases water excretion • Treat hypertension and fluid overload	candesartan (Atacand) losartan (Cozaar) olmesartan (Benicar) valsartan (Diovan)
Nitrates • Vasodilators • Treat angina, MI	isosorbide mononitrate (Imdur) nitroglycerin
Statins • Decrease "bad" cholesterols (LDL, triglycerides), and increase "good" cholesterol (HDL) • Treat hyperlipidemia	atorvastatin (Lipitor) pravastatin (Pravachol) rosuvastatin (Crestor) simvastatin (Zocor)
• Dissolve clots • Treat PE, MI, ischemic stroke	tPA (tissue plasminogen activator)
Prothrombotic • Promote blood clots • Reverse major bleeding caused by warfarin (Coumadin)	prothrombin complex concentrate (Kcentra)
Anticoagulant ("blood thinners") • Inhibit some part of the clotting cascade • Treat MI, ischemic stroke, DVT/PE, arrhythmia	apixaban (Eliquis) dabigatran (Pradexa) enoxaparin (Lovenox) heparin rivaroxaban (Xarelto) warfarin (Coumadin) or (Jantoven)
Antiplatelet • Prevent platelets from participating in clotting • Treat MI, ischemic stroke, DVT/PE, arrhythmia	acetylsalicylic acid (Aspirin) clopidogrel (Plavix) ticagrelor (Brilinta)

CHF, Congestive heart failure; *DVT,* deep vein thrombosis; *MI,* Myocardial infarction.

CASE STUDY 15.1

Dr. Marsh has been practicing internal medicine for over 15 years, and he has never been busier. The physician's office where he is employed is part of the regional hospital system, with eight other physicians and five physician assistants at his location alone. In the past year the administrators have begun hiring medical scribes to help the physicians document their patient encounters. Dr. Marsh appreciates the helping hands very much, not only because he can spend less time charting, but it also allows him to do his job better. Because he is not staring at the computer screen during the patient visit, he is able to focus his attention on the patient.

The scribe, Marta Perez, accompanies Dr. Marsh for his 2:00 pm appointment, a physical examination for a 55-year-old restaurant manager whose problem list includes hyperlipidemia and hypertension. The medical assistant recorded a normal body temperature of 98.6 °F, blood pressure 140/95, and heartrate 90 bpm; the EHR calculated the patient's BMI as 33.4. Dr. Marsh spends some time discussing with the patient the late nights and stress of working in the restaurant industry. The patient admits he feels tired, and confides that because he does not get home until after midnight, he usually cannot fall asleep until after 2:00 am. He also said that he fainted at work last month, but that he figured it was just because he had not eaten all day. He denies chest pain and his only complaint is that he is out of breath whenever he has to go down the stairs to the restaurant's walk-in cooler.

Dr. Marsh listened carefully to the patient's heart and announced "no murmurs." He then had the patient lie down on the exam table, and elevated the head of the bed 45 degrees. Dr. Marsh observed the patient's jugular vein and said it was normal. He felt the carotid arteries on the patient's neck and

Continued

CASE STUDY 15.1 —cont'd

announced there was no diminution of pulse. The physician counseled the patient on the importance of a healthy diet and they discussed the possibility of starting a statin.

QUESTIONS

1. What is in the patient's problem list?
2. How was the patient's hyperlipidemia diagnosed?
3. How and where does Marta document the patient's fainting episode?
4. How and where does Marta document the patient's shortness of breath?
5. What other symptoms should Marta document?
6. Which of the patient's problems would the statin treat?

Practice Questions

1. The _____ valve separates the left atrium and ventricle.
2. The _____ is the muscular layer of the heart.
3. The four _____ carry blood from the lungs to the heart.
4. _____ is/are the result of arterial expansion and can be palpated.
5. A 52-year-old male patient presents to the emergency department with a several-hour history of chest pain that shoots into his left arm. He has been sweating profusely, is short of breath with any activity, and even passed out earlier in the day. He did fall when he passed out but denies hitting his head. He is also having a pins and needles sensation in both hands and in his feet, and states that he has been feeling on edge and worried for the past several days. No fevers or chills. How should this be documented in the review of systems?
6. On physical exam the emergency department notes that this is an obese man who appears to be in moderate distress. There is no trauma visible to his head and no focal neurologic deficits. He is visibly diaphoretic. Pallor is also noted. His heart is tachycardic and there is a 2/6 systolic ejection murmur present. Pulses are diminished in all four extremities and he has 1+ pitting bilateral lower extremity edema. No jugular venous distension. How should this be documented in the physical exam?
7. The patient reports that he has had tubes placed in the arteries of his heart before to keep them open. What procedure should be documented?
8. The patient has many risk factors for a myocardial infarction (heart attack), which include high blood pressure and high cholesterol. How should these be documented in the medical history?
9. This patient will receive many medications in the course of his care for the myocardial infarction that was confirmed with ECG. One of these medications will be a beta blocker. From the following list, which is a beta blocker?
   a. diltiazem (Cardizem)
   b. propranolol (Inderal)
   c. enalapril (Vasotec)
   d. losartan (Cozaar)

Respiratory System

1. Use medical terminology to document medical issues involving the respiratory system.
2. Describe the anatomy and physiology of the respiratory system.
3. Document respiratory system symptoms related during a review of systems.
4. Document signs related by the provider during a physical exam of the respiratory system.
5. Document operations and procedures for the respiratory system.
6. Document the respiratory system clinical impressions, diagnoses, and signs and symptoms commonly found in a problem list.
7. Document relevant drug classes and medications for the treatment of problems associated with the respiratory system.

KEY TERMS

Acidosis	Croup	Parietal pleura
Alkalosis	Cyanosis	Pleural cavity
Alveoli	Cystic fibrosis	Pneumothorax
Apex	Diaphragm	Rales
Apnea	Dyspnea	Rhonchi
Aspiration	Expiration	Sarcoidosis
Asthma	Hemoptysis	Spirometry
Base	Hyperventilation	Stridor
Bronchiole	Hypoxia	Tachypnea
Bronchoscopy	Inspiration	Thoracentesis
Bronchus	Intubation	Thoracostomy
Chronic obstructive	Lung	Trachea
pulmonary disease	Obstructive sleep apnea	Tripod position
(COPD)	(OSA)	Visceral pleura
Clubbing	Orthopnea	Wheezing
Consolidation		

Anatomy and Physiology

The respiratory system is a series of hollow tubes that connect the oral and nasal cavities to the lungs in the thoracic cavity, where gas exchange occurs (Fig. 16.1).

Upon *inspiration*, air travels from the oral and nasal cavities through the pharynx into the **trachea**, which is a hollow cartilaginous tube situated between the two lungs. The trachea divides into the left and right **bronchi** (**bronchus**, singular) which enter the left and right **lungs**.

The lungs are situated with their bases resting on the diaphragm, and the apices (**apex**, singular) cephalad (Fig. 16.2). The bronchi diverge into smaller tube-like **bronchioles**, and terminate at the **alveoli (alveolus**, singular). These are essentially sacs of air in which gas exchange actually occurs (Fig. 16.3).

Below is a diagram illustrating the *respiratory tree*:

oral/nasal cavity → trachea → bronchi → bronchioles → alveoli

NOTE

As you can see in Fig. 16.2, healthcare professionals have several landmarks useful in describing the lungs. The oblique fissure separates the upper and lower lobes of the left lungs. The three lobes of the right lung are separated by the oblique fissure as well as the horizontal fissure. The top or most superior segment of the lung is the **apex** (plural *apices*), and the **bases** are inferior. *Bibasilar* is a term used to describe something that pertains to both bases of the lungs; the term *biapical* refers to both apices.

There are two pleural membranes in the thoracic cavity associated with the lungs. The **parietal pleura** lines the thoracic cage, and the **visceral pleura** lines the lungs. The space between the two pleura is the **pleural cavity**, which is filled with *pleural fluid* that reduces friction (Fig. 16.4).

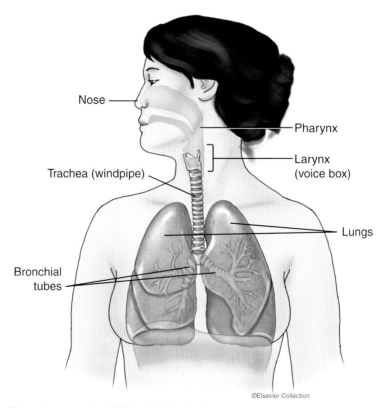

©Elsevier Collection

Fig. 16.1   The respiratory system. (© Elsevier Collection.)

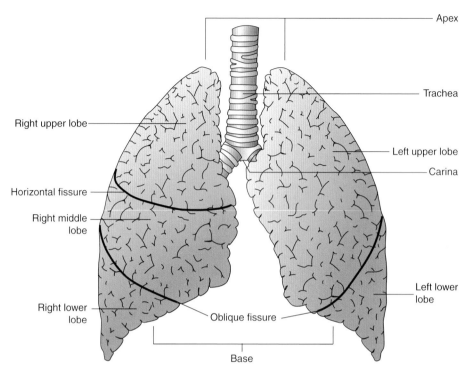

Fig. 16.2 The lobes of the lungs. (From Hicks GH: *Cardiopulmonary anatomy and physiology*, Philadelphia, 2000, WB Saunders.)

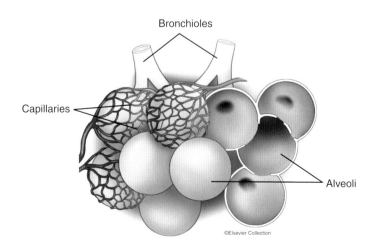

Pulmonary parenchyma

Fig. 16.3 Alveoli of the lungs. (© Elsevier Collection.)

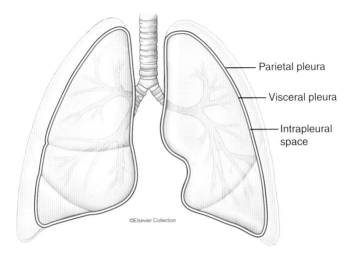

©Elsevier Collection

Fig. 16.4   Pleura of the lungs. (© Elsevier Collection.)

The **diaphragm** is a large muscle that separates the thoracic and abdominal cavities. It plays a major role in increasing and decreasing lung volumes. The pressure gradient within the pleural cavity changes with contraction and relaxation of the diaphragm. Without going into too much detail about pressure gradients: during **inspiration** (or inhalation), the diaphragm contracts and increases lung volume, essentially "pulling" oxygenated air into the lungs. During **expiration** (or exhalation), the diaphragm relaxes and decreases lung volume, "pushing" air carrying carbon dioxide out of the lungs (Fig. 16.5).

Other muscles in the chest and abdomen also participate in changing lung volume, but to a lesser degree and often only in respiratory distress (when one is having difficulty breathing normally). These muscles may be referred to as *accessory muscles*.

The respiratory system and cardiovascular system work closely together to perform gas exchange. In fact, they are sometimes referred to as the *cardiopulmonary system*. The lungs are the site at which reoxygenation occurs: deoxygenated blood gets rid of carbon dioxide to be exhaled as waste, and instead picks up oxygen to deliver to the body's tissues. Because of this interrelatedness between the two systems, if one system is not functional, the other is often not functional either.

Review of Systems

The review of systems for respiratory complaints will have any number of colloquialisms (lay terms) that the scribe will want to translate into medical language. For example, if a patient says they are coughing up blood, the scribe should document **hemoptysis**. Another common colloquialism is "shortness of breath with exercise," which translates into *dyspnea on exertion (DOE)*. A very important medical term distinction is identifying the source of what the patient may call "spit" or "phlegm" or "mucous." The provider will want to determine if this material is being coughed up from the airway (as opposed to draining from the sinuses or being vomited, for example). If it is coming from the lungs or respiratory tree, it is rightly labeled "sputum" in the medical record.

Symptoms that can be placed in multiple systems have been designated as such in italics. Remember to always maximize the number of systems that are included in the review of systems so that the chart can be billed at higher levels (if desired). For example: if a patient is having hemoptysis and dyspnea, it would be best to include hemoptysis in "*hematologic/lymphatic*" and dyspnea in "*respiratory*" (two billable systems), as opposed to including hemoptysis and dyspnea in "*respiratory*" (one billable system).

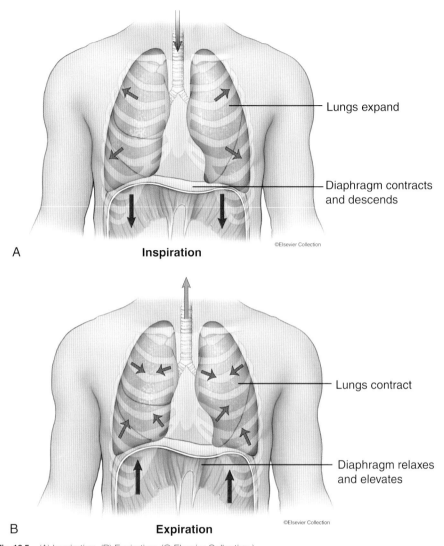

Fig. 16.5 (A) Inspiration. (B) Expiration. (© Elsevier Collection.)

Cough—productive (with sputum) or nonproductive (without sputum)
Dyspnea (*cardiovascular*)—shortness of breath
Dyspnea on exertion (DOE) (*cardiovascular*)—exertional shortness of breath
Hemoptysis (*hematologic/lymphatic*)—productive cough with blood
Orthopnea (*cardiovascular*)—shortness of breath that worsens supine
Paroxysmal nocturnal dyspnea (PND) (*cardiovascular*)—sudden awakening at night with shortness of breath
Platypnea (*cardiovascular*)—shortness of breath worsening with sitting
Pleuritic chest pain (*musculoskeletal*)—chest pain with inspiration
Posttussive chest pain (*musculoskeletal*)—chest pain after coughing
Wheezing—whistling sound produced during expiration

Medical Terminology Word Parts for the Respiratory System

Combining Forms

spir/o	to breathe
trache/o	trachea
thorac/o pector/o	chest
pulmon/o pneumon/o pneum/o	lung
bronch/o bronchi/o	bronchus
bronchiol/o	bronchiole
alveol/o	alveolus
apic/o	apex
bas/o	base
lob/o lobul/o	lobe
pleur/o	pleura
viscer/o	viscera
pariet/o	wall
diaphragm/o diaphragmat/o phren/o	diaphragm
hem/o	blood
orth/o	straight
noct/o	night
tuss/o	cough
cyan/o	blue
phon/o	sound
eg/o	goat-like
ox/o	oxygen
loqui/o	speak
capn/o carb/o	carbon dioxide
laryng/o	larynx
rhin/o	nose
sin/o	sinus

Prefixes

ex-	out
in-	in
inter-	between
para-	near, during
re-	again
dys-	difficult
platy-	flat
oxy-	sharp, acute, oxygen
post-	after
tachy-	fast
hyper-	excessive
brady-	slow
a-	without
hypo-	deficient

Suffixes

-um	structure
-atory -al -ic -ive	pertaining to
-pnea	breathing
-ptysis	spitting
-itis	inflammation
-osis	abnormal condition
-scopy	process of viewing
-ectomy	removal
-metry	process of measuring
-centesis	surgical puncture
-stomy	new opening
-tomy	incision
-ectasis	dilation

Physical Exam

When a patient is in respiratory distress, they may be observed with ***pursed lipped breathing*** (exactly as it sounds), in a **tripod position** (leaning forward with hands on the bed or legs,

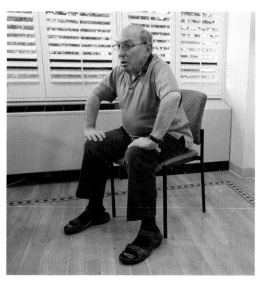

Fig. 16.6   The patient in a tripod position to ease dyspnea. (From Yoost BL, Crawford LR: *Fundamentals of nursing: active learning for collaborative practice*, St. Louis, 2020. Elsevier.)

Fig. 16.6), using accessory muscles (discussed above), and with **cyanosis** (blue discoloration from hypoxia, Fig. 16.7). They may present with **tachypnea** (breathing rapidly), or **hyperventilation** (breathing rapidly and inefficiently).

Apnea—cessation of breathing

Arterial oxygen saturation (SaO2)—percent of oxygen dissolved into arterial blood (normal is 95%–100% for nonsmokers)

Bradypnea—slow breathing rate (<12 breaths per minute for most)

Clubbing—club-shaped nail deformity associated with chronic hypoxia related to cardiopulmonary disease (Fig. 16.8)

Cyanosis—blue or purple discoloration of the skin from hypoxia (see Fig. 16.7)

Consolidation—an area of the lung in which the air has been replaced by fluid and other material

Egophony (E to A egophony)—increased resonance of voice sounds during auscultation (goat-like sounds), usually due to lung consolidation. The patient will be asked to say "ee," (a long E) but a positive finding will make it sound like "ay" (a long A), hence "e to a."

Hyperventilation—rapid and inefficient breathing that decreases CO_2

Hypoxia—oxygen deprivation

Pectus excavatum—congenital depression of the sternum

Rales (crackles)—crackling, rattling, or clicking noises heard during inspiration caused by small airway collapse. Often these are described by location heard such as basilar (at the bottom or bases of the lungs; or bibasilar if bilateral) or apical (at the tops or apices of the lungs).

Rhonchi—rattling noises caused by secretions within the bronchi

Stridor—high-pitched breath sound heard during inspiration, usually caused by upper airway obstruction or narrowing

Tachypnea—rapid breathing rate (>20 breaths per minute)

Tracheal deviation—tracheal displacement from normal position

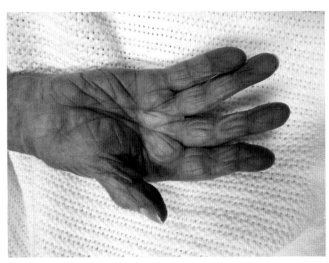

Fig. 16.7 Cyanosis in the fingertips. (James Heilman: CC BY-SA 3.0, https://commons.wikimedia.org/w/index.php?curid=17978808.)

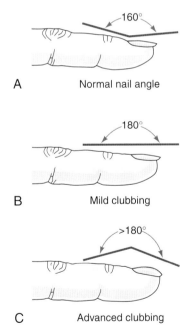

Fig. 16.8 Clubbing of fingers. (A) Normal fingernail angle is 160 degrees. (B) Early mild clubbing appears as a flattened angle between nail and skin (180 degrees). (C) Advanced clubbing shows a rounded (clubbed) fingertip and nail. (From Copstead LC, Banasik JL: *Pathophysiology*, ed 5, Philadelphia, 2012, Elsevier.)

Whispered pectoriloquy—magnified volume of whispering during auscultation of the lungs, usually due to consolidation

Operations/Procedures

Any of the patient's prior surgical history (including major operations or minor procedures) may be discussed in the context of a patient's medical history. Patients often do not know the name of the operation and will describe their understanding of the procedure in lay terms. It is the scribe's duty to translate the patient's procedural description into the equivalent medical term. For example, if a patient says they had a lung lobe removed, the scribe should record that the patient had an "lobectomy".

Bi-level positive airway pressure (Bi-PAP)—ventilation that reduces work of breathing

Bronchial lavage (BAL)—fluid is injected into a part of the lung and collected for examination

Bronchoscopy—endoscopic visualization of the airways

Continuous positive airway pressure (C-PAP)—ventilation that keeps airways open

Extubation—removing a tube from the trachea

Intubation—placing a tube in the trachea to help with respiration

Lobectomy—surgical removal of a lung lobe

Lung transplant—diseased lungs are partially or totally replaced

Lung volume reduction surgery (LVRS)—removing damaged parts of the lungs to give the healthier parts more functionality

Pulmonary function test (PFT)—evaluation of respiratory function

Spirometry—testing of the ability to move air through the respiratory system quickly (Fig. 16.9)

Thoracentesis—hollow needle inserted to the thorax to remove fluid, blood or pus from the pleural space (Fig. 16.10)

Thoracostomy—small incision/opening in the chest wall created for draining the pleural cavity of abnormal collections of air, fluid, blood or pus, usually accomplished with a thin tube, the thoracostomy tube

Thoracotomy—incision into the pleural space to access the thorax

Problem List

Remember to maintain the problem list as an up-to-date listing of all current clinical impressions, diagnoses, and signs and symptoms.

Patients often will instead describe the problem to their provider and not be aware of the correct medical term. It is the scribe's duty to translate the lay terms into medical terminology. For example, the patient may say that they have a history of a collapsed lung, in which case the scribe should document "pneumothorax."

Acidosis—increased acidity (H+) of blood/tissues

Acute respiratory distress syndrome (ARDS)—acute fluid accumulation in alveoli, causing collapse and respiratory distress

Alkalosis—decreased acidity (H+) of blood/tissues

Aspiration—foreign materials are inhaled and trapped within the bronchial tree or lungs

Asthma—long-term inflammatory disease of the airway that causes bronchial narrowing and difficulty breathing

Bronchitis—inflammation of the bronchi of the lungs

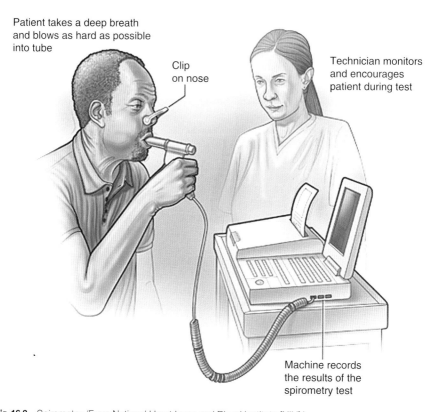

Patient takes a deep breath
and blows as hard as possible
into tube

Clip
on nose

Technician monitors
and encourages
patient during test

Machine records
the results of the
spirometry test

Fig. 16.9   Spirometry. (From National Heart Lung and Blood Institute [NIH].)

Bronchiectasis—chronic lung disease with scarring and enlargement of airways causing difficulty clearing mucous secretions

Bronchiolitis—disease of young children and infants with blockage of small airways (bronchioles) due to viral infection

Bronchospasm—constriction of muscles in the bronchioles that narrows the airway and causes difficulty breathing

Chronic obstructive pulmonary disease (COPD)—chronic lung inflammation causing bronchial narrowing, difficulty breathing, and eventually lung scarring

Croup—also called laryngotracheobronchitis, a viral infection affecting the upper airway resulting in a "barking" type of cough and sometimes stridor

Cystic fibrosis—an inherited disorder that causes abnormally thick body secretions leading to problems throughout the body and especially the lungs

Hypercapnia or hypercarbia—elevated blood carbon dioxide

Hypercarbia—elevated blood carbon dioxide

Interstitial lung disease (ILD)—group of lung diseases causing scarring of the lung interstitium (lung tissue)

Laryngitis—inflammation of the larynx

Laryngospasm—vocal cord spasm causing difficulty breathing/speaking

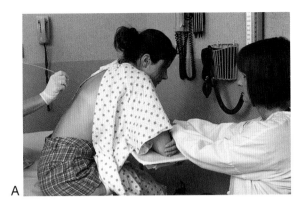

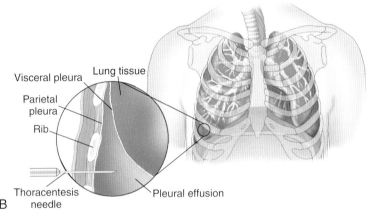

Visceral pleura
Lung tissue
Parietal pleura
Rib
Thoracentesis needle
B
Pleural effusion

Fig. 16.10 Thoracocentesis. (A) Common position for thoracentesis. (B) The insertion site depends on the location of the fluid. (A, From Harkreader H, Hogan ML: *Fundamentals of nursing*, ed 3, St. Louis, 2007, Elsevier Saunders; B, From Leonard PC: *Quick & easy medical terminology*, ed 9, St. Louis, 2020.)

Obstructive sleep apnea (OSA)—intermittent airway collapse during sleep that causes episodes of apnea

Pleural effusion—fluid accumulation in the pleural cavity

Pneumonia—inflammation of alveoli (usually from an infectious etiology) causing them to fill with fluid and become nonfunctional

Pneumothorax—partial or completely collapsed lung (Fig. 16.11)

Pulmonary edema—fluid accumulation in the lungs

Pulmonary embolism (PE)—obstruction of a lung artery by an embolus (foreign substance) that can cause cardiopulmonary arrest

Respiratory failure—inadequate gas exchange in the respiratory system resulting in failure of the respiratory system

Rhinitis—the "runny nose," also called "coryza," may be infectious (viral generally) or allergic

Sarcoidosis—inflammatory granulomatous disease of the lungs

Sinusitis—inflammatory condition of the sinuses which could have an infectious or allergic cause

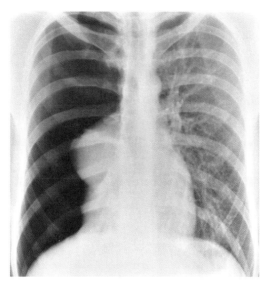

Fig. 16.11   Pneumothorax: the chest x-ray (radiograph) shows a complete collapse of the patient's right lung. (From Johnson NM, Eisenberg RL: *Comprehensive radiologic pathology*, ed 7, St. Louis, 2021, Elsevier.)

Stridor—an abnormal breath sound heard during inspiration and caused by narrowing of the upper airway (as in croup for example)

Upper respiratory infection (URI)—an infection of the upper respiratory tree

Wheezing—an abnormal breath sound heard during expiration and caused by narrowing of the lower airway (as in asthma for example)

NOTE

In December 2019, a novel (new) coronavirus was identified in China, named SARS-CoV-2. The virus causes the disease called COVID-19, and it spread quickly throughout the world, reaching pandemic status in March 2020. Like other infectious respiratory diseases, COVID transmits through respiratory droplets released into the air when an infected person coughs or sneezes.

SARS-CoV-2 attacks the epithelial lining of the lungs, hampering their ability to clear debris. The reduced function can cause pneumonia, ARDS, or sepsis (a blood infection). In addition to respiratory problems, medical researchers discovered that the virus is able to damage the heart and cardiovascular system.

CASE STUDY 16.1

Twenty-one-year-old Jameis Meyer presented to the emergency department (ED) at 8:00 a.m. with right-sided chest pain and difficulty breathing due to increased pain during respiration. He said his symptoms began around midnight with shortness of breath, and the accompanying pain got worse as the night went on. At the advice of his girlfriend, around 3:00 a.m. he took a hot bath and applied Vicks menthol rub without relief. Mr. Meyer was unable to sleep and rated his pain at a 4 overall, but a 10 if he were to lay on his right side. The triage nurse assigned the patient an ES2 acuity score.

After an electrocardiogram (ECG) revealed normal sinus rhythm, an AP chest radiograph (see Fig. 16.11) showed complete collapse of the patient's right lung. The consulting surgeon ordered Percocet

Continued

for pain. Bedside ultrasound was used to visualize the tube placement. A local anesthetic was applied to the skin at the 5th intercostal space, mid-axillary line on the right. The surgeon inserted an 18-gauge needle into Mr. Meyer's pleural space and aspirated air to verify placement, then inserted a guide wire and removed the needle. He next inserted a 14 Fr Arrow pigtail chest drain into the pleural space through a 0.5 cm incision and connected the drain to Pleur-Evac suction. The tube connected to a one-way valve and was sutured in place. Mr. Meyer complained of nausea during the procedure, which was otherwise well tolerated, and there were no complications. EBL (estimated blood loss) was 10 cc.

QUESTIONS

1. How should the scribe document the chief complaint?
2. What type of "note within a note" might be used in documenting this encounter?
3. What is the duration, timing, and onset of the patient's symptoms?
4. Based on the information given, what is Mr. Meyer's diagnosis, and what procedure was performed?
5. What information does the scribe need to know about the local anesthetic the patient was administered?

Medications

Many drugs are related to other drugs in both function and chemical composition. These drugs would be considered to be in the same drug class (Table 16.1). This gives options within a class to choose different drugs with slightly different profiles (actions and side-effects).

A scribe should be able to diligently record the patient's medication list, which includes the drug name (generic or brand), dose, frequency, and indication (reason for taking the drug).

TABLE 16.1 ■ Selected Respiratory System Medications

Drug Class and Uses	Generic Name (Brand Name)
Short-acting beta agonists (SABA) • Rapid bronchodilation • These are known as "rescue inhalers" • Acute treatment for inflammatory airway disease (e.g. asthma or COPD)	albuterol (Proventil) epinephrine (EpiPen) isoproterenol levalbuterol (Xopenex) pirbuterol (Maxair) terbutaline (Brethine)
Long-acting beta agonists (LABA) • Prophylactic bronchodilation • These are known as "preventative inhalers" • Long-term maintenance therapy for inflammatory airway disease	budesonide formoterol (Symbicort) salmeterol (Serevent)
Anticholinergics • Reduces parasympathetic tone (bronchodilation) and bronchospasm • Used to treat airway inflammation	aclidinium (Pressair) ipratropium bromide (Atrovent) tiotropium bromide (Spiriva)
Antitussive • Not a class • Used to prevent cough	dextromethorphan (Robitussin)

Continued

TABLE 16.1 ■ Selected Respiratory System Medications —cont'd

Drug Class and Uses	Generic Name (Brand Name)
Glucocorticoids • Immunosuppressive and anti-inflammatory • Used to prevent airway inflammation or as treatment for acute and severe inflammation	**Inhaled** beclomethasone (Beclovent) budesonide (Pulmicort) fluticasone propionate (Flovent) triamcinolone (Azmacort) **Oral or parenteral** dexamethasone methylprednisolone prednisone
Combinations (of the above)	albuterol PLUS ipratropium (Duoneb) helium PLUS oxygen (Heliox)

Practice Questions

1. The _____ is a cartilaginous tube situated between the lungs.
2. The _____ is a large muscle that changes lung volumes.
3. The _____ reduces friction between the two layers of pleura.
4. _____ are sacs of air at which gas exchange occurs.
5. A 31-year-old female patient presents to her pulmonologist for evaluation of shortness of breath and wheezing that began several days ago. She also has been coughing up white and clear mucous. She has a history of seasonal allergies in the spring and has noticed that her symptoms have worsened since spring has begun and her allergies worsened. She denies any lightheadedness, numbness or tingling, or passing out. No fevers or chills. How should this be documented in the review of systems?
6. On physical exam the patient appears to be in mild respiratory distress. Heart rate is tachycardic but no murmurs, gallops, or rubs are auscultated. She is tachypneic and oxygen saturation is 91% on room air. No stridor is noted. There is bibasilar expiratory wheezing. No clubbing or cyanosis. She has clear rhinorrhea and nasal turbinates are swollen. Cobblestoning is noted in the oropharynx. How should this be documented in the physical exam?
7. The patient reports that as a child she was diagnosed with an inflammatory airway disease that would cause her to have similar "attacks" of shortness of breath and wheezing. She was given an emergency inhaler but stopped using this long ago. What diagnosis should be documented?
8. Because of her inflammatory airway disease, in the past she has required a tube down her throat to help her breathe. How should this procedure be documented in the surgical/operative history?
9. What *rescue* inhaler was the patient likely given as a child?
   a. salmeterol (Serevent)
   b. fluticasone propionate (Flovent)
   c. dextromethorphan (Robitussin)
   d. albuterol (Proventil)

CHAPTER 17

Gastrointestinal System

1. Use medical terminology to document medical issues involving the gastrointestinal system.
2. Describe the anatomy and physiology of the gastrointestinal system.
3. Document gastrointestinal system symptoms related during a review of systems.
4. Document the signs related by the provider during a physical exam of the gastrointestinal system.
5. Document operations and procedures for the gastrointestinal system.
6. Document the gastrointestinal system clinical impressions, diagnoses, and signs and symptoms commonly found in a problem list.
7. Document relevant drug classes and medications for the treatment of problems associated with the gastrointestinal system.

Anorexia	Duodenum	Melena
Anus	Dyspepsia	Mesentery
Appendix	Dysphagia	Oral cavity
Ascending colon	Emesis	Pancreas
Ascites	Esophageal varices	Paracentesis
Barrett's esophagus	Esophagus	Peristalsis
Bolus	Gallbladder	Peritoneum
Cecum	Hemorrhoid	Polydipsia
Celiac disease	Hepatomegaly	Rectum
Cholecystectomy	Hernia	Reflux
Cirrhosis	Ileum	Sigmoid colon
Colon	Ileus	Small intestine
Colostomy	Irritable bowel syndrome	Splenomegaly
Descending colon	(IBS)	Stomach
Distension	Jejunum	Transverse colon
Diverticulitis	Laparoscopy	Ulcerative colitis (UC)
Diverticulosis	Liver	

Anatomy and Physiology

The digestive system or gastrointestinal system consists of a series of participating organs that work together to absorb nutrients from the food we eat and ultimately expel the waste as stool (Fig. 17.1). Most of these organs are hollow tubes, which allow food to pass through the body. The solid digestive organs (such as the liver and pancreas) typically produce substances that aid in digestion.

After entering the **oral cavity**, food is swallowed and then passed through the **esophagus** into the stomach. The **stomach** begins the digestive process by releasing enzymes and acids, and mechanically breaks down the food using **peristalsis** (wavelike contractions of the muscle).

The food **bolus** then passes into the **small intestine** which is the primary site of food absorption and consists of three parts: the **duodenum**, **jejunum**, and the **ileum**. Enzymes and bile are released from the **pancreas** and **gallbladder**, respectively, into the small intestine to facilitate digestion. The **liver** synthesizes the bile, which is then stored in the gallbladder.

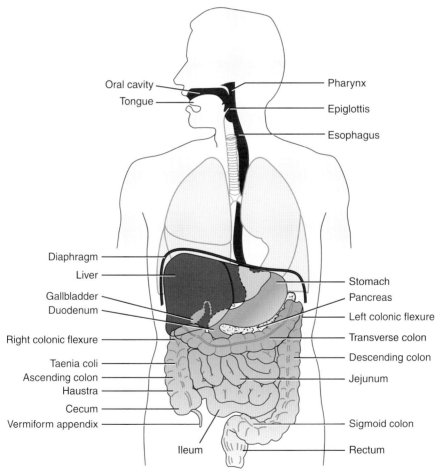

Fig. 17.1 Gastrointestinal system. (From Koersterman JL: *Buck's step-by-step medical coding*, ed 2021, St. Louis, 2021, Elsevier.)

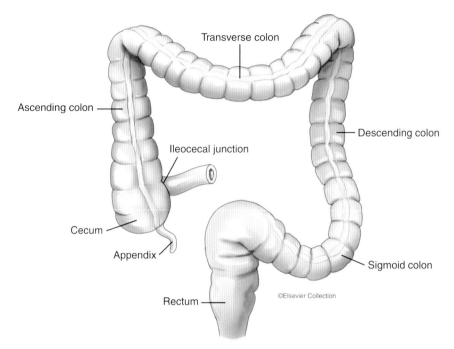

Fig. 17.2   Sections of the large intestine. (© Elsevier Collection.)

The food bolus next passes into the cecum of the **colon**, which absorbs water from the digested contents. The colon is divided into the **ascending colon, transverse colon, descending colon, sigmoid colon**, and the **rectum**. The **cecum** is the first portion of the ascending colon (Fig. 17.2).

After the bolus passes through the entire colon, the contents of the colon are emptied into the rectum as stool before expulsion through the **anus**.

Below is a diagram illustrating the sequence of travel for food, from ingestion to expulsion:

oral cavity → esophagus → stomach → small intestine (*duodenum   jejunum   ileum*) → colon
(*ascending   transverse   descending   sigmoid*) → rectum → anus

With the exception of the oral cavity and esophagus, all the organs of the gastrointestinal system are found in the abdominopelvic cavity. The abdominopelvic cavity is lined by a membrane called the **peritoneum**. Two layers comprise the peritoneum: the *parietal layer*, which lines the cavity walls, and the *visceral layer*, which lines the organs. Extensions of the visceral layer called the *greater* and *lesser omenta* fix the abdominal organs in place. The peritoneum's two layers meet at a fold called the **mesentery**, which attaches to the posterior wall of the abdominal cavity on a diagonal line from the superior left at the second lumbar vertebra down to the right at the sacroiliac joint.

Several organs in the digestive system have functions other than digestion. The **liver** metabolizes wastes and toxins, participates in metabolic cycles, processes nutrients absorbed during digestion, and synthesizes cholesterol and blood clotting proteins. The pancreas is both an exocrine and an endocrine organ. It synthesizes enzymes for digestion and participates in endocrine regulation of blood glucose. The **appendix** is a vestigial organ at the end of the cecum with a debated function.

Medical Terminology Word Parts for the Gastrointestinal System

Combining Forms

or/o	mouth, oral cavity
stom/o	
stomat/o	
esophag/o	esophagus
gastr/o	stomach
bol/o	bolus
intestin/o	intestines
enter/o	small intestine
duoden/o	duodenum
jejun/o	jejunum
ile/o	ileum
pancreat/o	pancreas
cholecyst/o	gallbladder
hepat/o	liver
col/o	large intestine, colon
colon/o	
sigmoid/o	sigmoid colon
rect/o	rectum
cec/o	cecum
an/o	anus
proct/o	rectum and anus
appendic/o	appendix
append/o	
fec/a	feces
peritone/o	peritoneum
umbilic/o	umbilicus, navel
orex/o	appetite
hemat/o	blood
dips/o	thirst
phag/o	swallow

Prefixes

epi-	above, upon
supra-	above
a-	without
an-	
dys-	bad, abnormal, difficult
dia-	through
poly-	much, many, excessive
para-	near, beside, abnormal
intra-	within

Suffixes

-stalsis	contraction
-phagia	condition of swallowing or eating
-pepsia	digestive condition
-rrhea	flow, discharge
-algia	pain
-emesis	vomiting
-itis	inflammation
-ia	condition
-megaly	enlargement
-scopy	viewing
-ectomy	removal
-stomy	forming an opening
-centesis	surgical puncture
-osis	abnormal condition

Review of Systems

It is the duty of the scribe to translate the patient's interpretation of their symptoms into medical lingo. For example, if a patient says they are vomiting blood the scribe should document "hematemesis."

Symptoms that can be placed in multiple systems have been designated as such in italics. Remember to always maximize the number of systems that are included in the review of systems so that the chart can be billed at higher levels (if desired). For example, if a patient is having anorexia and nausea, it would be best to include anorexia in "*constitutional*" and nausea in "*digestive*" (two billable systems), as opposed to including anorexia and nausea in "*digestive*" (one system).

Abdominal pain—pain or discomfort in the abdomen
Anorexia (*constitutional, endocrine, psychiatric*)—loss of appetite
Bloating—sensation of abdominal fullness
Constipation—difficult or infrequent bowel movements
Diarrhea (*endocrine*)—loose or watery stools
Distension—abdominal protrusion
Dyspepsia—indigestion
Dysphagia (*neurologic*)—difficulty swallowing
Emesis—vomiting
Eructation—belching
Fecal incontinence (*neurologic*)—involuntary bowel movement
Flatulence—gas
Hematemesis (*hematologic/lymphatic*)—vomiting blood
Hematochezia (*hematologic/lymphatic*)—stools with bright red blood
Melena (*hematologic/lymphatic*)—black and tarry stools
Nausea—urge to vomit
Obstipation—inability to pass stool or gas
Polydipsia (*constitutional, endocrine*)—excessive thirst
Polyphagia (*constitutional, endocrine*)—excessive hunger

Physical Exam

During the physical exam, the abdomen is sometimes divided into four *abdominopelvic quadrants* (Fig. 17.3), or nine *abdominopelvic regions* (Fig. 17.4). Remember to consider anatomical position when naming the quadrants: the patient's left will appear on the examiner's right, and vice versa.

The nomenclature of the four quadrants is designated based on laterality (left versus right), and direction (upper versus lower). Facing the patient and starting in the *left upper quadrant (LUQ)* is the 1 o'clock position, and moving clockwise, there is the *left lower quadrant (LLQ)* at 5 o'clock, the *right lower quadrant (RLQ)* at 7 o'clock, and the *right upper quadrant (RUQ)* at 11 o'clock.

When describing location of the abdomen using the regional system with its nine regions instead of the simpler quadrant system with its four quadrants, the provider will use different nomenclature to describe these smaller areas. The upper outer regions are called the *right hypo-chondriac* and *left hypochondriac* regions. The lower outer regions are the *right iliac* and *left iliac* regions. The central regions are named based on other structures that are nearby. The *epigastric* region is located directly overlying the stomach; the *umbilical* region is located around the umbilicus (also called the belly button or navel in lay language); the *suprapubic* or *hypogastric* region is located superiorly to the *symphysis pubis* (pubic bone). The *left lumbar* and *right lumbar* regions, also sometimes referred to as the *left* and *right gutter*, are the middle most lateral regions. These terms are less commonly used.

Anal fissure—tear in the skin of the anal canal
Ascites—accumulation of fluid in the peritoneal cavity (Fig. 17.5)
Blumberg's sign (rebound)—abdominal pain with rapid removal of pressure
Guaiac test—checks for hidden (occult) blood in stool
Heel tap sign—test for abdominal inflammation in which the examiner taps the bottom of both feet (positive test will elicit pain)
Hemorrhoids—vascular structures in the anal canal that may become swollen, painful, and inflamed
Hepatomegaly—liver enlargement
Hernia—organ protruding through a fascial layer that normally contains it, commonly into the abdominal wall

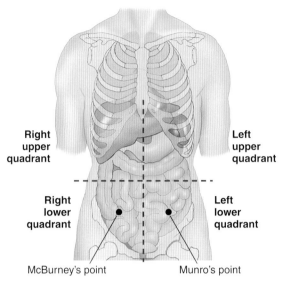

Fig. 17.3 Abdominopelvic quadrants. (From Shiland, BJ: *Medical terminology and anatomy for coding*, ed 4, St. Louis, 2021, Elsevier.)

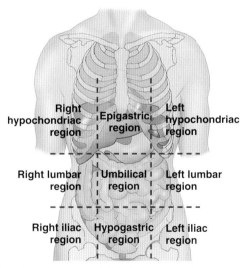

Fig. 17.4 Abdominopelvic regions. (From Shiland, BJ: *Medical terminology and anatomy for coding*, ed 4, St. Louis, 2021, Elsevier.)

McBurney's point—pain at this location in the right lower quadrant may indicate a possible appendicitis (see Fig. 17.3)

Murphy's sign—test for cholecystitis in which the examiner pushes the right upper quadrant as the patient inhales (positive test will elicit pain)

Obturator sign—test for appendicitis in which the examiner flexes and internally rotates the right leg or hip (positive test will elicit pain)

Organomegaly—both spleen and liver enlargement

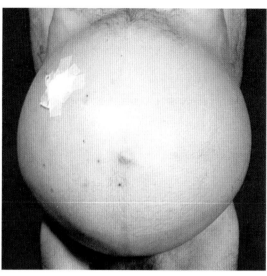

Fig. 17.5   Ascites. (From Morse SA, Holmes KK, Ballard RC, Moreland AA: *Atlas of sexually transmitted diseases and AIDS*, ed 4, Philadelphia, 2010, Saunders Elsevier, p 213, Fig. 12.16.)

Psoas sign—test for appendicitis in which the examiner flexes the right leg or hip (positive test will elicit pain)

Rectal prolapse—rectal walls protrude and can be seen outside the body

Rovsing's sign—test for appendicitis in which the examiner palpates the left lower quadrant (positive test will elicit right lower quadrant pain)

Splenomegaly—spleen enlargement

Operations/Procedures

Any of the patient's prior surgical history (including major operations or minor procedures) may be discussed in the context of a patient's medical history. Patients often do not know the name of the operation and will describe their understanding of the procedure in lay terms. It is the scribe's duty to translate the patient's procedural description into the equivalent medical term. For example, if a patient says they had their appendix removed, the scribe should record that the patient had an "appendectomy."

Appendectomy—removal of the appendix

Banding—elastic bands used for constriction of part of the gastrointestinal tract (GIT)

Cholecystectomy—removal of the gallbladder

Colectomy—removal of part (hemi-) or the entire colon

Colonoscopy—visualizing the lower GI tract with a flexible fiberoptic device called an endoscope (Fig. 17.6)

Colostomy—forming an opening (stoma) by bringing a part of the intestine through an incision (Fig. 17.7)

Esophagogastroduodenoscopy (EGD)—visualizing the upper GI tract with an endoscope

Gastrectomy—removal of the stomach

HIDA scan—a nuclear medicine test to evaluate for gallbladder disease

Ileostomy—stoma formation in the ileum of the small intestine

Laparoscopy—performing an abdominal operation through small incisions with a camera

Paracentesis—collecting peritoneal fluid using a needle inserted into the peritoneal space

Polypectomy—removal of colorectal polyp(s) to prevent them from turning cancerous (see Fig. 17.6)

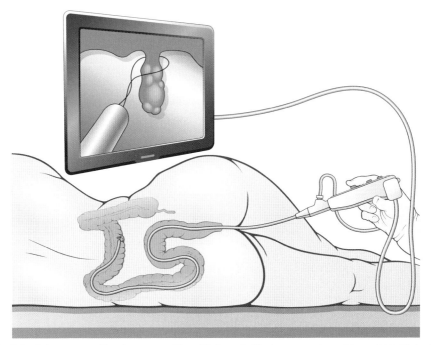

Fig. 17.6 Colonoscopy with polypectomy. (From Chabner D: *The language of medicine*, ed 12, St. Louis, 2021, Elsevier.)

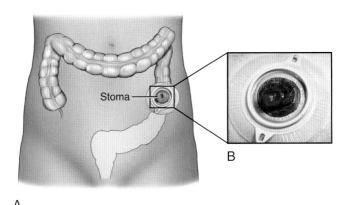

Fig. 17.7 Colostomy. (A) Location of the stoma on the sigmoid colon. (B) The stoma. (From Potter PA, Perry AG: *Fundamentals of nursing*, ed 7, St Louis, 2011, Mosby.)

Problem List

Pain in different quadrants can be indicative of certain medical conditions. Pain in the RUQ may be a gallbladder problem, and often radiates into the back just below the right scapula. Pain in the RLQ may be an issue with the appendix. Pain in the LLQ is often because of a condition called diverticulitis (inflammation of diverticula in the colon), or constipation.

Pain in various regions can also provide a hint regarding the possible underlying problem. Pain in the epigastric region may be related to the stomach, or sometimes the heart. Pain in the umbilical region may be an evolving appendicitis (classically, begins here and migrates to the RLQ). Pain in the suprapubic region is frequently a bladder problem.

Patients often do not know the name of a specific diagnosis, but will instead describe it to their provider. It is the scribe's duty to translate the lay terms into medical terminology. For example, if the patient says they have liver scarring, the scribe should document "cirrhosis."

Abdominal adhesions—scar tissue in the abdominal cavity

Appendicitis—appendix inflammation

Autoimmune hepatitis—autoimmune liver disease

Barrett's esophagus—change in cell type of the lower esophagus that represents a precancerous state (usually a result of chronic acid **reflux**, the abnormal flow of stomach acid into the esophagus)

Celiac disease—autoimmune hypersensitivity to gluten

Cholecystitis—gallbladder inflammation

Cholelithiasis—gallbladder stones

Cirrhosis—liver scarring, often but not always caused by alcoholism

***Clostridium difficile* colitis (*C. diff*)**—colitis from a bacterial infection with *C. difficile*

Crohn's disease—inflammatory bowel disease that causes ulcers in the GI tract

Diverticulitis—infection and inflammation of diverticula (pouches) in the colon wall (Fig. 17.8)

Diverticulosis—presence of small pouches in the colon wall (see Fig. 17.8A)

Esophageal varices—bleeding veins in the lower part of the esophagus

Esophagitis—esophageal inflammation

Fatty liver disease—accumulation of fat in the liver

Gastric ulcer—stomach ulcers

Gastritis—stomach inflammation

Gastroesophageal reflux disease (**GERD**; heartburn)—gastric acid is refluxed through the esophageal sphincter and causes discomfort

Helicobacter pylori—bacterial infection by *H. pylori* causing peptic ulcer disease

Hepatitis A, B, or C—infectious liver disease caused by the hepatitis A, B, or C virus

Hyperbilirubinemia—high blood bilirubin

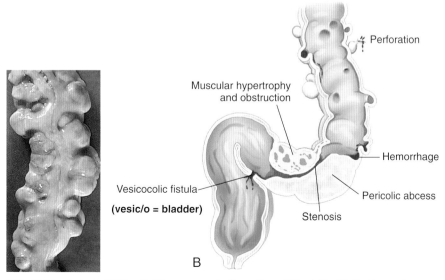

Fig. 17.8 (A) Diverticulosis. (B) Diverticulitis and complications. (From Shiland, BJ: *Medical terminology and anatomy for coding*, ed 4, St. Louis, 2021, Elsevier.)

Ileus—pseudo-obstruction in the GI tract caused by failure of peristalsis
Irritable bowel syndrome (IBS)—chronic GI symptoms with no other identifiable cause
Pancreatitis—pancreatic inflammation
Peptic ulcer disease (PUD)—ulcers in the esophagus, stomach, or duodenum
Splenic rupture—rupture of the spleen
Ulcerative colitis (UC)—inflammatory bowel disease that causes ulcers in the colon

Medications

Many drugs are related to other drugs in both function and chemical composition. These drugs would be considered to be in the same drug class, as shown in Table 17.1. This gives the provider options within a class to choose different drugs with slightly different profiles (actions and side effects). Although knowing the drug class mechanism of action is not essential to become a great scribe, having familiarity with the mechanism can facilitate faster and more accurate documentation. This is because within a class, the generic names tend to sound similar. This is usually a good way to identify a drug class from a generic name. For example, in the proton pump inhibitor class, all of the drug names end in "azole."

TABLE 17.1 ■ Selected Gastrointestinal System Medications

Drug Class and Uses	Generic Name (Brand Name)
Proton pump inhibitor (PPI) • Reduces gastric acid production • Used to treat reflux	dexlansoprazole (Dexilant) esomeprazole (Nexium) lansoprazole (Prevacid) or (Levant) omeprazole (Prilosec) pantoprazole (Protonix)
H_2 blockers • Block stomach acid secretion • Used to treat reflux	cimetidine (Tagamet) famotidine (Pepcid) nizatidine (Axid) ranitidine (Zantac)*
Anticholinergics • Used to treat GIT spasm	dicyclomine (Bentyl)
Peripheral opioid receptor agonist • Used as an anti-diarrheal	loperamide (Imodium)
Glucocorticoid • Anti-inflammatory • Many indications	dexamethasone (Decadron) prednisone (Deltasone)
Antiemetics • Not a drug class • Used to prevent vomiting	metoclopramide (Reglan) ondansetron (Zofran) prochlorperazine (Compazine) promethazine (Phenergan)
Tetracyclic antidepressant • Occasionally useful in some GI disorders	mirtazapine (Remeron)
Laxatives • Loosen stools to help induce a bowel movement • Used to treat constipation	magnesium citrate polyethylene glycol (Golytely) or (MiraLAX)

*The U.S. Food and Drug Administration removed ranitidine (Zantac) from the market in April 2020.

A scribe should be able to diligently record the patient's medication list, which includes the drug name (generic or brand), dose, frequency, and indication (reason for taking the drug).

CASE STUDY 17.1

Jason is a scribe working in the Hawkins Inflammatory Bowel Disease Center, a nationally-recognized facility dedicated to the study and treatment of inflammatory bowel diseases, including celiac disease, Crohn's disease, and ulcerative colitis. The team of 22 physicians treat both adults and children, and many patients travel long distances to obtain their expert care.

The gastroenterologists at the center see patients in the office and also perform general and endoscopic surgery. Jason's skills are best employed in the examination room, however, creating an accurate and comprehensive record in the EHR. This aspect of the documentation is especially important because many times, patients seek the resources at Hawkins IBDC after they have not had success treating their problems elsewhere.

Today, Jason is working with Dr. Ma, whose 11 a.m. appointment is Julie Goss, a new patient seeking a second opinion. Ms. Goss initially saw her primary care provider (PCP) over a year ago for "really bad gas," and the advice at the time was to make dietary changes. About two months ago, while the gas symptoms persisted, Julie began to have diarrhea that would not go away. She made another appointment with her PCP, who ordered abdominal x-rays. When the imaging came back normal, Julie was referred to a GI doctor in her hometown, who arranged for a colonoscopy just last month. He found severe inflammation throughout Julie's colon and ulceration around her ileocecal valve. Julie awoke from the colonoscopy procedure with a surprising diagnosis of Crohn's disease.

The doctor prescribed Julie the steroid prednisone to control her symptoms until they could decide on another treatment, such as an immunosuppressant or biological to reduce the inflammation in her bowels. "But it's just some really smelly gas and diarrhea," Julie told Dr. Ma. "It seems aggressive to go through all that, and I'm not sure about the side effects of these medications. So I'm here to see what the experts say."

"How are you feeling today?" Dr. Ma asked.

"Fine!" Julie said. "The steroids really control my symptoms."

"Any pain today?" the physician asked.

"No, I never had any pain throughout all this. Just the bad gas and more recently the diarrhea. And certainly a sense of fullness."

"What about any heartburn or reflux?"

"No."

"Any bloody stool?"

Julie hesitated. "No, I don't think so," she said, "I noticed some blood on the toilet paper this week, but I think it might be from a hemorrhoid."

"Smoker?" asked the physician.

"No, I quit 10 years ago," Julie said.

"Congratulations," Dr. Ma said. "Do you drink alcohol?"

"Oh my, yes." Julie answered.

"What kind and how much?" Dr. Ma asked.

"Almost always beer—I love craft beers," Julie said, "My husband and I try something new every week. I'll usually have three or four every other night or so."

"OK, do you take ibuprofen?" asked Dr. Ma.

"Sometimes—when I drink too much craft beer!" Julie laughed.

Dr. Ma asked Julie to sit on the exam table while he listened to her heart and breath sounds with a stethoscope. He then asked her to lie down and felt different areas of her abdomen. He asked if she felt any pain; she said no.

Dr. Ma explained that he would like to see the biopsy slides from her recent colonoscopy, so he would have her local hospital's pathology department forward them. He and the other physicians at Hawkins would look at her medical records, laboratory results, and pathology slides as a team before making any decisions about care. "We may want to do another colonoscopy, too." Dr. Ma said. He added that she should not take any ibuprofen for the time being.

QUESTIONS

1. What should Jason record under gastrointestinal for the ROS?
2. What is the *duration* of Julie's "bad gas"?
3. What is the *duration* of Julie's diarrhea?
4. What physical examination technique did Dr. Ma perform when he felt Julie's abdomen?
5. What medications should Jason record in the HPI?
6. In what drug class is the steroid prednisone?

Practice Questions

1. The _____ stores bile that is synthesized by the liver.
2. The _____ produces digestive enzymes.
3. The _____ region is located above the stomach.
4. The first portion of the small intestine is the _____.
5. A 60-year-old male patient presents to his GI specialist for follow-up of his liver disease. He reports having worsened right upper abdominal pain and the sensation of abdominal fullness. He is feeling the urge to vomit and has also been vomiting more than normal. No blood in his vomit. He has had a loss of appetite and has had some indigestion. No chest pain or sweating. How should this be documented in the review of systems?
6. On exam the patient is cachectic and appears older than his stated age. Scleral icterus is noted and he has generalized jaundice. Normal rhythm and rate, with no murmurs gallops, or rubs. Breath sounds are normal. There is hepatomegaly with tenderness in the right upper quadrant and abdominal ascites. 4+ pitting edema in both lower extremities. Thready pulses in both legs. How should this be documented in the physical exam?
7. The patient has required a procedure multiple times in the past to drain fluid from his peritoneum. What is this called?
8. This patient has a history of liver scarring related to alcoholism. What is this diagnosis?
9. The GI specialist decides to give the patient a medication to help with his reflux. Which medication would be an option?
   a. loperamide (Imodium)
   b. pantoprazole (Protonix)
   c. ondansetron (Zofran)
   d. magnesium citrate

CHAPTER 18

Genitourinary (Reproductive System and Urinary System)

1. Use medical terminology to document medical issues involving the genitourinary system.
2. Describe the anatomy and physiology of the genitourinary system.
3. Document genitourinary system symptoms related during a review of systems.
4. Document signs related by the provider during a physical exam of the genitourinary system.
5. Document operations and procedures for the genitourinary system.
6. Document the genitourinary system clinical impressions, diagnoses, and signs and symptoms commonly found in a problem list.
7. Document relevant drug classes and medications for the treatment of problems associated with the genitourinary system.

Abortion
Adnexa
Amenorrhea
Benign prostatic hyperplasia (BPH)
Bladder
Cervix
Chlamydia
Circumcision
Clitoris
Costovertebral angle
Cryptorchidism
Cystocele
Cystoscopy
Dilatation and curettage (D&C)
Dysmenorrhea

Dysuria
Eclampsia
Ejaculate
Ejaculatory duct
Endometriosis
Epididymis
Fallopian tube
Flank region
Genitourinary system
Glans
Gonorrhea
Gravid
Hematuria
Hemodialysis
Hysterectomy
Introitus
Kidney

Labia majora
Labia minora
Leukorrhea
Lithotripsy
Malodorous
Multigravida
Multiparous
Nulligravida
Nulliparous
Oliguria
Ova
Ovary
Parous
Peritoneal dialysis
Pre-eclampsia
Prepuce
Primigravida

Continued

Anatomy and Physiology

The **genitourinary system** is a combination of both male and female reproductive systems and the **renal** or urinary system. Although traditionally these are thought of as two separate systems, they are counted as one system together in review of systems and physical exam for billing.

It should be noted that often the scribe will be asked to leave the room prior to a genital exam. This is because the scribe is non essential personnel, and the patient's comfort and privacy is always prioritized. In some instances, however, the scribe, if female, may be asked to remain in the room during the examination of a female patient to act as a chaperone—a witness that no inappropriate behaviors took place during the exam. Either way, the scribe will be provided with the information necessary to complete the history and physical in this area.

MALE REPRODUCTIVE SYSTEM

The externally visible portion of the male reproductive system (Fig. 18.1) includes the **glans**, or head of the **penis**. The glans may be covered by the **prepuce** (foreskin) unless surgically removed by **circumcision**. At the tip of the glans is the **urethral meatus**, which is the urethral opening.

Also visible externally is the **scrotum**, two pouches that hold the **testicles** or **testes** (**testis**, singular). The **testes** are the organs which produce **sperm**, the male reproductive cell that fertilizes female eggs (ova). Mature sperm travel from the testes through the **epididymis** to the **vas deferens** (a duct). The vas deferens joins with the **seminal vesicle**, a gland which contributes to the composition of **semen**, to form the **ejaculatory duct**. This becomes the *prostatic duct*, where the **prostate gland** also contributes to the composition of semen. Urine and **ejaculate** (a mixture of sperm and nutritional fluids) are expelled through the **urethra** and urethral meatus.

FEMALE REPRODUCTIVE SYSTEM

The female reproductive system (Fig. 18.2) is designed to receive sperm from the male to fertilize an **ova** (egg). The fertilized egg is then developed into a fetus and ultimately a living child.

The **introitus** is the opening into the **vaginal canal** and the **vaginal vault**, the most internal portion of the vagina. Posteriorly are the **vaginal fornices** (**fornix**, singular). These *vaginal spaces*, or *vaginal recesses*, are in the posterior vagina above and below the uterine cervix. The **cervix** is the inferior portion of the uterus and contains the **cervical os**. This is the cervical opening leading into the **uterus**, the hollow muscular organ that houses the fetus during pregnancy. The **fallopian tubes** are located in the superior uterus bilaterally. These are hollow tubes that connect the uterus to the ovaries. The **ovaries** are two organs situated above the uterus that produce ova. **Adnexae** (**adnexa**, singular) is the ovarian region adjacent to the uterus.

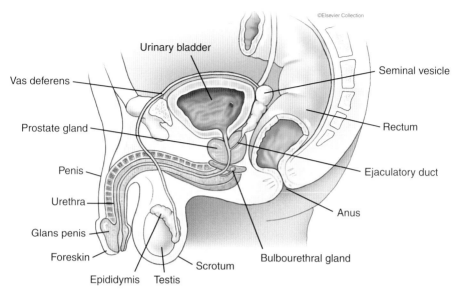

©Elsevier Collection

Fig. 18.1   Male reproductive organs. (© Elsevier Collection.)

Externally, the introitus is surrounded by two pairs of labia: **labia minora** (medial) and **labia majora** (lateral; Fig. 18.3). Anteriorly to the introitus is the opening of the urethra, which expels urine from the bladder. The most anterior structure is the **clitoris**, which is erectile tissue analogous to the glans penis.

URINARY (RENAL) SYSTEM

The urinary system is comprised of the pair of kidneys that are connected to a series of tubes which ultimately terminate outside the body (Fig. 18.4). The two **kidneys** are located in the posterior abdominal cavity. The kidneys filter blood and pass the waste products and excess fluid into the ureters as **urine**. They also play a role in electrolyte regulation and water resorption (letting water be taken back into the body). The **ureters** are hollow tubes that drain the urine into the urinary **bladder**, which is a muscular pouch that stores the urine until it is expelled through the body via the urethra.

Review of Systems

It is the duty of the scribe to translate the patient's interpretation of their symptoms into medical lingo. For example, if a patient says they have burning pain with urination the scribe should document **dysuria**.

Note: Symptoms that can be placed in multiple systems have been designated as such in italics. Remember to always maximize the number of <u>systems</u> that are included in the review of systems so that the chart can be billed at higher levels (if desired). For example, if a patient is having hematuria and dysuria, it would be best to include hematuria in "*hematologic/lymphatic*" and dysuria in "*genitourinary*" (two billable systems), as opposed to including hematuria and dysuria in "*genitourinary*" (one billable system).

Abortion—loss of pregnancy secondary to premature expulsion of the fetus from the uterus; an abortion may be spontaneous (miscarriage) or induced (intentionally caused)

Amenorrhea (*endocrine*)—absence of menses

Anuria—no urine production

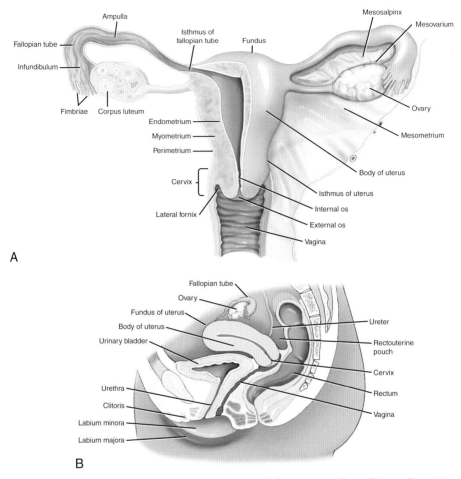

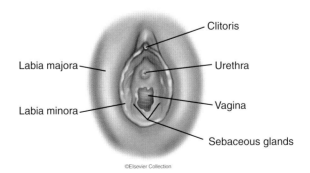

Fig. 18.2   Female reproductive organs. (A) Frontal view. (B) Sagittal view. (From Shiland, BJ: *Medical terminology and anatomy for coding*, ed 4, St. Louis, 2021, Elsevier.)

Fig. 18.3   Female external genitalia. (© Elsevier Collection.)

Dysmenorrhea—painful menses

Dysuria—pain with urination (often described as "burning")

Flank pain—pain in the region between the ribs and the thoracic vertebrae that lies atop the kidneys

G(#) P(#) Ab(#)—gravida (# of pregnancies), para (# of viable pregnancies), abortions (# of miscarriages/abortions)

Gravid—the condition of being pregnant; derivative words include **nulligravida** (having had no pregnancies), **primigravida** (having a first pregnancy) and **multigravida** (a pregnant woman having had at least one prior pregnancy)

Hematuria (*hematologic/lymphatic*)—blood in urine

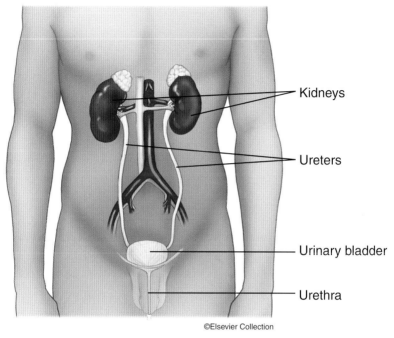

©Elsevier Collection

Fig. 18.4   Urinary system. (© Elsevier Collection.)

Medical Terminology Word Parts for the Genitourinary System

Combining Forms			
ren/o	kidney	test/o testicul/o orchi/o orchid/o orch/o	testis
genit/o	genital		
urin/o	urine urinary system	sperm/o spermat/o	sperm
balan/o	glans penis	epididym/o	epididymis
phall/o	penis	vas/o	vas deferens
preputi/o posth/o	prepuce/foreskin	scrot/o	scrotum

Continued

Medical Terminology Word Parts for the Genitourinary System—cont'd

vesicul/o	seminal vesicle		dys-	bad, abnormal, difficult
semin/i	semen		dia-	through
prostat/o	prostate		crypt-	hidden
urethr/o	urethra		poly-	much, many, excessive
meatu/o	meatus			
o/o ov/o ov/i ovul/o	ovum		para-	near, beside, abnormal
			intra-	within
colp/o vagin/o	vagina		hypo-	below
			hyper-	excessive
cervic/o	cervix		circum-	around
hyster/o metri/o metr/o uter/o	uterus		primi-	first
			nulli-	none
			multi-	many
salping/o	fallopian tube		ec-	out
labi/o	labia			
clitorid/o	clitoris		***Suffixes***	
oophor/o ovari/o	ovary		-spadias	tear
			-plasia	formation
nephr/o ren/o	kidney		-cele	protrusion
			-rrhea	flow, discharge
ur/o urin/o	urine		-rrhagia	bursting forth
			-algia	pain
ureter/o	ureter		-cision	process of cutting
cyst/o vesic/o	bladder		-itis	inflammation
			-ia	condition
men/o	menstruation		-uria	urine condition
gravid/o	pregnancy		-ectomy	removal
olig/o	scanty		-scopy	viewing
leuk/o	white		-pexy	fixation, suspension
hemat/o	blood		-stomy	forming an opening
lith/o	stone		-tripsy	crushing
hydr/o	water		-osis	abnormal condition
gon/o	seed		-para	delivery
top/o	place		-al -ic	pertaining to
Prefixes			-plasia	formation
epi-	above, upon			
supra-	above			
a- an-	without			

Hot flash (*constitutional, endocrine*)—feeling warm and sweaty

Incomplete voiding—not completely emptying the bladder

Last menstrual period (LMP)—the date of a woman's last menses

Last normal menstrual cycle (LNMP)—the date of a woman's last normal menses if she has irregular or abnormal menstrual cycles

Leukorrhea—white or yellow vaginal discharge

Malodorous—foul smelling

Menometrorrhagia—prolonged or excessive and irregular menses

Menopause—not having a menses (older age or after uterine removal)

Menorrhagia—abnormally heavy or prolonged bleeding during menses

Metrorrhagia—menses at irregular intervals or spotting between menses

Oliguria—small amount of urine production

Parous—the condition of having children; derivative words include **nulliparous** (having birthed no children) and **multiparous** (having birthed more than one child)

Pelvic pain—pain of the pelvic floor

Penile discharge—any drainage from the male urethral opening of an unusual color or odor

Polyuria (*endocrine*)—excessive urine production

Testicular pain—pain in either or both testicles

Testicular swelling or mass

Urinary frequency—urinating more frequently than normal

Urinary incontinence (*neurologic*)—involuntary loss of urinary control

Urinary urgency—sudden, compelling urge to urinate

Vaginal discharge—any vaginal discharge of an unusual color or odor

Physical Exam

Superficially, the kidneys are in the **flank region** of the back. If there is a kidney problem, sometimes there will be tenderness to percussion in the **costovertebral angle**, an area between the ribs and vertebrae in the flank region (Fig. 18.5). Most likely this will be from a urinary tract infection that traveled from elsewhere in the urinary tract to the kidneys.

Adnexal tenderness—pain with palpation of the adnexa

Bladder distension—a filled bladder that can be felt with palpation of the lower abdomen

Chandelier sign—marked cervical motion tenderness on pelvic exam

Costovertebral angle (CVA) tenderness—tenderness to percussion over the kidney that may indicate kidney infection (see Fig. 18.5)

Discharge—fluid or discharge from the urethral opening or vagina that can be normal or abnormal

External inguinal ring—area palpated frequently in male exam looking for inguinal hernia (Fig. 18.6)

Flank tenderness—tenderness in the flank region (which lies atop the kidneys but is a broader region than the CVA)

Suprapubic tenderness—pain with palpation of the lower abdomen just above the pubic symphysis

Operations/Procedures

Patients often do not know the name of the operation and will describe their understanding of the procedure in lay terms. It is the scribe's duty to translate the patient's procedural description into the equivalent medical term. For example, if a patient says they had their uterus removed, the scribe should record that the patient had a "partial hysterectomy."

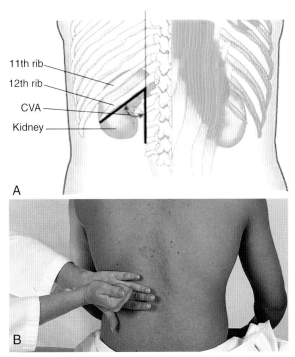

Fig. 18.5 (A) Costovertebral angle. (B) Indirect fist percussion of the costovertebral angle (*CVA*). (In Lewis SL, Dirksen SR, Heitkemper MM, Bucher L, Harding MM: *Medical-surgical nursing: assessment and management of clinical problems*, ed 11, St. Louis, 2020, Elsevier. From Jarvis C: *Physical examination and health assessment*, ed 7, St. Louis, 2016, Saunders.)

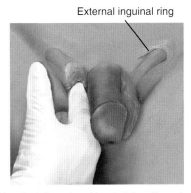

Fig. 18.6 Palpation for inguinal hernia at the external inguinal ring. (From Jarvis C: *Physical examination and health assessment*, ed 8, St. Louis, 2016, Elsevier.)

Arteriovenous (AV) fistula—abnormal or surgical passage connecting an artery to a vein (often surgically created for hemodialysis)

Cesarian section—surgically removing child(ren) from the uterus through an incision in the abdominal wall and uterus

Circumcision—surgical removal of the male prepuce or foreskin

Cystoscopy—endoscopy of the urinary bladder

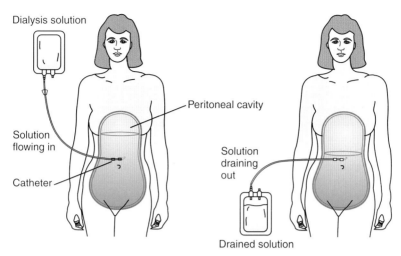

Fig. 18.7 Peritoneal dialysis. The solution is infused into the abdominal cavity and later drained. (From Heimgartner NM, Workman ML, Rebar CR, Ignatavicius DD: *Medical-surgical nursing: concepts for interprofessional collaborative care*, ed 10, St. Louis, 2021, Elsevier.)

Dilatation and curettage (D&C)—dilation of the cervix and removal of uterine contents (could be done after miscarriage or abortion)

Hemodialysis—filtering the blood and removing waste products of a person with renal dysfunction

Hysterectomy (complete)—removal of the uterus, fallopian tubes, and ovaries

Hysterectomy (partial)—removal of the uterus only

Lithotripsy—destruction of kidney stones with lasers, ultrasound waves, or mechanically

Oophorectomy—surgical removal of one or both ovaries

Orchiectomy—surgical removal of one or both testes

Orchiopexy—surgical fixation of the testis (to correct cryptorchidism)

Peritoneal dialysis—dialysis that uses the peritoneum in the abdomen as a membrane (as opposed to a machine; Fig. 18.7)

Tubal ligation—tying off the fallopian tubes to prevent eggs from reaching the uterus (an effective way to prevent pregnancy)

Uterine ablation—removal or destruction of the endometrial lining of the uterus

Vasectomy—severance of the vas deferens to prevent sperm from being ejaculated (an effective way to prevent pregnancy)

Problem List

Patients often do not know the name of a specific diagnosis, but will instead describe it to their provider. It is the scribe's duty to translate the lay terms into medical terminology. For example, if the patient says they have prostate enlargement that is benign, the scribe should document "benign prostatic hyperplasia."

Acute kidney injury (AKI)—acute loss of kidney function

Bacterial vaginosis (BV)—excessive growth of normal vaginal bacteria that causes itching and discharge

Benign prostatic hyperplasia (BPH)—benign (noncancerous) prostate enlargement that may cause urinary retention

Cervicitis—inflammation of the uterine cervix

Chlamydia—common STI that is known to cause white penile or vaginal discharge, dysuria, and abdominal pain

Chronic kidney disease (CKD)—progressive loss of kidney function

Cryptorchidism—the condition of having undescended testicles

Cystitis—lower urinary tract infection

Cystocele—bladder herniation into the vagina (Fig. 18.8)

Dysfunctional uterine bleeding (DUB)—abnormal uterine bleeding without pathology

Eclampsia—advanced complications of preeclampsia with seizures

Ectopic pregnancy—embryo attaches outside the uterus and the pregnancy cannot be carried to term (dangerous for the mother)

Endometrial cancer—cancer of the endometrial cells in the uterus

Endometriosis—endometrial tissue grows outside the uterus (Fig. 18.9)

End-stage renal disease (ESRD)—the most advanced renal disease

Epididymitis—epididymal inflammation

Erectile dysfunction (impotence)—the inability to maintain an erection

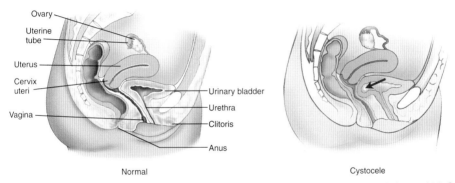

Fig. 18.8 Cystocele. (From Leonard PC: *Building a medical vocabulary: with Spanish translations*, ed 10, St. Louis, 2017, Elsevier.)

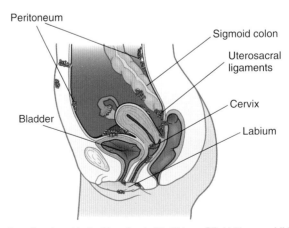

Fig. 18.9 Common sites of endometriosis. (From Lewis SL, Dirksen SR, Heitkemper MM, Bucher L, Harding MM: *Medical-surgical nursing: assessment and management of clinical problems*, ed 11, St. Louis, 2020, Elsevier.)

Gestational diabetes mellitus (GDM)—developing diabetes during pregnancy with no prior diabetic history

Glomerulonephritis—inflammation of the glomeruli in the kidneys

Gonorrhea—STI that can cause green penile or vaginal discharge

Hydrocele—an accumulation of fluid within a sac around the testicle

Hypercalcemia—elevated blood calcium (Ca^{2+})

Hyperkalemia—elevated blood potassium (K^+)

Hypernatremia—elevated blood sodium (Na^+)

Hypocalcemia—low blood calcium (Ca^{2+})

Hypokalemia—low blood potassium (K^+)

Hyponatremia—low blood sodium (Na^+)

Hypospadias—congenital condition where the urethral meatus opens somewhere along the underside of the penis as opposed to opening at the tip of the glans penis

Interstitial cystitis—chronic inflammation of the bladder

Miscarriage (spontaneous as opposed to induced **abortion**)—termination of pregnancy before viable fetal age

Nephrolithiasis—stones formed in the kidneys

Ovarian cancer—cancer of one or both ovaries

Ovarian cysts—fluid-filled sac in the ovaries

Polycystic ovary syndrome (PCOS)—variety of symptoms caused by elevated androgenic (male) hormones in women

Pre-eclampsia—pregnancy complication with high blood pressure, proteinuria, and swelling

Prostate cancer—cancer of the prostate gland

Prostatitis—inflammation of the prostate gland

Proteinuria—excessive protein content in the urine

Pyelonephritis—upper urinary tract infection that may cause inflammation of the kidneys

Renal failure—kidney failure

Trichomoniasis—STI that can cause yellow/green frothy discharge

Ureterolithiasis—urinary stone found in the ureter

Urinary tract infection (UTI)—infection of the urinary tract

Uterine fibroids—benign tumors of the uterus

Vaginitis—vaginal inflammation

Medications

Many drugs are related to other drugs in both function and chemical composition. These drugs would be considered to be in the same drug class. This gives options within a class to choose different drugs with slightly different profiles (actions and side effects).

A scribe should be able to diligently record the patient's medication list, which includes the drug name (generic or brand), dose, frequency, and indication (reason for taking the drug).

Drug Class and Uses	Generic Name (Brand Name)
Alpha antagonists • Treat urinary retention	tamsulosin (Flomax)
Antimuscarinics • Treat urinary incontinence	oxybutynin (Ditropan) tolterodine (Detrol)
PDE5 inhibitors • Treat erectile dysfunction	tadalafil (Cialis) sildenafil (Viagra) vardenafil (Levitra)

Continued

Drug Class and Uses	Generic Name (Brand Name)
Contraceptives • Prevent pregnancy • Regulate menstrual cycles	**Progestin only** drospirenone (Yaz) etonogestrel contraceptive implant (Nexplanon) levonorgestrel intrauterine device (Mirena) medroxyprogesterone acetate injection (Depo-Provera) **Progestin + estrogen** drospirenone-ethinyl estradiol (Yasmin) ethinyl estradiol/etonogestrel vaginal ring (Nuvaring) **Non-hormonal** copper intrauterine device (Paragard)
Hormones • Replace normal female hormones after a hysterectomy or menopause	estrogen (Premarin)
• Increase fluid resorption by the kidneys	vasopressin (Vasostrict)

CASE STUDY 18.1

Ozzie is an energetic 10-year-old who has spent his summer swimming at the neighbor's pool and exploring the nearby wooded area. Nearly every evening Ozzie would recount to his parents the day's amazing happenings—tales of the swamp monster he and a friend heard in the storm drain, or the impossible "hangtime" he achieved on the skateboard jump. But although Ozzie tends to exaggerate, his parents took Ozzie seriously when he told them what had happened in the bathroom. "I peed blood!" he reported. His mother noted that he did not seem to be urinating much and when he did, she was able to confirm that the urine had a bloody appearance.

The pediatrician, Dr. Snow, saw Ozzie the next day in the office. She noted that the boy was well developed and well nourished, and that he appears his age. Although he did not have a fever, Ozzie's blood pressure was elevated. Dr. Snow noted edema around the boy's eyelids and face, and said "1+" as she squeezed his foot above the medial malleolus. She said that his neck was supple, his thyroid felt good, and that there was no remarkable lymphadenopathy. When Dr. Snow palpated his abdomen, Ozzie admitted it hurt a little at all four quadrants, and he also indicated mild bilateral flank pain. Ozzie's mother said that his appetite did seem diminished, but she had not noticed until now. Examination of Ozzie's genitals revealed that both testes were descended and no penile lesions were found.

Dr. Snow ordered a urinalysis and blood tests for Ozzie. Ozzie's urine was dark. Lab results showed albuminuria and hyperlipidemia, and antibodies to a streptococcal bacteria. Dr. Snow's impression is poststreptococcal glomerulonephritis, a type of kidney disease that can develop after infection of the group A strep bacteria. She believes Ozzie will get better on his own, but wants to continue periodic 24-hour urine tests to monitor his kidney function.

QUESTIONS

1. As the scribe, how would you record Ozzie's chief complaint?
2. What is the medical term for diminished amounts of urine?
3. How and where would you record Ozzie's mother's observation that his appetite is diminished?
4. What information would you record under constitutional in the physical exam portion of the note?
5. Where in the physical exam would you place the following signs?
   a. + edema
   b. – lymphadenopathy
   c. – thyromegaly
   d. Tender abdomen
   e. Bilateral flank tenderness

Practice Questions

1. _____ are the male organs which produce sperm.
2. _____ are the female organs which produce eggs.
3. _____ filter the blood and excrete waste as urine.
4. Urine is expelled from the body via the _____ opening.
5. An 87-year-old female patient presents to her gynecologist for evaluation of a several week history of pain with urination. She also describes having to suddenly urinate frequently throughout the day, and admits that she does not always make it to the bathroom on time. No blood in her urine. She has had a low-grade fever with chills at home. She is also having some discomfort above her bladder, especially when she urinates, that occasionally travels into her back (she points to the flank region). The patient is postmenopausal but is still having hot flashes. She has had two pregnancies with one vaginal full-term birth and one miscarriage. How should this be documented in the review of systems?
6. On exam there is suprapubic tenderness to palpation. A pulsatile mass is present around the umbilicus and there is a well-healed incision in the lower abdomen. There is right costo-vertebral angle tenderness to percussion. Dorsal kyphosis is noted. Mucous membranes are dry. The patient appears cachectic. How should this be documented in the physical exam?
7. The patient is asked about the scar in the lower abdomen and she reports that it was from a surgery to remove both of her ovaries. What should be documented in the surgical history?
8. At the end of the exam the patient mentions that she is prone to urinary tract infections, and in the past has had to be hospitalized for an infection that travelled to her kidneys. What should be included in her medical history?

CHAPTER 19

Hematology and the Lymphatic and Immune System

Anatomy and Physiology

Hematology (the study of blood) and the lymphatic and immune systems are all interconnected. **Bone marrow** is housed inside many bones, particularly those that are centrally located such as the ribs, sternum, cranium, vertebrae, and pelvis. **Hematopoietic stem cells** reside in the bone marrow and give rise to all three classes of cells found within the blood: **erythrocytes** (red blood cells [**RBCs**]), **thrombocytes** (platelets), and **leukocytes** (white blood cells; Fig. 19.1). Blood comprises these formed elements and a liquid portion, called **plasma** (Fig. 19.2).

Erythrocytes are the **heme** (iron) carrying cells of the blood that are responsible for oxygen and carbon dioxide transportation. Erythrocytes pick up oxygen at the lungs and deliver it to the body's tissues in exchange for carbon dioxide, which is then transported back to the lungs for exhalation (Fig. 19.3).

Thrombocytes (platelets) are the cells that participate in the clotting cascade, which prevents abnormal bleeding.

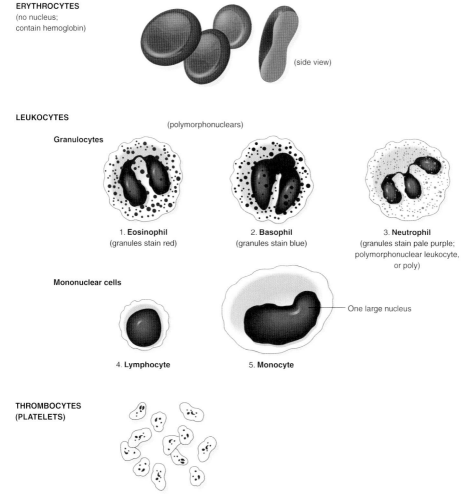

Fig. 19.1   Types of blood cells. (From Chabner D: *The language of medicine*, ed 12, St. Louis, 2021, Elsevier.)

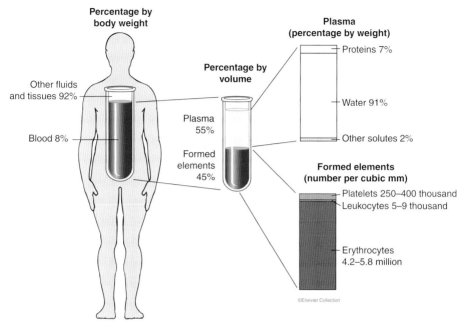

Fig. 19.2 Composition of whole blood. (© Elsevier Collection.)

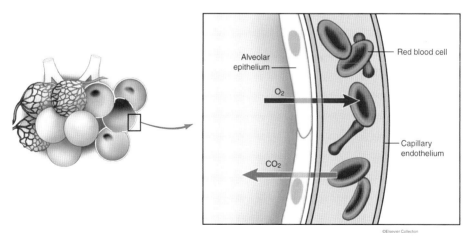

Fig. 19.3 Gas exchange via the erythrocytes in the lungs. (© Elsevier Collection.)

Leukocytes (white blood cells [WBCs]) are the cells that are responsible for proper immune function and host defense against pathogens and other foreign materials. There are many types of white blood cells with various functions, as shown in Fig. 19.1. Each cell type participates in either or both branches of the immune system.

The *innate immune system* includes all existing defense mechanisms against pathogens. This branch of the immune system is the first line of defense against a foreign invader: it is rapidly activated and has broad effects. Some examples of innate defense mechanisms include the skin (physical barrier), chemicals and enzymes in the mouth and digestive tract (chemical barrier), and certain types of leukocytes (e.g. macrophages, which are scavenger cells).

The *adaptive immune system* is the branch of the immune system that is generated in response to the presence of a certain pathogen. This branch of the immune system is the second line of defense against a foreign invader: it is slow to act but it is targeted toward a specific pathogen. Certain types of leukocytes participate in this branch of the immune system (e.g. lymphocytes).

Neutrophils and **monocytes** (which develop into **macrophages**) are considered to be scavenger cells, as they phagocytose (eat) foreign materials and other dead cells and tissues. These cells are part of the innate immune system.

Lymphocytes are the functional unit of the adaptive immune system, and include many cell types. **B cells** produce antibodies against an **antigen** (foreign protein). **Antibodies** are proteins that attach to their target and mark it for destruction by other cell types, like macrophages. There are several types of **T cells**, but the two most important include CD4 T cells and CD8 T cells. *CD4 T cells* (*T helper cells*) activate other T cells and B cells, and then regulate their activity. *CD8 T cells* (*cytotoxic T cells*) destroy the antigen they are instructed to attack. The last type of lymphocyte is the **natural killer (NK) cell**, which primarily attacks tumor cells or virally infected cells.

All leukocytes travel in the body via the circulatory system and the lymphatic system. **Lymphatic vessels** are a series of vessels that terminate in open-ended tubes in the **interstitium**, akin to blood capillaries (Fig. 19.4). These tubes collect interstitial fluid, which becomes **lymphatic fluid** as it enters the lymphatic system.

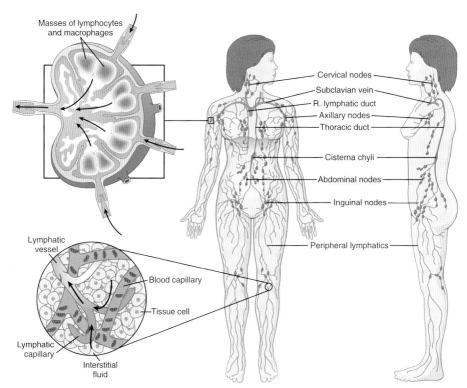

Fig. 19.4 The lymphatic system. (From Hall JE, Hall ME: *Guyton and Hall textbook of medical physiology*, ed 14, Philadelphia, 2021, Elsevier.)

Lymphatic vessels increase in size until they join the venous circulation via *lymphatic trunks*, which empty their contents at the junction of both subclavian veins.

Lymph nodes are areas of lymphatic tissue scattered throughout the body that filter the blood for foreign antigens. They are also the site where many cell types interact when an immune response is being generated. The sites of major lymph nodes are depicted in Fig. 19.4.

The **spleen**, an organ located in the left upper quadrant of the abdominal cavity (Fig. 19.5), is comparable to a large lymph node. It also filters the blood to screen for foreign antigens.

Medical Terminology Word Parts for the Hematologic, the Lymphatic and the Immune Systems

Combining Forms		poly-	much, many
hem/o	blood	pan-	all
hemat/o			
		Suffixes	
myel/o	bone marrow	-al	pertaining to
erythr/o	red	-ior	
thromb/o	clot	-ia	condition of
leuk/o	white	-logy	study of
neutr/o	neutral	-poesis	formation
phag/o	eat, swallow	-cyte	cell
lymph/o	lymph	-gen	producing
lymphat/o		-pathy	pertaining to disease
lymphaden/o	lymph gland	-itis	inflammation
lymphangi/o	lymph vessel	-rrhea	discharge, flow
splen/o	spleen	-penia	deficiency
rhin/o	nose	-emia	blood condition
purpur/o	purple	-emesis	vomiting
bi/o	life	-osis	abnormal condition
Prefixes		-cytosis	abnormal increase in cells
a-	without		
mono-	one	-opsy	process of viewing
marco-	large	-ectomy	removal
anti-	against	-oma	tumor, mass

Review of Systems

Remember that it is the duty of the scribe to translate the patient's interpretation of their symptoms into medical lingo. For example, if a patient says they have black and tarry stools, the scribe should document "melena."

In the review of systems, *hematologic/lymphatic* symptoms are billed as one system and *allergic/immunologic* symptoms are billed as one system.

Symptoms that can be placed in multiple systems have been designated as such in italics in the list below. If a patient is having lymphadenopathy and bruising, it would be best to include

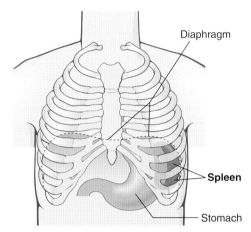

Fig. 19.5   Location of the spleen. (From Chabner D: *The language of medicine*, ed 12, St. Louis, 2021, Elsevier.)

lymphadenopathy in "*hematologic/lymphatic*" and bruising in "*integumentary*" (two billable systems), as opposed to including lymphadenopathy and bruising in "*hematologic/lymphatic*" (one system).

HEMATOLOGIC/LYMPHATIC

Bruising (*integumentary*)—blue, purple, yellow, or green discoloration, usually from trauma
Epistaxis (*HEENT*)—nose bleed
Hematemesis (*digestive*)—vomiting blood
Hematochezia (*digestive*)—stools with bright red blood that can be due to GI bleed in the lower GI tract
Hematuria (*genitourinary*)—blood in urine
Hemoptysis (*respiratory*)—coughing blood
Lymphadenopathy—swollen lymph nodes
Lymphatic streaking (lymphangitis)—red streaking, normally up an extremity, due to a distal infection
Melena (*digestive*)—black and tarry stools from a bleed in the upper GI track

ALLERGIC/IMMUNOLOGIC

Congestion *(HEENT)*—swelling and/or irritation of the nasal tissues that causes the sensation of not being able to inhale through the nasal cavity
Fever (*constitutional*)—a temperature greater than 100.4 °F (38°C)
Postnasal drainage *(HEENT)*—mucus drainage down the throat that causes voice clearing, a sore throat, and hoarseness
Pruritus (*integumentary*)—sensation of itchiness
Rash (*integumentary*)—any abnormal change in the skin
Recent illnesses (*constitutional*)—any recent illnesses (e.g. upper respiratory infection or urinary tract infection)
Rhinorrhea *(HEENT)*—runny nose

Sinus pain/pressure *(HEENT)*—facial pain or pressure

Anemia, a deficiency in RBCs, can cause many signs and symptoms. Symptoms are often related to hypoxia caused by the deficiency, and can include dizziness, palpitations, fatigue, and shortness of breath. **Thrombocytopenia** is a deficiency in platelets that affects the ability of blood clots to form. Extremely low levels of platelets may cause spontaneous and unexplained bleeding, such as **hematemesis** (vomiting blood), **hematochezia** (rectal blood), and **epistaxis** (nose bleeding).

Physical Exam

Physical findings may at times be appropriately placed in a different body system than what is listed, but less often than in the review of systems.

Hematologic/lymphatic/immunologic are billed as one system.

Abscess—collection of pus in body tissues

Contusion—bruise

Discharge—any fluid exuded from the skin described as purulent (pus-like), sanguinous (bloody), clear, serosanguinous (blood + clear)

Ecchymosis—skin discoloration from bruising or bleeding internally (Fig. 19.6)

Erythema (rubor)—redness

Hematoma—collection of blood within the skin, usually due to trauma that ruptures capillaries

Lymphadenopathy—swollen lymph nodes caused by a variety of things that increase immune function (like infection or autoimmune disease)

Lymphangitis—inflammation of lymphatic vessels that look like streaking, typically seen up a limb as a result of spreading infection from a distal location (Fig. 19.7). Symptoms can include redness, warmth, and lymphadenopathy.

Lymphedema—extremity swelling from damage to the lymphatic system (differentiated from cardiovascular edema because lymphedema is usually unilateral, versus bilateral swelling seen in cardiovascular edema)

Paronychia—bacterial or fungal infection where the nail and skin meet, causing redness, swelling, and pain

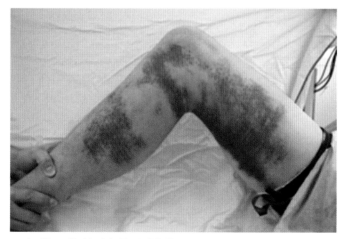

Fig. 19.6 Ecchymosis. (From Chahla J, LaPrade RF: *Evidence-based management of complex knee injuries: restoring the anatomy to achieve best outcomes*, St. Louis, 2021, Elsevier.)

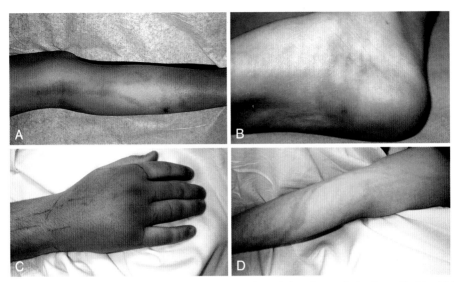

Fig. 19.7   Lymphangitis. (A) An insect bite was the source of inoculation of group A streptococci in this child, who subsequently suffered secondary cellulitis and lymphangitis. The erythematous streaks coursing up the leg were tender and slightly indurated. (B) Three distinct lymphangitic streaks are seen coursing up the instep from an area of cellulitis surrounding a puncture wound of the foot. Pseudomonas was the causative organism. (C and D) In this child irregular lymphatic streaks are seen coursing up the arm from a cellulitic area involving the dorsum of his hand. (From Zitelli BJ, Nowalk AJ, McIntire SC: *Zitelli and Davis' atlas of pediatric physical diagnosis*, ed 7, St. Louis, 2018, Elsevier.)

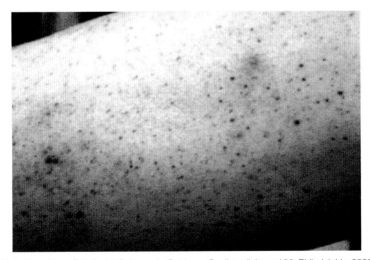

Fig. 19.8   Petechiae. (From Schafer AI, Goldman L: *Goldman-Cecil medicine*, ed 26, Philadelphia, 2020, Elsevier.)

Petechiae—pinpoint erythematous rash often caused by superficial capillaries under the skin that rupture and bleed (Fig. 19.8)

Purpura—itchy purplish rash often caused by superficial capillaries under the skin that rupture and bleed (Fig. 19.9)

Urticaria (hives)—welt-like rash notable for red, raised, pruritic bumps that is often due to an allergen

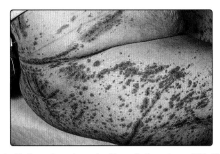

Fig. 19.9 Purpura in a patient with thrombocytopenia. (From Ardren-Jones MR, Gawkrodger DJ: *Dermatology: an illustrated colour text*, ed 7, Amsterdam, 2020, Elsevier.)

Lymph nodes can become swollen and sometimes painful during infection as inflammatory messengers and cells gather as they prepare to fight the perceived threat. **Lymphadenopathy** (swollen lymph nodes) may be palpable on exam (), and typically enlarge near the site of infection.

For the anemic patient on exam, **pallor** (paleness) is often noted. This can be observed in the skin, mucous membranes, and conjunctiva. A patient with thrombocytopenia may present with **petechiae** and **purpura** (small spots of bleeding visible on the skin) on exam.

Operations/Procedures

Any of the patient's prior surgical history (including major operations or minor procedures) may be discussed in the context of a patient's medical history. Patients often do not know the name of the operation and will describe their understanding of the procedure in lay terms. It is the scribe's duty to translate the patient's procedural description into the equivalent medical term. For example, if a patient says they had their spleen removed, the scribe should record that the patient had a "splenectomy."

Bone marrow biopsy—analysis of bone marrow for diagnostic purposes

Splenectomy—removal of the spleen

Problem List

Patients often do not know the name of a specific diagnosis, but will instead describe it to their provider. It is the scribe's duty to translate the lay terms into medical terminology. For example, if the patient says they have a history of low red cells, the scribe should document "anemia."

Acquired immunodeficiency syndrome (AIDS)—progression of HIV with T4 cell destruction below a set lower limit, and increasing frequency of severe opportunistic infections (e.g. with fungi and bacteria that do not normally affect healthy individuals)

Anemia—decrease in the number of RBCs or hemoglobin

Human immunodeficiency virus (HIV)—virus that destroys T4 cells causing immunodeficiency and frequent infections potentially leading to AIDS

Leukemia—group of cancers of the blood/bone marrow that cause leukocytosis of abnormally developed and malfunctional WBCs

Leukocytosis—increase in the number of WBCs

Leukopenia—decrease in the number of WBCs

Lymphoma—group of blood cell tumors that develop from WBCs

Pancytopenia—decrease in the number of RBCs, WBCs, and platelets

Polycythemia—increase in the number of RBCs

Thrombocytopenia—decrease in the number of platelets

Thrombocytosis—increase in the number of platelets

Medications

A scribe should be able to diligently record the patient's medication list, which includes the drug name (generic or brand), dose, frequency, and indication (reason for taking the drug). Table 19.1 lists drugs related to hematology, lymphatic, and immune disorders.

TABLE 19.1 ■ Selected Hematology, Lymphatic, and Immune System Medications

Drug Class	Generic Name (Brand Name)
Antihistamines • Treat allergies	cetirizine (Zyrtec) diphenhydramine (Benadryl) fexofenadine (Allegra) hydroxyzine (Vistaril) loratadine (Claritin)
Leukotriene antagonists • Bronchodilators • Treat airway inflammation (e.g. in allergies)	montelukast (Singulair)
Antifungals • Not a class • Group of drugs used for fungal infections	fluconazole (Diflucan) nystatin (Mycostatin)
Antivirals • Not a class • Group of drugs used for viral infections	acyclovir (Zovirax) - *herpes simplex and herpes zoster* oseltamivir (Tamiflu) - *influenza virus* valacyclovir (Valtrex) - *herpes simplex and herpes zoster*

Antibiotics
• Not a class
• Group of drugs used for bacterial infections
	Penicillins
	amoxicillin (Amoxil)
	ampicillin-clavulanate (Augmentin)
	ampicillin-sulbactam (Unasyn)
	penicillin V potassium (Pen VK)
	piperacillin-tazobactam (Zosyn)
	Macrolides
	   azithromycin (Zithromax or Z Pak)
	Cephalosporins
	   cefazolin (Ancef) or (Kefzol)
	   ceftriaxone (Rocephin)
	   cephalexin (Keflex)
	Fluoroquinolones
	   ciprofloxacin (Cipro)
	   levofloxacin (Levaquin)
	Sulfa
	   trimethoprim-sulfamethoxazole (Bactrim DS)
	Tetracyclines
	   doxycycline (Vibramycin)
	   minocycline (Minocin)
	Glycopeptides
	   vancomycin (Vancocin)
	Miscellaneous
	   clindamycin (Cleocin)
	   metronidazole (Flagyl)
	   nitrofurantoin (Macrobid)

Continued

TABLE 19.1 ■ Selected Hematology, Lymphatic, and Immune System Medications—cont'd

Drug Class	Generic Name (Brand Name)
Steroidal anti-inflammatories • Immunosuppressants • Reduce inflammation	methylprednisolone (Medrol) prednisone
Non-steroidal anti-inflammatory drugs (NSAIDs) • Inhibit the COX enzyme (**COX inhibitor**), reducing inflammatory molecules • Reduce inflammation, pain (**analgesic**), and fever (**antipyretic**)	aspirin/acetylsalicylic acid (Bayer) celecoxib (Celebrex) diclofenac (Voltaren) ibuprofen (Motrin) or (Advil) ketorolac (Toradol) meloxicam (Mobic) nabumetone (Relafen) naproxen (Aleve) or (Naprosyn)

Although knowing the drug class mechanism of action is not essential to become a great scribe, having familiarity with the mechanism can facilitate faster and more accurate documentation. This is because within a class, the generic names tend to sound similar. This is usually a good way to identify a drug class from a generic name. For example, in the penicillin class, all of the drug generic names end in "cillin."

CASE STUDY 19.1

Jack Jackson, a 35-year-old helicopter pilot, enters the ED with swollen lymph nodes in his neck and underarms, and night sweats. With his busy flight schedule, he has not had time to see his PCP. Jack says he felt sluggish for several weeks but thought he had a lingering cold or maybe the flu. He states his night sweats began around the same time, and noticed the swollen lymph nodes soon after. He admits to a vague abdominal pain, rating it a 3 on the pain scale, but has not felt nauseous, has not had diarrhea, does not feel out of breath, and has not experienced chest pain. He took his temperature earlier in the week and it was elevated, and it was still elevated yesterday. The triage nurse recorded 101.1 °F. He has been drinking a cup of Theraflu at night before bed, which helps him sleep, but his symptoms have persisted. Jack has to be ready for the traffic report in the morning and wants some kind of medication to make him feel better.

Upon abdominal palpation, the physician detected splenomegaly and hepatomegaly. The ED physician orders a CXR, CBC, ESR, LFT, kidney function test, and arranges for lymph and bone marrow biopsies. All his blood cell counts are low, and his LFT shows decreased levels of albumin. Microscopy of the biopsies reveals cancer cells.

QUESTIONS
1. How would the scribe report the chief complaint for Mr. Jackson?
2. How would the scribe record the HPI for Mr. Jackson?
3. In the ROS, what could be reported under Constitutional for this patient?
4. Under which system would the scribe record Mr. Jackson's lymphadenopathy?
5. What is the term for decreased levels of all types of blood cells?
6. What is the term for cancer that arises from white blood cells?

Practice Questions

1. _____ produce antibodies specific for an antigen.
2. _____, which are located throughout the body, filter the blood.
3. _____, located within the bones, produces the three classes of cells in the blood.

4. _____ are the type of blood cells that participate in the clotting cascade.

5. A 32-year-old male patient presents to an immunologist for evaluation of recurrent infections. He reports having frequent bouts of bronchitis and pneumonia, the last illness about a week ago. He has intermittent fevers and swollen lymph nodes. The patient also has recurrent unexplained nosebleeds, episodes of a cough productive of blood, and occasionally has a bowel movement with bright red blood. He states he awakes and notices unexplained bruising over various areas of his body. How should this be documented in the review of systems?

6. On exam the patient is noted to have bruising in various stages of healing over all four extremities. He has swollen nasal turbinates, and cobblestoning with erythema of the posterior oropharynx. Lymphadenopathy in the cervical chain bilaterally and of the posterior auricular nodes. Breath sounds are normal. Heart rate and rhythm are normal. Abdomen is soft and nontender. The patient overall appears frail. How should this be documented in the physical exam?

7. The immunologist would like to send the patient to have some of his bone marrow taken out for analysis. What is the name of this procedure?

8. On the patient's last lab work a complete blood count demonstrated low erythrocytes, leukocytes, and thrombocytes. What is this called?

9. Until the results of the biopsy return, the immunologist would like to start the patient on a prophylactic antibiotic for the recurrent infections. Which is an antibiotic?
   a. acyclovir (Zovirax)
   b. nystatin (Mycostatin)
   c. amoxicillin (Amoxil)
   d. cetirizine (Zyrtec)

CHAPTER 20

Endocrine System

LEARNING OBJECTIVES

1. Use medical terminology to document medical issues involving the endocrine system.
2. Describe the anatomy and physiology of the endocrine system.
3. Document endocrine system symptoms related during a review of systems.
4. Document signs related by the provider during a physical exam of the endocrine system.
5. Document operations and procedures for the endocrine system.
6. Document endocrine system clinical impressions, diagnoses, and signs and symptoms commonly found in a problem list.
7. Document relevant drug classes and medications for the treatment of problems associated with the endocrine system.

KEY TERMS

Adenohypophysis
Adrenal glands
Adrenaline (epinephrine)
Adrenocorticotropic hormone (ACTH)
Alopecia
Blood tonicity
Cortisol
Diabetes insipidus (DI)
Diabetes mellitus (DM)
Endocrine
Endocrine system
Exocrine
Exophthalmos

Glucagon
Glucocorticoids
Hirsutism
Hormone
Hyperthyroidism
Hypothalamus
Hypothyroidism
Insulin
Neurohypophysis
Noradrenaline (norepinephrine)
Pancreas
Parathyroid gland
Parathyroid hormone

Pituitary gland
Polydipsia
Polyphagia
Polyuria
Renin-angiotensin-aldosterone system (RAAS)
Thyroid gland
Thyroid stimulating hormone (TSH)
Thyroid storm
Thyromegaly (goiter)
Thyroxine (T4)
Triiodothyronine (T3)

Anatomy and Physiology

The **endocrine system** (Fig. 20.1) is a group of organs and glands that produce **hormones**, which are chemical messengers that travel through the blood to other parts of the body to exert an effect. Each hormone has a different function and target, and they are regulated in various ways.

The **hypothalamus** is a structure in the brain (neural tissue) that makes a connection to and regulates the **pituitary gland**, which is part of the endocrine system (Fig. 20.2). The pituitary gland is comprised of two functionally different components: the **adenohypophysis** (anterior

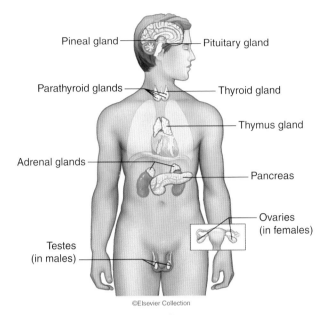

Fig. 20.1   The endocrine system. (© Elsevier Collection.)

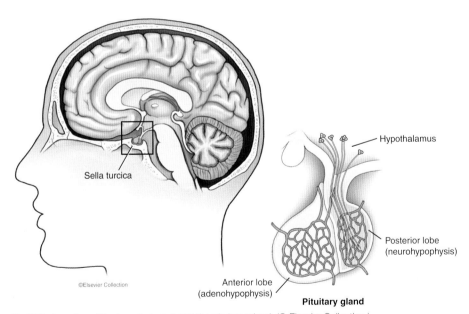

Fig. 20.2   Location of the hypothalamus and the pituitary gland. (© Elsevier Collection.)

pituitary) which is an endocrine gland, and **neurohypophysis** (posterior pituitary) which is still part of the nervous system. The hypothalamus produces *releasing and inhibiting hormones*, which act on the pituitary gland to modulate the production and release of other hormones that travel elsewhere in the body to exert their effects.

For a scribe it is not important to know the specifics of this process (other than what was provided above) or the details about each of the many hormones regulated by the hypothalamus and pituitary gland. However, three of the most important hormones will be discussed below.

Antidiuretic hormone (ADH)/vasopressin is regulated by the hypothalamus/pituitary gland and exerts its effects primarily on the kidneys to regulate **blood tonicity** (concentration of solutes). This is accomplished by changing the rate of water reabsorption versus excretion through urine. In short, increasing water reabsorption increases blood volume and produces dilution (decreases blood viscosity). Contrarily, increasing water excretion decreases blood volume and increases blood viscosity.

Thyroid stimulating hormone (TSH) is produced by the pituitary gland and exerts its effects on the **thyroid gland**, a butterfly-shaped gland in the anterior neck (Fig. 20.3) that produces the thyroid hormones **triiodothyronine (T3)** and **thyroxine (T4)**. T3 and T4 regulate the body's metabolic activity. Increased thyroid hormones produce increased metabolic activity, and vice versa.

Adrenocorticotropic hormone (ACTH) is also produced by the pituitary gland and acts on the **adrenal glands**, which sit atop the kidneys (Fig. 20.4) and produce many hormones. The hormones that are most affected by ACTH are the **glucocorticoids**, such as **cortisol**. Cortisol is often produced in times of stress (hence it is known as the "stress hormone") and affects metabolism and is an immunosuppressant.

The **renin-angiotensin-aldosterone system (RAAS)** is a chain of hormones that are affected by ACTH. The complete system is too complex to explain fully in the scope of this text, but essentially it acts to regulate blood volume and electrolyte composition.

The adrenal glands produce other hormones that are not greatly affected by ACTH but are primarily regulated in different ways. **Adrenaline/noradrenaline (epinephrine/norepinephrine)** are produced by the adrenal glands in times of stress, regulated by the sympathetic nervous system. These hormones have many effects throughout the body, including increasing heart rate, producing sweat, and dilating the pupils.

There are other organs in the body that are part of the endocrine system, but are not regulated by the hypothalamus and pituitary gland. The **parathyroid gland** is actually a set of four small glands that are located behind the thyroid gland in the neck (Fig. 20.5). This gland produces

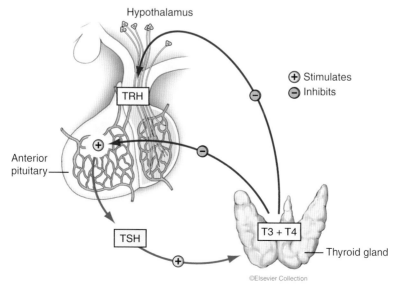

©Elsevier Collection

Fig. 20.3 Interrelationship of the pituitary and thyroid glands. The anterior pituitary secretes thyroid-stimulating hormone (*TSH*) also called thyrotropin, prompting the thyroid to produce T3 and T4. Increased T3 levels inhibit the hypothalamus from producing thyrotropin-releasing hormone (*TRH*). (© Elsevier Collection.)

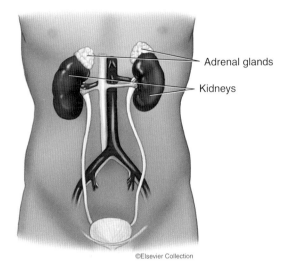

Fig. 20.4 Location of the adrenal glands. (© Elsevier Collection.)

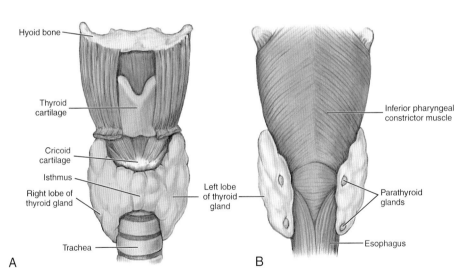

Fig. 20.5 Thyroid gland with parathyroid glands noted from an anterior view (A) and from a posterior view (B). (From Herring SW, Fehrenbach MJ: *Illustrated anatomy of the head and neck*, ed 6, St. Louis, 2021, Elsevier.)

parathyroid hormone, which regulates the levels of serum calcium and phosphate. Levels of these minerals affect bone mineral composition and density.

The **pancreas** is an organ in the abdominal cavity that is considered to be both an **endocrine** (glandular) and an **exocrine** (digestive) organ. Its endocrine functions include the modulation of blood glucose via two hormones with oppositional actions:

- **Insulin,** which decreases blood glucose when levels are too high, and
- **Glucagon,** which increases blood glucose when levels are too low.

Fig. 20.6 shows the role of the pancreas in regulating blood glucose levels.

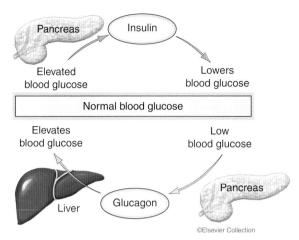

©Elsevier Collection

Fig. 20.6   The pancreas' regulation of the blood glucose. (© Elsevier Collection.)

Medical Terminology Word Parts for the Endocrine System

Combining Forms

crin/o	secrete
hormon/o	hormone
aden/o	gland
phys/o	growing
pituitar/o	pituitary gland; hypophysis
neur/o	nerve
thyr/o, thyroid/o	thyroid gland
cortic/o	cortex, outer region
adrenal/o	adrenal gland
parathyroid/o	parathyroid gland
gluc/o	sugar
glyc/o	sugar
pancreat/o	pancreas
calc/o, calci/o	calcium

Prefixes

endo-	within, inside
hypo-	below
exo-	outer
para-	near, beside, abnormal
a- an-	without
dia-	through
poly-	much, many
hyper-	excessive

Suffixes

-phoresis	sweating
-rrhea	flow, discharge
-dispia	condition of thirst
-phagia	condition of eating, swallowing
-ia	condition
-uria	urine condition
-megaly	enlargement
-ectomy	removal
-itis	inflammation
-osis	abnormal condition
-al -ic	pertaining to
-penia	deficiency

Review of Systems

It is the duty of the scribe to translate the patient's interpretation of their symptoms into medical lingo. For example, if a patient says they are extremely and frequently thirsty, the scribe should document "polydipsia."

Symptoms that can be placed in multiple systems have been designated as such in italics. Remember to always maximize the number of <u>systems</u> that are included in the review of systems so that the chart can be billed at higher levels (if desired). For example, if a patient is having alopecia and palpitations, it would be best to include alopecia in "*endocrine*" and palpitations in "*cardiovascular*" (two billable systems), as opposed to including alopecia and palpitations in "*endocrine*" (one billable system).

Alopecia—hair loss

Amenorrhea (*genitourinary*)—absence of menses

Anorexia (*constitutional, digestive, psychiatric*)—loss of appetite

Diaphoresis (*cardiovascular, integumentary*)—sweating

Diarrhea (*digestive*)—loose or watery stools

Dry skin (*integumentary*)—also called ***xeroderma***

Fatigue (*constitutional*)—feeling excessively tired

Hot flash (*constitutional, genitourinary*)—feeling warm and sweaty

Palpitations (*cardiovascular*)—heart beats that are abnormal (such as beats that are irregular, hard, racing, fast, skipped, etc.)

Polydipsia (*constitutional, digestive*)—excessive thirst

Polyphagia (*constitutional, digestive*)—excessive hunger

Polyuria (*genitourinary*)—excessive urine production

Temperature intolerance—intolerance to hot/cold temperatures

Physical Exam

Physical findings may at times be appropriately placed in a different body system than what is listed, but less often than in the review of systems.

Exophthalmos—protrusion of the eyes due to excessive thyroid hormone (Fig. 20.7)

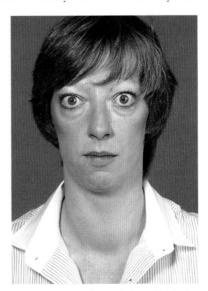

Fig. 20.7 Woman with exophthalmos and goiter. (From Forbes CD, Jackson WF: *Colour atlas and text of clinical medicine*, ed 3, London, 2003, Mosby.)

Hirsutism—excessive hairiness on women caused by overproduction of androgenic hormones (male sex hormones)

Hyperpigmentation—darkening of an area of skin or nails

Thyromegaly (goiter)—thyroid gland enlargement caused by malfunction of the thyroid gland (see Fig. 20.7)

Thyromegaly (**goiter**, see Fig. 20.7) is an enlarged thyroid gland that can be palpated as a swelling in the anterior neck on exam. It can be associated with **hyperthyroidism** (excessive thyroid hormone production), or **hypothyroidism** (inadequate thyroid hormone production).

Operations/Procedures

It is the scribe's duty to translate the patient's procedural description into the equivalent medical term. For example, if a patient says they had their thyroid gland removed, the scribe should record that the patient had an "thyroidectomy."

Parathyroidectomy—removal of parathyroid glands

Thyroidectomy—removal of the thyroid gland

Problem List

It is the scribe's duty to translate the lay terms into medical terminology. For example, if the patient says they have a history of low bone mineral density, the scribe should document "osteopenia."

Addison disease—adrenal glands do not produce enough glucocorticoids (like cortisol)

Cushing disease—a cause of Cushing's syndrome that is due to overproduction of ACTH

Cushing syndrome—disorder caused by prolonged cortisol exposure, resulting in central obesity, a round "moon" face, and high blood pressure (Fig. 20.8)

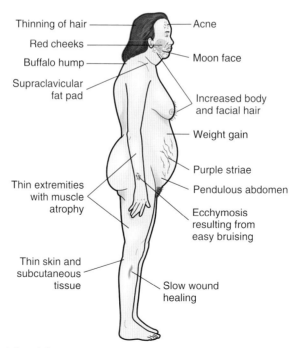

Fig. 20.8 Characteristics of Cushing syndrome. (From Lewis SL, Dirksen SR, Heitkemper MM, Bucher L, Harding MM: *Medical-surgical nursing: assessment and management of clinical problems*, ed 11, St. Louis, 2020.)

Diabetes insipidus (DI)—excessive thirst and secretion of large amounts of urine due to abnormal production or response to vasopressin

Diabetes mellitus type I (DM I)—autoimmune destruction of insulin-producing cells in the pancreas causing high blood glucose over a prolonged period

Diabetes mellitus type II (DM II)—chronically elevated blood glucose level that causes insulin resistance and results in the inability to utilize dietary glucose

Graves disease—autoimmune disease affecting the thyroid and causing hyperthyroidism

Hashimoto's thyroiditis—autoimmune destruction of the thyroid gland causing hypothyroidism

Hypercalcemia—elevated blood calcium (Ca^{2+})

Hyperglycemia—elevated blood glucose

Hyperthyroidism—excessive production of thyroid hormone

Hypocalcemia—low blood calcium (Ca^{2+})

Hypoglycemia—low blood glucose

Hypothyroidism—thyroid hormone deficiency

Osteopenia—low bone mineral density, not to the point of osteoporosis but still increases risk of fracture

Osteoporosis (OP)—decreased bone mineral density that significantly increases risk of fracture

Thyroid storm—complication of hyperthyroidism in which T3 and T4 are overproduced and cause a dangerous increase in metabolism

Medications

A scribe should be able to diligently record the patient's medication list, which includes the drug name (generic or brand), dose, frequency, and indication (reason for taking the drug). Table 20.1 lists selected drugs for the endocrine system.

TABLE 20.1 ■ Selected Endocrine System Medications

Drug Class and Uses	Generic Name (Brand Name)
Diabetic • Not a class • Used to treat diabetes	glipizide (Glucotrol) glyburide (Glynase) or (Diabeta) glyburide + metformin (Glucovance) insulin (Humulin R) insulin aspart (Novolog) insulin glargine (Lantus) insulin lispro (Humalog) metformin (Glucophage) sitagliptin (Januvia)
Hormone replacement • Not a class • Used to replace thyroid hormones	levothyroxine (Synthroid)
Vasopressin hormone replacement • Not a class • Used to replace vasopressin (decreases water excretion as urine)	vasopressin (Vasostrict) desmopressin (DDAVP)

CASE STUDY 20.1

Thirty-five-year-old Beth comes to her family physician with what she feels are bizarre symptoms. She has been drinking gallons of water every day, and urinating so frequently that her urine is always completely clear. At first she thought it was healthy to crave water so much, although she started to suspect there was a problem when she was awakening in the middle of the night with a pounding heart, dying of thirst. "The wakeups started about Friday of last week, about 4 days ago," she said, "but I've been drinking a lot of water for 3 or 4 weeks." Besides that, Beth thinks she has been irritable, and she sometimes feels lightheaded at work.

The physician asked whether she has experienced any nausea or vomiting, and Beth confirmed that she has been queasy more than usual. The physician asked about blurred vision, and Beth remembered a time last week when she was snacking in front of the television and soon was not able to focus on the screen.

The physician suspects Beth may have diabetes insipidus, so she ordered labs. The results showed low levels of vasopressin. Beth was referred to an endocrinologist for care.

QUESTIONS

1. How might the scribe construct an HPI for Beth?
2. How would the scribe document this patient's review of systems?
3. Antidiuretic hormone (ADH)/vasopressin is regulated by the hypothalamus/pituitary gland and exerts its effects primarily on the _____ to regulate the concentration of solutes.
4. The physician's _____ is diabetes insipidus.
5. Beth's episode of blurred vision may have been caused by _____, due to losing more fluids than she could replace through drinking water.

Practice Questions

1. The "butterfly" gland in the neck that produces T3 and T4 is the _____.
2. The _____ regulates blood glucose with two main hormones.
3. _____ is a hormone that decreases blood glucose.
4. The _____ glands sit atop the kidneys and produce cortisol.
5. A 60-year-old female patient presents to an endocrinologist for evaluation of many symptoms that have worsened over the past few months. She has had unexplained weight loss accompanied by excessive hunger, and episodes of a racing heart and breaking into a sweat. No shortness of breath with this. She has had a lot of hair loss and her nails are brittle and break easily. She has muscle aches, heat intolerance, and is more irritable than normal. How should this be documented in the review of systems?
6. On exam the patient appears anxious and is diaphoretic. Her hair is thinning in various places and her skin is dry and flaky. Exophthalmos is present and mucous membranes are dry. Thyroid exam shows goiter. Heart sounds are irregular and tachycardic. Breath sounds are normal. Abdomen is soft and nontender. No calf tenderness. Slight resting tremor in both hands and hyperreflexia is present in both lower extremities. She overall appears cachectic. How should this be documented in the physical exam?
7. This patient may need to have her thyroid gland removed. What is this procedure called?
8. When the pending lab work returns it shows significantly elevated thyroid hormones. What is this called?
9. If this patient has her thyroid gland removed, she will have to be on thyroid replacement therapy permanently. Which of the following is an appropriate medication?
   a. levothyroxine (Synthroid)
   b. glipizide (Glucotrol)
   c. metformin (Glucophage)
   d. vasopressin (Vasostrict)

Practical Application

CHAPTER 21

Anticipating Pertinent Questions for Chief Complaints

1. Document signs and symptoms to support a diagnosis.
2. This chapter is a very brief summary of some of the questions that may be asked by a provider while assessing patients with certain chief complaints. A new scribe may believe these questions to be random or unrelated to the chief complaint. However, if a scribe is able to anticipate these very relevant questions they will become more efficient at documentation.
3. Accompanying each chief complaint is a differential of possible diagnoses that a provider might consider during an encounter. With each diagnosis is a list of associated questions that are specific to that diagnosis. These questions may make that specific diagnosis less or more likely, depending on whether they become pertinent negatives or positives.
4. It is not necessary to memorize the differential of each chief complaint or any of the risk factors associated with certain diagnoses. This chapter is simply a guide to help with efficacy and efficiency.

Abdominal Pain

Differential: Think gallbladder, appendix, ulcers, intestinal cramps, liver disease, vascular problems (ischemia), urinary issues (infections, stones, obstructions), infectious diarrhea, autoimmune disease (Crohn's or ulcerative colitis), skin disorder (shingles), intestinal obstruction (from tumor or adhesions), or gynecologic issues (tumors, infections, ovarian cysts, ectopic or normal pregnancy, endometriosis)

Gallbladder (stones or obstruction):
HPI: Right upper quadrant abdominal pain radiating to the back or chest, triggered by fatty meals
ROS: Abdominal bloating, nausea, vomiting, indigestion
PMHx: Gallbladder disease or stones (recurrent problem more likely)

Appendix (appendicitis):
HPI: Gradual onset with migratory pain from periumbilical area to the right lower quadrant (classic presentation)
ROS: Low grade fevers

Ulcers:
HPI: Epigastric pain, intolerance to spicy food, relief with antacids
ROS: Dyspepsia, melena, "coffee ground" emesis
SHx: History of alcoholism

Intestinal cramps:
  HPI: Intermittent, severe, cramping in varying locations
  ROS: Change in bowel movements, often constipation
Liver:
  HPI: Constant pain in the right upper quadrant
  ROS: Jaundice, fatigue, weight loss, anorexia, abdominal distension
  PMHx: Hepatitis (risk factor for cirrhosis or recurrence)
  SHx: Alcohol use (cirrhosis risk factor), IV drug use (Hepatitis C risk factor)
Vascular issues (ischemia):
  HPI: Severe or mild and intermittent pain (degree of ischemia)
  PMHx: Diabetes or hypertension (risk factors for vascular disease). History of atrial fibrillation (embolism of small clots)
Urinary (infections, stones, obstructions):
  ROS: Fever (infection), pain radiating to the flank (kidney involvement), urinary symptoms (dysuria, hematuria, urgency, frequency)
  PMHx: Prostate problems (urinary retention/inability to urinate)
Infectious diarrhea:
  ROS: Fever, diarrhea, blood or mucus in stool, vomiting
  SHx: Recent travels or suspicious foods (exposure to infection)
Autoimmune disease (Crohn's or ulcerative colitis):
  HPI: Right lower quadrant pain common
  ROS: Low grade fevers, diarrhea, bloody stools or stools with mucus
  PMHx: Inflammatory bowel disease (recurrent problem more likely)
Skin (shingles):
  ROS: Rash or burning sensation
  PMHx: Chickenpox, shingles, or immunosuppression (risk factors)
Intestinal obstruction (from tumor or adhesions):
  HPI: Generalized abdominal pain that is crampy in nature
  ROS: Nausea, vomiting (food or fecal material), no recent bowel movement, weight loss, anorexia, abdominal bloating or distention
  PMHx: Prior surgeries (scarring/adhesions that can cause obstruction)
Gynecologic (tumors, infections, ovarian cysts, ectopic or normal pregnancy, endometriosis):
  HPI: Lower abdominal pain (ovarian cyst or ectopic)
  ROS: Last known menstrual period and normalcy of cycle, menorrhagia or menometrorrhagia (endometriosis or ectopic pregnancy), unexpected weight changes (malignancy), fever or chills (infection), abnormal discharge (infection), or breast swelling and nausea (pregnancy)
  PMHx: History of sexually transmitted diseases (STD or ectopic), or prior pregnancies
  SHx: Number of sexual partners (infection), birth control (pregnancy)

Back Pain

Differential: Think arthritis, malignancy (primary bone or metastatic disease), abdominal aortic aneurysm, gynecologic source (tumors, pelvic inflammatory disease), muscular strain, spinal infection, or renal disease (kidney infection or stones)
Arthritis:
  HPI: Chronic and gradual onset
  ROS: Polyarticular involvement
  PMHx: Arthritis (history of similar may explain current) or autoimmune disease (often leads to arthritis)

Malignancy (primary or metastatic disease):
 ROS: Unexplained weight loss, night sweats, anorexia. Loss of bladder or bowel control, leg weakness or pain, saddle anesthesias (if tumor impinges on lower spinal canal)
 PMHx: Malignancy (recurrence or metastasis more likely)
 FHx: Malignancy (risk factor)
Abdominal aortic aneurysm:
 HPI: Sudden onset, "tearing" in nature (classic for dissecting aneurysm)
 ROS: Lightheadedness or syncope (hypovolemia/internal blood loss), abdominal pain, or cold leg/foot (loss of peripheral circulation)
 PMHx: Long-standing hypertension (risk factor)
 SHx: Smoking history (worsens vascular disease)
Gynecologic (tumors, pelvic inflammatory disease):
 ROS: Abnormal vaginal discharge or bleeding, pelvic floor pain
 PMHx: Prior infection, ectopic pregnancy, endometriosis, or uterine fibroids (recurrent problem more likely)
 PSHx: Gynecologic malignancy or ovarian cyst surgery
Muscular strain:
 HPI: Recent sports or work injury or other accident or trauma
 ROS: Lack of findings to indicate other causes (diagnosis of exclusion)
 PMHx: Other injuries to the same area (weak or susceptible muscle)
Spinal infection:
 HPI: Gradual onset
 ROS: Fever. Back pain. Lower extremity paresthesias
 PMHx: Immunocompromised due to steroids, chemotherapy, immunodeficiency disease (higher risk of infection)
 SHx: IV drug abuse (risk factor for spinal abscess)
Renal (kidney infection or stones):
 HPI: Sudden onset (kidney stone) or gradual (infection). Location is flank (not midline). Pain is constant and waxes/wanes in severity
 ROS: Urinary symptoms (dysuria, hematuria, urinary frequency, and urgency) or abdominal pain
 PMHx: Kidney stones or urinary tract infections (recurrent issue likely)

Chest Pain

Differential: Think cardiac (myocardial infarction), pulmonary (pneumonia or pulmonary embolism), gastrointestinal (esophageal spasm or ulcer), musculoskeletal (rib injury or inflammation), skin (shingles)
Cardiac (myocardial infarction):
 HPI: Pain is exertional, pressure-like, or may radiate to an arm or jaw
 ROS: Nausea, diaphoresis, shortness of breath
 PMHx: Hypertension, hyperlipidemia, diabetes (coronary artery disease risk factors), coronary artery disease (myocardial infarction risk factor)
 FHx: Coronary artery disease at a young age (risk factor for CAD)
 SHx: Smoking (risk factor for coronary artery disease)
Pulmonary (pneumonia or pulmonary embolism):
 HPI: Pain is pleuritic or sharp
 ROS: Cough, shortness of breath, fever (pneumonia or bronchitis)

PMHx: Pulmonary issues like asthma or COPD (pulmonary etiology likely). Prior deep venous thrombosis, pulmonary embolism, or hypercoagulable state (risk factors for pulmonary embolism)

SHx: Recent prolonged immobilization like travel, surgery or illness (risk factors for pulmonary embolism); smoking (infection risk factor)

Gastrointestinal (esophageal spasm or ulcer):

HPI: Pain is associated with swallowing

ROS: Acid-like taste in mouth (GERD/reflux)

PMHx: GERD or ulcers (history of similar may explain symptoms)

Musculoskeletal (rib injury or inflammation):

HPI: Pain is associated with movement and is alleviated with rest

ROS: Recent known trauma

Skin (shingles):

ROS: Rash or burning sensation

PMHx: Chickenpox, prior shingles, or immunosuppression (shingles)

Eye Complaints

Differential: Think glaucoma, amaurosis fugax (stroke warning), corneal abrasion, retinal detachment or vascular occlusion (central venous or arterial)

Glaucoma:

ROS: Eye pain, nausea, visual clouding, gradual or acute loss of vision beginning in the periphery

PMHx: Diabetes or prolonged steroid use (risk factors)

Amaurosis fugax (stroke warning):

ROS: Temporary loss of vision that is unilateral and painless

PMHx: Stroke, hypertension, or diabetes (risk factors for stroke)

Corneal abrasion:

HPI: Constant unilateral eye pain

ROS: Foreign body sensation, eye pain or discomfort, tearing, redness, photophobia, headache or blurred vision

SHx: Occupation or activities (risk for foreign body exposures)

Retinal detachment:

HPI: Onset after trauma (risk factor)

ROS: Floaters, light flashes or "curtain" of visual field loss

Vascular occlusion:

ROS: Vision loss: painful (venous) or painless (arterial)

Fall

Differential: Think syncope (most likely cardiac but also dehydration, anemia, malnutrition or seizures), disequilibrium (intracranial hemorrhage, stroke, or inner ear problem), weakness (malignancy, dehydration, anemia, or stroke), mechanical fall, abuse, or infectious process

Syncope (most likely cardiac, but also dehydration, anemia, malnutrition, or seizures):

HPI: Sudden, without prior warning (suggests cardiac) or gradual onset (suggests dehydration, anemia, or malnutrition)

ROS: Palpitations (drop in blood pressure), dizziness or lightheadedness (drop in blood pressure from dehydration or anemia), shortness of breath (pulmonary embolism), chest pain (pulmonary embolism or myocardial infarction), sensory changes (malnutrition), tongue biting or urinary/stool incontinence (seizures), last meal (hypoglycemia)

SHx: Recreational drug use (altered mental status with loss of consciousness, especially overdose). New medicine prescribed or change in dosage of medications (drop in blood pressure)

Disequilibrium (intracranial hemorrhage, stroke, inner ear):

ROS: Headache (intracranial bleed), visual changes, imbalance, or abnormal gait (cerebellar), focal weakness (stroke), tinnitus (inner ear)

Weakness (malignancy, dehydration, anemia, or stroke):

ROS: Weight loss or anorexia (malignancy), decreased fluids (dehydration), recent illness (dehydration), bleeding (anemia), focal weakness (stroke)

PMHx: Diabetes (dehydration or stroke), known malignancy (recurrent problem is more likely), or malnutrition (dehydration and general weakness from deconditioning)

Mechanical fall:

HPI: Falls due to tripping, slipping, or stumbling

PMHx: Neurologic conditions (difficulty with gait and creates fall risk)

Abuse:

ROS: Recent injuries

SHx: Home safety ("where" is home and "who" are housemates)

Infection:

ROS: Fever, urinary symptoms, cough, diarrhea, red skin (leads to weakness, increasing chance of falls)

Headache

Differential: Think migraines, tension headaches, intracranial hemorrhage, sinus problems, meningitis, or malignancy

Migraines:

HPI: Unilateral throbbing headache, similar to prior migraine headaches

ROS: Photophobia, phonophobia, nausea, vomiting, light flashes or other visual auras (often seen in classic migraines)

PMHx: History of migraines (recurrent problem more likely)

FHx: History of migraines (risk factor for migraines)

Tension headache:

HPI: Bilateral headache, located frontally, radiating to the occiput

ROS: No focal complaints, such as unilateral extremity weakness or facial droop. Neck pain frequently. Increased life stressors

Intracranial hemorrhage:

HPI: Sudden onset (thunderclap), severe, triggered by another event usually exertional (such as during sexual intercourse or exercise)

ROS: Nausea, vomiting, focal weakness, dizziness, altered level of consciousness, seizures

Medications: Anticoagulation (bleeding more likely)

Sinus problems:

HPI: Headache is frontal, pressure-like, with discolored sinus drainage

ROS: Fever and chills, facial pain and pressure, nasal symptoms. No associated neurologic deficits

PMHx: Allergies or prior sinusitis (recurrent problem more likely)

Meningitis:

HPI: Gradual onset of febrile illness that has progressed to headache and neck stiffness (classic presentation)

ROS: Fever, neck stiffness, rash, photophobia, altered consciousness

PMHx: Immunocompromised due to steroids, chemotherapy, or immunodeficiency (more prone to infections). Meningitis vaccine (makes infection less likely)

SHx: Exposure to meningitis (infection more likely)

Malignancy:

HPI: Gradual onset, not easily relieved with nighttime symptoms or waking up in the morning with a headache

ROS: Slow onset of neurologic findings such as focal weakness, confusion or somnolence. Fever, weight loss, and anorexia

PMHx: Malignancy (metastatic disease more likely)

Pregnancy Complications

Differential: Think miscarriage or ectopic pregnancy

Miscarriage:

HPI: Gravida/para/abortus (GPA), Rh factor ("Rh negative" increases risk), or prior pregnancy complications (recurrent problem more likely)

ROS: Vaginal bleeding (with type [bright red, dark, clots] and amount of blood), pelvic or abdominal pain or cramping, vaginal discharge

PMHx: Diabetes, hypertension, or lupus (risk factors)

SHx: Alcohol, smoking, or recreational drugs (risk factors)

Ectopic pregnancy:

HPI: Last known menstrual period (diagnosed in early pregnancy)

ROS: Vaginal bleeding, abdominal pain or cramping. Lightheadedness or syncope (due to internal bleeding and hypovolemia)

PMHx: Sexually transmitted infections (causes scarring and increases risk) or prior ectopics (recurrent problem more likely)

SHx: Sexual history (risky sexual behaviors make ectopic more likely)

PSHx: Tubal ligation (ectopic more likely)

Shortness of Breath

Differential: Think infection (pneumonia), chronic lung disease (COPD/emphysema), airway spasm (asthma), heart disease (congestive heart failure), malignancy (primary lung or metastatic disease), hypercoagulable state (pulmonary embolism), or aspiration (foreign body in lungs)

Infection (pneumonia):

ROS: Productive cough or fever (infectious)

PMHx: Immunocompromised due to steroids, chemotherapy, or other immunodeficiency (risk factors for infection)

SHx: Exposure to infectious causes (risk factor for infection)

Chronic lung disease (COPD/emphysema):

HPI: Exposure to respiratory irritants (worsens underlying disease)

PMHx: COPD/emphysema (recurrent problem more likely)

SHx: Smoking or occupational exposure (risk factors for chronic lung disease); poor compliance with home medications (recurrent symptoms)

Airway spasm (asthma):

HPI: Recent exposure to possible allergen (worsens underlying disease)

ROS: Sneezing, watery or itchy eyes, rhinorrhea, or wheezing (allergic)

PMHx: Asthma or known allergies (recurrent problem more likely)

Heart disease (CHF):
ROS: Orthopnea, leg swelling, weight gain
PMHx: Coronary artery disease causing myocardial infarction, hypertension, hyper-
lipidemia, diabetes (risk factors for CHF)
FHx: Coronary artery disease in a relative at a young age (risk factor for myocardial infarction)
SHx: Smoking or recreational drugs (risk factors for myocardial infarction or CHF)
Malignancy (primary lung malignancy or metastatic disease):
ROS: Unexplained weight loss, night sweats, or anorexia
PMHx: Malignancy (metastatic or recurrent disease more likely)
SHx: Smoking (risk factor for malignancy)
Hypercoagulable state (pulmonary embolism):
HPI: Sudden onset
ROS: Pleuritic chest pain (hallmark), unilateral leg pain/swelling (DVT)
PMHx: Prior DVT, PE, or hypercoagulable state (risk factors for PE)
FHx: Hypercoagulability (risk factor for DVT/PE)
SHx: Recent prolonged immobilization like travel, surgery, illness (risk factor for DVT/PE)
Medications: Hormones (hypercoagulability risk factor), anticoagulants (clotting less likely)
Aspiration (foreign body in lungs):
ROS: Fever, cough, or shortness of breath
PMHx: Stroke or Alzheimer's dementia (difficulty swallowing, making aspiration more
likely)

Trauma

Differential: Think: why did this happen? Was this caused by a medical issue that will need to
be evaluated in addition to the injuries, such as syncope causing a fall? What is injured and
will the patient require surgery? The differential for trauma is a little different than the other
examples. General questions that will arise in trauma are the following:
Trauma (general):
HPI: Mechanism of injury (knife, gun, fall, or motor vehicle accident). Use of seat belts or
air bag deployment if motor vehicle accident (suggests certain possible injuries). Last
meal (an empty stomach is preferred before surgery to avoid vomiting and aspiration)
Medications: Last tetanus shot (if open skin). Anticoagulants (bleeding may be more
difficult to stop)
SHx: Drug use (may affect mental status)

Weakness

Differential: Think anemia, electrolyte disturbance, dehydration, cardiac problem, malignancy,
nutritional issue, renal disease, stroke, depression, or occult infection
Anemia:
ROS: Hematochezia, melena, heavy menses, epistaxis, dyspnea (anemia)
PMHx: Nutritional deficiency (inability to produce adequate hemoglobin or RBCs)
Medications: Anticoagulants (bleeding difficult to stop)
SHx: Gastric bypass (malnutrition)
FHx: Anemias or mediterranean descent (certain gene-linked entities)
Electrolyte disturbance:
ROS: Nausea, vomiting, or diarrhea (loss of fluids and electrolytes)
PMHx: Endocrine problems such as diabetes (alters electrolytes)
Medications: Diuretic use (electrolyte imbalances)

Dehydration:
  ROS: Nausea, vomiting, diarrhea, or poor fluid intake
  PMHx: Diabetes (polyuria from excessive glucose)
Cardiac problem:
  ROS: Chest pain, palpitations, unexplained nausea or dyspnea on exertion, leg swelling or orthopnea (heart failure). Low blood pressure
Malignancy:
  ROS: Unexplained weight loss, loss of appetite, lumps or bumps, rectal bleeding, or new pain
  PMHX: Routine screening exams such as pap smears, self breast exams, colonoscopies or prostate exams (regular screening reduces risk)
  FHx: Malignancy (risk factor)
Nutritional issue:
  PMHx: Gallbladder or pancreas problems, or malignancy
  SHx: Weight loss programs or fad diets, or alcohol use
  PSHx: Any kind of gastric bypass
Renal disease:
  PMHx: Hypertension, diabetes, or recurrent kidney infections (risk factors for renal disease)
Stroke:
  ROS: Focal weakness, headaches, or altered mental status
  Medications: Anticoagulation (stroke less likely if blood is thin)
Depression:
  ROS: Loss of interest, lack of participation in activities, history of suicidal thoughts, poor appetite or sleep habits, worsening school grades
  FHx: Depression (risk factor for depression)
Infection:
  ROS: Fever, chills, cough, sore throat, urinary symptoms (frequency, dysuria, new onset incontinence)

Practice Questions

For questions 1 to 4, complete the sentence with the possible diagnosis for a patient with abdominal pain.

1. _____ cause(s) right upper quadrant pain that may radiate into the right shoulder blade, bloating, and fatty food intolerance.

2. _____ cause(s) a sudden "tearing" pain that radiates into the back and is accompanied by syncope and hypotension.

3. _____ cause(s) flank pain radiating to the groin along with blood in the urine.

4. _____ cause(s) jaundice and is seen in chronic alcoholics.

Match the cause of dyspnea to its diagnosis.

_____ 5. infection   A. pulmonary embolism

_____ 6. airway spasm   B. asthma

_____ 7. heart disease   C. pneumonia

_____ 8. hypercoagulable state   D. congestive heart failure

Match the clinical condition to its characteristic.

_____ 9. right sided weakness   A. hepatitis

_____ 10. crushing chest pain   B. myocardial infarction

_____ 11. jaundice   C. congestive heart failure

_____ 12. stiff neck   D. asthma

_____ 13. wheezing   E. stroke

_____ 14. orthopnea   F. meningitis

CHAPTER 22

Practice Exercises

1. Document the patient's history of present illness (HPI), review of systems (ROS) templates, and physical exam.

This chapter offers additional opportunity to practice some of the skills taught throughout this text. The practice is logistically limited without access to an electronic medical record. However, the six cases within this chapter enable you (the reader) to practice writing a history of present illness (HPI), completing documentation elements and review of systems (ROS) templates, and also documenting a physical exam for each case.

Blank forms have been provided at the end of each case for you to complete. Because many healthcare facilities have transitioned to the electronic health record, however, using a template or form on a computer would most closely simulate a real scribing situation. You can complete a template into which you can document the visit on this title's Evolve website at http://evolve. elsevier.com/Kwiatek.

The following is a step-by-step explanation describing how to best utilize the practice cases in the upcoming pages:

1. A dialogue from a fictional encounter between a patient and a provider will be given. Synthesize an HPI from this dialogue. Each dialogue will be based on one of the chief complaints discussed in detail in Chapter 21, Chief Complaints and Pertinent Questions.

   The first sentence of the HPI should provide the patient's age, sex, and chief complaint. The second sentence should then say: "*The patient (or other historian) states/reports....*"

2. With the information in the written history, place the documentation elements in the proper locations within the documentation elements template.

3. Complete the ROS by placing the symptoms from the history into the proper locations within the review of systems template.

4. After the dialogue, a short list of physical exam findings will be given. Practice placing these findings into the correct system within the physical exam template.

NOTE

The "observable" physical exam findings will be excluded from our examples for several reasons. First, the use of these is completely provider dependent and should be clarified with each provider. Second, you should primarily focus on placing the given physical exam within the correct systems in the template. Adding the observables to this will confound the true intent of the exercise. And lastly, because this is a written exercise, using "observable" physical exam findings is impossible.

5. Compare the chart you have created with the one given in the "Answer Key." "Answer Key" is in quotations because every history by nature will be unique. However, there are key elements that should be included in the history you have created. These should be easy to identify because they have been emphasized throughout this text.

   Additionally, symptoms and signs in the review of systems and physical exam findings can sometimes be placed into multiple systems. If you have placed them in systems other than what is noted in the "Answer Key," you are not necessarily wrong for doing so. Refer to the pages discussing review of systems and physical exam within the systems-based chapters (Part III) for any clarification on this matter.

6. Read the *Key Points* section concluding each practice example. This section will explain the pertinent information that should have been included in the history, in addition to learning points about each case.

Case 1

The patient is a 68-year-old male with **abdominal pain**.

Patient: I've had this pain for months now (*points to right upper quadrant*). It's constantly there. I just hate going to the hospital so I've dealt with it the best I could.

Provider: Does the pain go anywhere else, or worsen after eating?

Patient: The pain is just in that one spot. And it doesn't get better or worse with anything. It just hurts.

Provider: How would you describe the pain?

Patient: I guess it's sharp. Maybe even stabbing.

Provider: Have you had fevers or chills? Nausea, vomiting, or diarrhea?

Patient: None of that. But I have lost a lot of weight here recently. About 65 pounds in the last year. I guess that could be because I haven't had an appetite. I also feel like my belly is swollen all the time. I know I'm not the smallest guy, but this is big even for me.

Provider: Have you noticed black or tarry stools that stick to the toilet bowl, or bright red blood in your stools?

Patient: No sir.

Provider: Have you been constipated?

Patient: I'm constipated most of the time. I guess my diet is probably not as good as it could be.

Provider: Do you drink alcohol?

Patient: Oh I drink about 6 or 8 beers a night and sometimes a fifth of liquor with that. I've been doing that for years now. Nothin' else to do.

Provider: Do you use any drugs?

Patient: I've smoked cigarettes for 40 years now, but I don't do any of that stuff on the streets.

Provider: Do you have a known history of liver failure or disease? Hepatitis? Cancer?

Patient: I don't really see doctors but nobody ever told me that I have any of those things.

Provider: Have you ever had any surgeries on your belly?

Patient: I had my appendix taken out when I was just a kid.

Provider: How have you been treating your symptoms at home?

Patient: I've been taking hot baths and those help for a bit. And I've been taking aspirin.

Provider: Do you have any changes in vision, a sore throat, shortness of breath or a cough, chest pain, urinary urgency or frequency, leg pain, weakness of one arm or leg, or new rashes?

Patient: I have shortness of breath because I'm a smoker, but it's gotten worse here lately.

Provider: Does it get worse when you exert yourself? Does it worsen when you lie down?

Patient: Mostly when I exert myself, but it's there all the time.

PHYSICAL EXAM FINDINGS: Well-developed but thin and cachectic appearing male. Scent of alcohol on his breath. Dry mucous membranes. Sclera are icteric. Jugular venous distension is present. Heart rate is irregularly irregular and tachycardic. There is a 2/6 systolic murmur heard best over the left sternal border and a S3 gallop. Breath sounds are diminished throughout and there are diffuse wheezes and crackles at the bases. Abdomen is soft and tender in the right upper quadrant with voluntary guarding, but no rebound. Hepatomegaly two finger breadths below the right costal margin. There is an ascitic wave. He has full body jaundice. 2+ pitting edema of the bilateral lower extremities and chronic stasis dermatitis changes. No calf tenderness. Faint distal pulses. No focal deficits. He is alert and cooperative.

ANSWER KEY

CASE 1: The patient is a 68-year-old male who presents with **abdominal pain**.

History of the Present Illness

The patient is a 68-year-old male with abdominal pain. The patient reports that for the past few months he has had constant non-radiating right upper quadrant abdominal pain. No modifying factors to pain, including worsening after eating, and he describes it as sharp and stabbing in nature. No nausea, vomiting, constipation or diarrhea. No melena or hematochezia. No fevers or chills. He has had a weight loss of about 65 pounds in the last year, which he attributes to a loss of appetite. He also has the sensation of abdominal bloating and distension. The patient has been taking hot baths at home and has taken aspirin with little relief. Otherwise, he has had a worsening of his chronic and exertionally related shortness of breath recently, but denies orthopnea, visual changes, a sore throat, chest pain, cough, urinary urgency or frequency, leg pain or swelling, unilateral weakness, or rashes.

No known history of liver failure or disease, hepatitis, or cancer but the patient does not follow a primary care physician regularly. He has a longstanding history of alcohol use, drinking six to eight beers daily plus an occasional fifth of liquor, and has smoked for 40 years. He denies any recreational drugs. Surgical history includes an appendectomy in childhood.

Descriptors (Documentation Elements)

Duration: A few months
Timing: Constant
Location: Right upper quadrant / **Radiation:** None
Character/Quality: Sharp and stabbing
Associated symptoms: Weight loss, anorexia, abdominal bloating and distension, dyspnea
Modifying factors: None/**Tx before arrival:** Hot baths and aspirin with little relief

Review of Systems

Constitutional: Positive weight loss and anorexia.
Integumentary: No rash.
Musculoskeletal: No leg pain.
HEENT: No sore throat or visual changes.
Nervous: No unilateral weakness.
Cardiovascular: No chest pain or orthopnea.
Respiratory: Positive dyspnea. No cough.
Digestive: No nausea, vomiting, diarrhea, or constipation. Positive abdominal pain and abdominal distension and bloating.
Genitourinary: No urinary urgency or frequency.
Allergic/Immunologic: No fever or chills.
Hematologic/Lymphatic: No melena or hematochezia.

Physical Exam

Constitutional: Well-developed but thin and cachectic appearing male. Scent of alcohol on his breath

Integumentary: Full body jaundice. Chronic stasis dermatitis changes.

Musculoskeletal: No calf tenderness.

HEENT: Dry mucous membranes. Sclera are icteric.

Nervous: No focal deficits. He is alert and cooperative.

Cardiovascular: Irregularly irregular and tachycardic. 2/6 systolic murmur heard best over the left sternal border and an S3 gallop. Jugular venous distension also present. 2+ pitting edema bilateral lower extremities and faint distal pulses.

Respiratory: Breath sounds are diminished throughout and there are diffuse wheezes and crackles at the bases.

Digestive: Soft and tender in the right upper quadrant with voluntary guarding but no rebound. Hepatomegaly two finger breadths below the right costal margin. There is an ascitic wave.

Key Points

This patient is presenting with ongoing right upper quadrant abdominal pain associated with significant weight loss, anorexia, and the sensation of abdominal fullness and distension. These symptoms are associated with a few risk factors that make some kind of liver disease a likely etiology for his symptoms.

First, let us review his risk factors. He does have a history of excessive alcohol use (risk factor for cirrhosis), but no formal diagnosis of liver failure or hepatitis (risk factor for cirrhosis). However, it is important to note that he does not regularly have any type of medical evaluation, meaning that he could have undiagnosed liver disease. He denies any IV drug use (risk factor for hepatitis). This is another great example to show how the pertinent questions can be used to direct the organization and flow of the written history.

The patient also is a 40-year smoker and has worsening shortness of breath. On physical exam, it was noted that he has pitting edema in both lower extremities, an S3 gallop, bibasilar crackles, and jugular venous distension. Thus this patient could also have some heart failure in addition to the probable liver disease. The complexity of this case is likely to be encountered in a scribing situation and the scribe must be able to organize the history in respect to each problem the patient may have. This kind of knowledge comes with experience.

Sometimes patients will give nonverbal cues describing their current condition. In this example, the patient indicated that his abdominal pain was in the right upper quadrant by pointing. In a real situation the scribe would be working on a computer as the provider and patient are interacting, but must remain mindful of these nonverbal cues.

Case 2

The patient is a 36-year-old female with **back pain**.

Patient: Two hours ago I woke with terrible stabbing pain in my right mid back. Sometimes it improves but it's always there.

Provider: Does the pain travel anywhere?

Patient: It's going into the right side of my stomach too.

Provider: Do you have any urinary urgency, frequency, burning, or blood in your urine?

Patient: A few days ago I started having burning and my urine has been pink. I've also been having low-grade fevers and chills.

Provider: Nausea or vomiting?

Patient: I've been nauseated but not vomiting.

Provider: Do you use street drugs? Specifically, do you inject anything?

Patient: I smoke marijuana occasionally but I don't do any of the others.

Provider: Do you have any loss of control of bowels or bladder, numbness when you wipe, or weakness?

Patient: None of that.

Provider: Any recent falls or other trauma?

Patient: Not recently.

Provider: Have you had similar symptoms before?

Patient: I've had kidney infections and stones in the past, but my pain has never been this severe.

Provider: How would you rate the pain on a scale of 1 to 10?

Patient: At its worst, an 8/10. Sometimes it improves to a 6/10.

Provider: Have you taken anything for your symptoms?

Patient: Tylenol and ibuprofen, but those didn't help much.

Provider: When was your last menstrual period?

Patient: I ended my cycle about a week ago. I have an IUD.

Provider: Do you have any other medical problems?

Patient: I have seasonal allergies and migraines, but that's it.

Provider: Otherwise have you had any light sensitivity, skin rashes or lesions, chest pain or palpitations, shortness of breath, a sore throat, headaches, or any other symptoms?

Patient: None of those.

PHYSICAL EXAM FINDINGS: This patient is a well-developed and slightly overweight female. Mucous membranes are somewhat dry. Normal heart rate and rhythm. No murmurs, gallops, or rubs. Breath sounds are normal and symmetric. Abdomen is soft and there is suprapubic tenderness. No pulsatile masses. Right CVA tenderness to percussion. No tenderness of the cervical, thoracic, lumbar, or sacral spine. No paraspinal tenderness. 2+ radial and dorsalis pulses in all four extremities and normal capillary refill. Alert and cooperative with no focal deficits.

ANSWER KEY

CASE 2: The patient is a 36-year-old female who presents with **back pain**.

History of the Present Illness

The patient is a 36-year-old female with back pain. The patient reports that 2 hours ago she awoke from sleep with constant, waxing and waning right flank pain radiating into the right side of her abdomen. She rates the pain as an 8/10 at its worst and as a 6/10 at its best, and describes it as stabbing. A few days ago, she began having dysuria and hematuria but no urinary urgency or frequency. She has had low-grade fevers and chills. She is nauseated but not vomiting. No urinary or bowel incontinence, saddle anesthesias, or weakness. No recent falls or other trauma. Last known menses ended about a week ago and she has an IUD. She has taken Tylenol and ibuprofen with little relief. Otherwise, she denies photophobia, skin rashes or lesions, chest pain or palpitations, dyspnea, sore throat, headaches, or any other symptoms.

Significant medical history includes kidney stones and infections. The patient states that her current symptoms are more severe. She occasionally smokes marijuana, but denies IV drug use.

Descriptors (Documentation Elements)

Duration: 2 hours
Timing: Constant, waxing and waning
Location: Right flank / **Radiation**: Right abdomen
Character/Quality: Stabbing

Intensity: 8/10 at its worst and 6/10 at its best

Associated symptoms: Dysuria, hematuria, fevers, chills, nausea

Context: Awakened from sleep by flank pain

Tx before arrival: Tylenol and ibuprofen with little relief

Review of Systems

Constitutional: No falls or other trauma.

Integumentary: No rash or lesions.

Musculoskeletal: No muscle weakness.

HEENT: No sore throat. No photophobia.

Nervous: No headaches. No incontinence or saddle anesthesias.

Cardiovascular: No chest pain or palpitations.

Respiratory: No dyspnea.

Digestive: Positive abdominal pain and nausea. No emesis.

Genitourinary: No urgency or frequency. Positive dysuria. Menses 1 week ago.

Allergic/Immunologic: Positive fever and chills.

Hematologic/Lymphatic: Positive hematuria.

Physical Exam

Constitutional: Well-developed and slightly overweight female.

Integumentary: Normal capillary refill.

Musculoskeletal: No tenderness of the cervical, thoracic, lumbar, or sacral spine. No paraspinal tenderness.

HEENT: Mucous membranes are somewhat dry.

Nervous: Alert and cooperative. No focal deficits.

Cardiovascular: Normal rate and rhythm. No murmurs, gallops, or rubs. 2+ radial and dorsalis pedis pulses in all four extremities.

Respiratory: Normal and symmetric breath sounds.

Digestive: Abdomen is soft and there is suprapubic tenderness. No pulsatile masses.

Genitourinary: Right CVA tenderness to percussion

Key Points

This patient is presenting with an acute onset of constant, waxing and waning flank pain associated with urinary symptoms and low-grade fevers that is likely to be renal in etiology (perhaps kidney stones or a kidney infection). She also has a history of kidney infections and stones in the past, making a recurrent problem more likely.

She does not have any of the risk factors for spinal infection (IV drug use), or any of the symptoms to suggest that this is a musculoskeletal (no trauma or falls) or a neurologic problem (urinary or bowel incontinence, saddle anesthesias, or weakness). This example demonstrates the importance of pertinent negatives. Denial of symptoms, signs, or risk factors makes certain diagnoses in the differential less likely.

The patient made a comment about having seasonal allergies and migraines. As the patient is not having any symptoms that could potentially be related to seasonal allergies or migraines this information was omitted from the history. If ever in doubt about whether or not something may be relevant it is best practice to include it in the history: it is easier for a provider to remove irrelevant information than to add it after the fact when it may have already been forgotten. Also, depending on the provider the scribe may be expected to update the medical history elsewhere in the chart. This is one of the duties that should be clarified prior to working with a new provider.

Case 3

The patient is a 53-year-old male with **chest pain**.

Provider: I've reviewed your ECG and I see some concerning changes. Tell me about your chest pain.

Patient: About an hour ago, I was shoveling snow and all of a sudden began having sharp chest pain *(points to sternum)*. I also had pain in my shoulder *(points left)* and jaw. I couldn't catch my breath and soaked my clothes with sweat. I had to go change my shirt before I called 911.

Provider: Did you feel sick to your stomach like you were going to throw-up? Have you had a cough recently? Fevers?

Patient: I have a cough normally because I smoke. But it hasn't changed and I don't cough anything up. I didn't feel like throwing-up and I haven't been having any fevers that I know about.

Provider: Does the chest pain worsen when you breathe?

Patient: No, but it did get worse when I continued to shovel snow.

Provider: Do you have diabetes, high blood pressure, or high cholesterol?

Patient: My family doctor says I have all of those but I've gotta' be honest with you doc. I don't take my medications, even though I tell my family doctor that I do.

Provider: Have you ever had a heart attack or heart disease?

Patient: No, I'm a healthy guy.

Provider: Does anyone in your family have heart problems?

Patient: My dad and his dad both had major heart attacks. And my uncle had diabetes, I think.

Provider: I was told that the paramedics gave you nitroglycerin when they picked you up. Did that relieve your pain at all?

Patient: It did! My pain is a 2/10 now, and before it was a 10/10.

Provider: Do you take any blood thinners? Aspirin?

Patient: I don't like taking any medications, so no.

Provider: Do you have any visual changes, a sore throat, abdominal pain, burning when you pee, leg pain or swelling, headaches, rashes, or any other symptoms?

Patient: None of that. Like I said—I'm a pretty healthy guy.

PHYSICAL EXAM FINDINGS: Well-developed and well-nourished obese male who is diaphoretic. Mucous membranes are dry. There is jugular venous distension. Heart is tachycardic and there is a 3/6 systolic ejection murmur. Breath sounds are normal but diminished throughout. No chest wall tenderness. Abdomen is soft and nontender. 1+ pitting edema bilaterally. No calf tenderness. Pulses are symmetric in all four extremities.

ANSWER KEY

CASE 3: The patient is a 53-year-old male with **chest pain**.

History of the Present Illness

The patient is a 53-year-old male with chest pain. The patient reports that about an hour ago he was shoveling snow and began to have an acute onset of sharp sternal chest pain radiating into his left jaw and shoulder. Pain is exertionally related, but there is not a pleuritic component that he can identify. He also became diaphoretic and short of breath, but denies nausea. He has a nonproductive cough which he attributes to his smoking history that sounds to be stable and chronic and he denies fevers. The patient was given nitroglycerin en route by paramedics and states that his pain improved from a 10/10 to a 2/10. Otherwise, he denies visual symptoms, a sore throat, abdominal pain, dysuria, leg pain or swelling, headaches, rashes, or any other symptoms.

Significant medical history includes diabetes, hypertension, and hyperlipidemia, all currently unmedicated due to patient's medication noncompliance. No personal history of CAD or MI. He is not anticoagulated. He also has a strong family history of cardiac disease, with reported MI in both his father and paternal grandfather.

Descriptors (Documentation Elements)

Duration: 1 hour
Onset: Acute / **Timing**: Improving after nitroglycerin
Location: Sternal / **Radiation**: Left jaw and shoulder
Character/Quality: Sharp
Intensity: 10/10 before nitroglycerin, and 2/10 after nitroglycerin
Associated symptoms: Diaphoresis, dyspnea, nonproductive cough
Context: Pain began while he was shoveling snow
Modifying factors: Pain exertionally worsened; no pleuritic component / **Tx before arrival**: Nitroglycerin with significant relief

Review of Systems

Constitutional: No fever.
Integumentary: Positive diaphoresis.
Musculoskeletal: No leg pain. Positive jaw pain and arm pain.
HEENT: No sore throat. No visual changes.
Nervous: No headaches.
Cardiovascular: No leg swelling. Positive chest pain.
Respiratory: Positive dyspnea and cough.
Digestive: No abdominal pain or nausea.
Genitourinary: No dysuria.
Allergic/Immunologic: No rash.

Physical Exam

Constitutional: Well-developed and well-nourished obese male.
Integumentary: Diaphoretic.
Musculoskeletal: No calf tenderness. No chest wall tenderness.
HEENT: Dry mucous membranes.
Cardiovascular: Tachycardic and 3/6 systolic ejection murmur. Jugular venous distension. 1+ pitting edema bilaterally. Pulses are symmetric in all four extremities.
Respiratory: Normal breath sounds but diminished throughout.
Digestive: Soft and nontender.

Key Points

This patient has many classic signs and symptoms that may indicate cardiac chest pain. He has exertional chest pain that is sternal and radiates into the left arm and the jaw, he is short of breath and diaphoretic, and his pain was relieved with nitroglycerin. He has many risk factors for heart disease including hypertension, hyperlipidemia, diabetes, tobacco abuse, and a strong family history of cardiac disease.

Sometimes patients will give nonverbal cues describing their current condition. In this case the patient indicated that his chest pain was sternal by pointing. In a real situation the scribe would be working on a computer as the provider and patient are interacting, but must remain mindful of these nonverbal cues.

Patients will often describe their medical problems in a manner that makes the most sense to them. The scribe must be able to interpret and translate the layman's terms into medical jargon. The patient said that he was shoveling snow when the chest pain began, but what should be taken away is that the chest pain is exertional. He also said that he soaked his shirt with his sweat, implying that the patient was diaphoretic.

Sometimes irrelevant information will be given during the course of a history-taking. This must be filtered out and excluded from the history. The comment made about the patient's uncle's diabetes is not relevant to his current complaints and was thus excluded from the history.

This patient said that he sees a family physician who prescribes medication for him for all of his diseases, but he is not taking any of them. This is important to note because the medication noncompliance is increasing this patient's risk for certain disease (in this case cardiac).

Case 4

The patient is a 26-year-old female with **dyspnea**.

Patient: I've had this respiratory infection for a few days now. A sore throat, a runny and stuffy nose, and a cough. Yesterday I was watching TV and all of a sudden couldn't seem to catch my breath. I wanted to see a doctor today because I didn't improve and I started to worry.

Provider: Do you have fevers, or have you been coughing anything up?

Patient: I've had a low-grade fever a few times with chills. The cough has been dry.

Provider: Do you have any chest pain or lightheadedness or dizziness?

Patient: I get sharp pains on the right side of my chest when I breathe, but it doesn't happen all the time. I also have some chest pain after coughing. I don't have any of the other things though.

Provider: Have you travelled recently? Any recent surgeries or illnesses?

Patient: I just returned from vacation in Jamaica about a week ago.

Provider: Do you have pain in your legs, or leg swelling?

Patient: None of those.

Provider: Do you have a history of cancer or autoimmune disease or blood clots in your legs or your lungs?

Patient: I've never been diagnosed with anything except asthma as a kid, but I haven't had problems with the asthma since I got older.

Provider: Does anyone in your family have a history of blood clots in their lungs or legs?

Patient: Not that I know of.

Provider: Are you on birth control or other hormones?

Patient: I take the daily birth control pill.

Provider: Do you smoke?

Patient: I've never smoked, but my mom always smoked in our house when I was growing up.

Provider: Just a few more routine questions. Do you have any visual changes, nausea, vomiting, diarrhea, burning with urination or blood in your urine, headaches, rashes, or any other symptoms?

Patient: None of those.

PHYSICAL EXAM FINDINGS: This is a well-developed and well-nourished female. Moist mucous membranes. Nose is congested and there is scant clear rhinorrhea. Posterior oropharynx is somewhat erythematous but no tonsillar swelling or exudates. No anterior cervical lymphadenopathy. Borderline tachycardia but with a regular rhythm. A few end expiratory wheezes but breath sounds are otherwise normal. No chest wall tenderness. Abdomen is soft and nontender. No calf tenderness. Negative Homan's sign. Strong dorsalis pedis and posterior tibial pulses and normal capillary refill. No focal neurological deficits and the patient is alert and cooperative.

ANSWER KEY

CASE 4: The patient is a 26-year-old female who presents with **shortness of breath**.

History of the Present Illness

The patient is a 26-year-old female with shortness of breath. The patient reports that for the past few days she has had a persistent sore throat, nonproductive cough, rhinorrhea and congestion, and an intermittent low-grade fever and chills. Yesterday she began having an acute onset of dyspnea while watching TV associated with pleuritic and posttussive chest pain. No lightheadedness or dizziness. No leg pain or swelling. Otherwise, she denies visual changes, nausea, vomiting, diarrhea, dysuria or hematuria, headaches, rashes, or any other symptoms.

The patient has a history of childhood asthma, now apparently resolved. No history of hypercoagulability, including cancer, lupus, deep venous thrombosis or pulmonary embolism. She is taking oral contraceptives. No family history of hypercoagulability. The patient is a non-smoker, but she had passive smoke exposure in childhood. She did return from vacation in Jamaica about a week ago.

Descriptors (Documentation Elements)

Duration: A few days
Onset: Acute / **Timing:** Persistent and worsening yesterday
Associated symptoms: Sore throat, rhinorrhea, congestion, nonproductive cough, fevers, chills, pleuritic and posttussive chest pain
Context: Symptoms began while she was watching TV
Modifying factors: Pleuritic and posttussive chest pain

Review of Systems

Constitutional: Positive fever and chills.
Integumentary: No rash.
Musculoskeletal: Positive posttussive chest pain. No leg pain.
HEENT: No visual changes.
Nervous: No headaches.
Cardiovascular: No leg swelling.
Respiratory: Positive cough, dyspnea, pleuritic chest pain.
Digestive: No nausea, vomiting, or diarrhea.
Genitourinary: No dysuria.
Allergic/Immunologic: Positive sore throat, rhinorrhea, congestion.
Lymphatic/Hematologic: No hematuria.

Physical Exam

Constitutional: Well-developed and well-nourished female.
Integumentary: Normal capillary refill to the lower extremities.
Musculoskeletal: No calf tenderness. Negative Homan's sign. No chest wall tenderness.
HEENT: Moist mucous membranes. Nose is congested with scant clear rhinorrhea. Posterior oropharynx somewhat erythematous, but no tonsillar swelling or exudates.
Nervous: No focal deficits. Alert and cooperative.
Cardiovascular: Borderline tachycardia. Regular rhythm. Strong dorsalis pedis and posterior tibial pulses.
Respiratory: Few end expiratory wheezes, but otherwise normal.
Digestive: Soft and nontender.
Hematologic/Lymphatic/Immunologic: No anterior cervical lymphadenopathy.

Key Points

This patient has many classic symptoms that may be indicative of pulmonary embolism. She had a sudden onset of shortness of breath with pleuritic chest pain (pain that worsens with inspiration). She has many risk factors, including a recent flight to Jamaica and back as well as daily oral contraceptive use. Although the patient doesn't smoke, she has had long-term passive exposure and this still constitutes a risk factor.

This patient also had symptoms and signs consistent with a respiratory infection: nasal congestion and rhinorrhea, a cough and posttussive chest pain, a sore throat, and fevers and chills. This type of case resembles a real patient encounter because rarely will encounters be "textbook." This is one of the many reasons why it is important for the scribe to do their due diligence and record a reliable history. This example also demonstrates that because a scribe (or the provider) may not know what is truly relevant to the patient case, it is better to include more historical information than less.

The patient reported a history of having childhood asthma, but is apparently asymptomatic in adulthood. Although the scribe is supposed to exclude irrelevant information from the history, since the patient is having shortness of breath associated with cold-like symptoms the remote history of asthma may be relevant so it was included.

Case 5

The patient is a 40-year-old male with a **headache**.

Patient: A few hours ago I was working at my computer and started having this throbbing headache on the right side of my head. I'm incredibly nauseous now and have vomited twice.

Provider: Did the headache come on suddenly, or did it gradually occur?

Patient: It was definitely gradual. At first it was just uncomfortable but it has gotten so much worse.

Provider: Does the headache move anywhere?

Patient: It stays on the right side of my head.

Provider: Do you have weakness of one arm or one leg, blurred or double vision, or a loss of balance or coordination?

Patient: No, I don't think so. But the bright lights in here are killing me.

Provider: Do sounds bother you too?

Patient: Not as much as the lights, but I think a quiet room would help.

Provider: Do you have any fevers or rashes? Neck stiffness?

Patient: None of those symptoms but I was diagnosed with a sinus infection a few weeks ago. My doctor gave me a Z-pak which cleared things up for me.

Provider: Do you have any facial pain or pressure, or nasal symptoms?

Patient: All of that improved with the antibiotic.

Provider: Did you have any symptoms before the headache began?

Patient: I saw some flashes of bright light. I wasn't sure what they were. I've never had them before.

Provider: Do you have a history of migraines? Or have you had any similar symptoms in the past?

Patient: No history of migraines, although my mom had them.

Provider: Do you have a cough, chest pain or palpitations, urinary urgency or frequency, joint pain or muscle aches?

Patient: None of those as of late.

PHYSICAL EXAM FINDINGS: This is a well-developed and well-nourished male in moderate distress. Moist mucous membranes. No sinus tenderness to percussion and nose appears normal. Few beats of horizontal nystagmus. Pupils are equal, round, and reactive to light and extraocular muscles are intact. There is some photophobia. No lymphadenopathy. Neck is supple. Regular rate and rhythm. No murmurs, gallops, or rubs. Breath sounds are normal. Abdomen is soft and nontender. Strong DP/PT pulses and no edema. No focal deficits and he is alert and oriented in all three dimensions. Extremity strength is 5/5 and symmetric in all four extremities. Sensation intact to light touch throughout. No pronator drift. Romberg's is unremarkable. No finger to nose ataxia and normal heel to shin testing. Negative Kernig's and Brudzinski's. Cranial nerves II through XII intact. Gait is normal.

ANSWER KEY

CASE 5: The patient is a 40-year-old male who presents with a **headache**.

History of the Present Illness

The patient is a 40-year-old male with a headache. The patient reports that a few hours ago he was working on a computer and developed a gradual onset of a progressively worsening non-radiating throbbing headache located on the right side of his head. He does have photophobia and phono-phobia, and has been nauseated and vomiting. He describes some visual aural symptoms preced-ing the headache. No personal history of migraines, although he does have a family history in his mother. No unilateral weakness, blurred vision or diplopia, or loss of balance or coordination. No fevers, rashes, or neck stiffness. He apparently was recently diagnosed with sinusitis a few weeks ago and was given a Z-pak by his family doctor but denies any nasal symptoms or facial pain or pressure. Otherwise, he denies palpitations, a cough, chest pain, urinary urgency or frequency, or arthralgias or myalgias.

Descriptors (Documentation Elements)

Duration: A few hours
Onset: Gradual / **Timing:** Progressively worsening
Location: Right head / **Radiation:** None
Character/Quality: Throbbing
Associated symptoms: Photophobia, phonophobia, nausea, vomiting, recent sinusitis
Context: Symptoms began while working on a computer
Modifying factors: Photophobia and phonophobia

Review of Systems

Constitutional: Positive recent sinusitis.
Integumentary: No rash.
Musculoskeletal: No arthralgias or myalgias.
HEENT: No blurred vision or diplopia. No facial pain or pressure or nasal symptoms.
Nervous: Positive headache, photophobia, phonophobia, visual aura. No unilateral weakness, loss of balance or coordination.
Cardiovascular: No chest pain or palpitations.
Respiratory: No cough.
Digestive: Positive nausea and vomiting.
Genitourinary: No urinary urgency or frequency.
Allergic/Immunologic: No fever.

Physical Exam

Constitutional: Well-developed well-nourished male. Moderate distress.
Musculoskeletal: Neck is supple.

HEENT: Moist mucous membranes. Few beats of horizontal nystagmus. PERRL. EOMI. Photophobia.

Nervous: Alert and oriented ×3. No focal deficits. Extremity strength is 5/5 and symmetric in all four extremities. Sensation intact to light touch throughout. No pronator drift. Negative Romberg's. No finger to nose ataxia. Normal heel to shin testing. Negative Kernig's and Brudzinski's. CN II-XII intact. Gait is normal.

Cardiovascular: Regular rate and rhythm. No murmurs, gallops, or rubs. Strong dorsalis pedis and posterior tibial pulses and no edema.

Respiratory: Breath sounds are normal.

Digestive: Soft and nontender.

Hematologic/Lymphatic/Immunologic: No lymphadenopathy.

Key Points

This patient is presenting with a gradual onset of a unilateral throbbing headache associated with nausea, vomiting, photophobia, and phonophobia. He also described flashing lights that precipitated the headache which seem to be consistent with a pre migrainous aura.

Patients will often describe symptoms or signs in a manner which makes sense to them, so the scribe should be cognizant of this while listening to a history. In this example the patient said that bright lights bothered him (photophobia), but when asked about sound sensitivity he stated that "a quiet room would help." This was a discrete cue that the patient does have sound sensitivity (phonophobia) as well.

The importance of pertinent negatives was demonstrated in this case. The patient's denial of fevers, rashes, and neck stiffness made meningitis less likely. The denial of unilateral weakness, visual disturbances, or loss of balance or coordination made stroke or transient ischemic attack less likely. Pertinent negatives should always be included within the history because they affect the provider's medical decision making process.

The patient did mention that he was recently treated for sinusitis with a Z-pak and is currently asymptomatic from that infection. Because the sinusitis occurred relatively recently, it may still be relevant to the patient's current headache and thus should be included within the history.

Case 6

The patient is a 22-year-old male who presents after a **motor vehicle accident**.

Patient: About an hour ago I was driving to school and this car ran a red light and t-boned me on the passenger side of my car.

Provider: How fast were you and he driving?

Patient: I was going about 35 miles per hour. The road was 35 miles per hour too but I'm not sure if he was driving within the speed limit.

Provider: What kind of cars were involved?

Patient: I was driving a sedan and he was in a pick-up truck.

Provider: Were you wearing a seat belt? Did the airbags deploy?

Patient: I was wearing my seatbelt and all of the airbags on the passenger's side went off.

Provider: Did you hit your head or lose consciousness?

Patient: I think I hit my head on the seat behind me, but I didn't pass out.

Provider: Are you on blood thinners?

Patient: The only medication I take is loratadine for springtime allergies.

Provider: Do you have a headache or changes in your vision, speech, or coordination?

Patient: I have a mild headache.

Provider: Do you have pain anywhere?

Patient: I hit my knees on the dash and they hurt now. My neck hurts and the back of my head hurts also.

Provider: Does anything make the pain better or worse?

Patient: Movement definitely makes everything hurt more.

Provider: Were you able to get out of the vehicle after the accident?

Patient: Yes I was. I helped the other guy out of his car and walked to the ambulance.

Provider: Do you have any fevers, chills, a sore throat, a cough or shortness of breath, palpitations, nausea, vomiting, diarrhea, burning with urination, rashes, or other symptoms?

Patient: None of that.

PHYSICAL EXAM FINDINGS: The patient is a well-developed and well-nourished male. There is a small hematoma on the posterior occiput. Pupils are equal, round, and reactive to light and extraocular muscles intact. Normal range of motion of the cervical spine and no midline tenderness. There is some left-sided paraspinal cervical tenderness. No midline tenderness, step off or deformity in the thoracic, lumbar, or sacral spine. Borderline tachycardia and normal rhythm. No murmurs, gallops, or rubs. Breath sounds are symmetric and clear. Abdomen is soft and non-tender. No seatbelt sign or other contusions. No chest wall tenderness. No bony tenderness in bilateral upper or lower extremities. Normal range of motion of all major joints. Abrasions to bilateral knees, but no bony tenderness. Both knees are stable to medial and lateral collateral stress. Normal anterior and posterior drawer signs. No effusions. 2+ dorsalis pedis and posterior tibial pulses and normal capillary refill in lower extremities. He is alert and oriented three times. No focal deficits noted. Cranial nerves II through XII intact. Extremity strength 5/5 and symmetric in all four extremities. Sensation to light touch intact throughout. Romberg's testing is unremarkable. No pronator drift. No finger to nose ataxia and normal heel shin testing. Gait is normal.

ANSWER KEY

CASE 6: The patient is a 22-year-old male who presents after a **motor vehicle accident**.

History of the Present Illness

The patient is a 22-year-old male who presents after a motor vehicle accident. The patient reports that about an hour ago he was the restrained driver of a sedan travelling around 35 mph that was t-boned on the passenger's side by a pick-up truck travelling on a road with a speed limit of 35 mph. The airbags on the passenger's side did deploy and he was restrained. The patient thinks he may have hit his posterior head on the seat, but he denies a loss of consciousness. No anticoagulation therapy. He has a mild headache now associated with neck pain and posterior head pain. No changes in his vision, speech, or coordination. He hit both knees on the dashboard and now has bilateral knee pain that is worsened with movement. He has been ambulatory since the accident. Otherwise he denies fevers, chills, a sore throat, cough, dyspnea, palpitations, nausea, vomiting, diarrhea, dysuria, rashes, or any other symptoms.

Descriptors (Documentation Elements)

Duration: 1 hour

Onset: Sudden

Associated symptoms: Head injury and head pain, headache, neck pain, knee pain

Context: Restrained driver of a sedan travelling around 35 mph that was t-boned on the passenger's side by a pick-up truck travelling on a road with a speed limit of 35 mph

Modifying factors: Pain worsened by movement

Review of Systems

Integumentary: No rash.

Musculoskeletal: Positive knee pain and neck pain.

HEENT: No sore throat or hearing changes. No visual changes. Positive head injury and pain.
Nervous: No changes in coordination or speech. Positive headache.
Respiratory: No dyspnea or cough.
Cardiovascular: No palpitations.
Digestive: No nausea, vomiting, or diarrhea.
Genitourinary: No dysuria.
Allergic/Immunologic: No fevers or chills.

Physical Exam

Constitutional: Well-developed and well-nourished male.
Integumentary: Normal distal capillary refill. Abrasions to both knees.
Musculoskeletal: Normal ROM of the cervical spine and no midline tenderness. Left paraspinal cervical tenderness. No midline tenderness, step offs or deformity to the thoracic,
   lumbar, or sacral spine. No chest wall tenderness. No bony tenderness in bilateral upper or
   lower extremities. No knee tenderness. No effusions. Both knees are stable to medial and
   lateral collateral stress. Normal anterior and posterior drawer signs. Normal range of motion
   of all major joints.
HEENT: Small hematoma on the posterior occiput. PERRL EOMI.
Nervous: A&O X3. No focal deficits. Cranial nerves II through XII intact. Extremity strength
   5/5 and symmetric in all four extremities. Sensation to light touch intact throughout. No
   pronator drift. Romberg's is unremarkable. No finger to nose ataxia and normal heel shin
   testing. Gait is normal.
Cardiovascular: Borderline tachycardia. Normal rhythm. No murmurs, gallops, or rubs.
   2+ DP/PT pulses bilaterally.
Respiratory: Breath sounds symmetric.
Digestive: Soft and nontender.
Hematologic/Lymphatic/Immunologic: No seatbelt sign or contusions.

Key Points

The content of a history for trauma cases varies depending on context. The patient in this case
was involved in a motor vehicle accident. Usually with this type of trauma, the following will be
discussed regarding the mechanism of injury: type of vehicles involved, how the vehicles impacted
one another and the speeds of each, where the patient was sitting in the vehicle, if the patient was
restrained or unrestrained, what airbags deployed (if any), damage to the vehicle, if the patient was
ambulatory after the accident, if they had to be extracted from the vehicle versus if they were able
to get out on their own, and more.

Any injury sustained because of the traumatic event should be documented in both the history
and physical exam. The types of injuries will vary depending on the type of trauma. In most cases,
head injuries will almost always be discussed. This could include whether the patient hit his or her
head, if there was a loss of consciousness, or if they are taking any blood thinners (makes bleeding
harder to stop and more likely to occur).

Trauma-focused physical exams are typically quite extensive, as seen in this example. Because
many traumas are high impact or occur at high velocity, many organ systems may be affected.
Thus the provider will examine everything, and the exam will (hopefully) mostly include pertinent
negatives.

Answers to Case Studies and Practice Questions

CHAPTER 1
CASE STUDY 1.1 QUESTIONS

1. Disorders of the ear, nose, and throat
2. Family physicians are primary care providers who see both adults and children.
3. history of the present illness (HPI)
4. electronic health record (EHR)
5. Certification ensures an individual has been trained, tested, and can be counted on to perform the job with competence.

PRACTICE QUESTIONS

1. provider
2. order
3. b
4. c
5. neurologist
6. cardiologist
7. urologist
8. psychiatrist
9. d

   The scribe should ask the provider for permission (d) because the patient may not be allowed any po (by mouth) intake for a variety of reasons. The scribe should not immediately get the patient a drink (a) because of this. The scribe should also not review the patient's test results (b) because they are non-clinical personnel and not certified to do this. The scribe should never ignore the patient's needs and merely excuse themselves from the situation (c).

CHAPTER 2
CASE STUDY 2.1 QUESTIONS

1. c
2. c
3. d
4. plaintiff; defendant
5. The audit trail

PRACTICE QUESTIONS

1. assault and battery
2. Malpractice
3. Implied
4. breach
5. a

   The Security Rule (a) specifically regulates electronic protected health information. The Portability Rule (b) does not exist. The Patient Safety Rule (c) applies specifically to those individuals who share patient information for safety analytic purposes. The Privacy Rule (d) regulates all forms of protected health information (including but not limited to electronic).

6. c

   Scribe companies employed by a hospital are business associates (c) and must adhere to HIPAA rules even though they are not directly the covered entity (b). The hospital would be the covered entity (b) under HIPAA.

7. Upcoding
8. conscience clause

CHAPTER 3

CASE STUDY 3.1 QUESTIONS

1. a
2. b
3. c
4. a
5. d

PRACTICE QUESTIONS

1. pathogen
2. personal protective equipment (PPE)
3. Transmission-based precautions
4. Occupational Safety and Health Administration (OSHA)
5. sterilization
6. sterile

CHAPTER 4

CASE STUDY 4.1 QUESTIONS

1. Revenue cycle
2. Neck pain with radiation to the left arm and difficulty sleeping
3. The provider's physical examination of the provider, namely "marked slowing and impairment of fine motor coordination in the left hand."
4. CPT, specifically E/M codes
5. ICD-10-CM, a diagnosis code
6. The provider's impression or assessment, and in the problem list.

7. The impression, cervicalgia, will be removed from the problem list and replaced with the new diagnosis.
8. The computerized physician order entry (CPOE)

PRACTICE QUESTIONS

1. continuum of care
2. diagnosis
3. litigation
4. third-party payer
5. outcomes
6. a
7. c
8. Health Insurance Portability and Accountability Act (HIPAA)

CHAPTER 5

CASE STUDY 5.1 QUESTIONS

1. Urinary frequency and lower back pain.
2. Social history
3. 4 days
4. The genitourinary section of the ROS, as "denies (or -) vaginal bleeding, denies (or -) gush of fluid"
5. Ausculation
6. Constitutional, cardiovascular, respiratory, and abdominal

PRACTICE QUESTIONS

1. f
2. e
3. d
4. a
5. c
6. b
7. d
   The chief complaint can include any reason for being seen by a medical provider.
8. a
   Answer (a) is correct; however, the history may be cloned from prior visits so long as it is altered so as to be current with any changes since last visit. Answer (b) is incorrect because a scribe is allowed to clone appropriate information (such as the results of testing). Answers (c) and (d) are incorrect because this is not an appropriate use of cloning.
9. d
   Answer (d) is correct because the patient is unable to provide a history due to their medical condition, and this is an acceptable reason for billing forgiveness. Answers (a) and (b) are incorrect because this is a high acuity visit. Answer (c) is incorrect because this patient will be unable to provide 10 systems for the review of systems.
10a. Past medical history
10b. Irrelevant
10c. Allergies

10d. Surgical history
10e. Social history
10f. Family history
These are definitional. The patient's stepfather's hypertension is irrelevant because they are unrelated.
11a. Branded/trademarked
11b. Generic
Brand names will always be capitalized. Generic names will be written in lowercase.
12a. true allergy
12b. contraindication
12c. intolerance
13a. heart rate (HR): normal adult 60–100 bpm
13b. blood pressure (BP): normal adult <130/80
13c. respiratory rate (RR): normal adult 12–18 bpm
13d. body temperature (BT): normal adult ~98.6°F
Oxygen saturation (SaO$_2$) would also be a valid answer.

CHAPTER 6

CASE STUDY 6.1 QUESTIONS

Duration: 3 hours
Onset: abrupt / Timing: constant and gradually worsening
Location: right naris/Radiation: Does not apply as a nose bleed does not radiate
Character/Quality: "pouring out like a faucet"
Intensity and severity do not particularly apply although it would not be wrong to say that severity is "severe" or "heavy."
Associated Symptoms: lightheadedness
Context: recent initiation of coumadin therapy 2 weeks ago
Modifying factors: None/Tx before arrival: nose pinching

PRACTICE QUESTIONS

1. c
   The history is sometimes limited, and the scribe should record the reason why so that the requirement for documenting elements can be forgiven. The historian will usually be the patient but could be any of several sources of history such as family member or police or EMS. The history is the subjective portion of the note and the physical exam the objective part. The history is always newly created and describes the current reason for the visit and should never be copied from a prior visit.

2. b
   Choice (b) is correct. This phrasing uses an objective speaking verb to begin the HPI, making it nonjudgmental and clearly documenting what was related to the provider. Choice (a) could be considered as straightforward, but there are negative connotations associated with the verb "complains." The use of the verb "insists" in choice (c) conveys that the documentarian has a reason not to believe the historian, making it subjective and even confusing. Choice (d) omits a speaking verb altogether, which misrepresents the facts: we do not ever know that the patient had a headache, but we do know that they *state* they had a headache. The correct language for choice (d) would therefore be, "The patient states that her headache began yesterday…"

3. The key is to use the verb *associates*, because the historian is identifying an inciting factor. One possible sentence is, "The patient associates her diarrhea with eating old leftovers."

4. The patient, his wife, and EMS are all historians in this case.
5. "The mother reports that the child has indicated possible pain in the right ear as he has been hitting at his ear since this morning."

CHAPTER 7

CASE STUDY 7.1 QUESTIONS

1. a
2. d
3. The patient was prepped from his chin to both feet. The sterile field would include this area and the space over it, the drapes surrounding the prepared skin, the scrubbed-in members of the surgical team, and all instrumentation and packages.
4. Informed consent
5. The patient was intubated and received general anesthesia, which is systemic. Local anesthesia affects only one part of the body.
6. The patient tolerated the procedure well.
7. rate; 100
8. The rhythm strip, an extension of lead II, is the most useful to examine rhythm.
9. The final impression
10. d

PRACTICE QUESTIONS

1. ELECTROCARDIOGRAM (ECG):
   Rate: 110 bpm
   Rhythm: Sinus tachycardia
   Axis: Normal
   Ectopy: Occasional PVCs
   Conduction: 1st degree AV block
   QRS complex: Narrow
   Q wave: No pathologic Q waves
   T wave: Normal
   ST segment: No acute changes
   Final impression: Sinus tachycardia with occasional PVCs and a 1st degree AV block. No acute changes.
   Comparison: Prior ECG on 3/22/2013 shows similar changes except rate is normal.
2. ELECTROCARDIOGRAM (ECG):
   Rate: 140 bpm
   Rhythm: Tachycardia
   Axis: Right axis deviation
   Conduction: New right bundle branch block in V1–V3
   P wave: Peaked in lead II
   QRS complex: Narrow
   Q wave: in the absence of comments on Q wave, scribe should verify with provider that there are none and then document "none."
   T wave: Inversions in V1–V3
   ST segment: Diffuse elevation
   Final impression: Changes consistent with acute pulmonary embolism and right heart strain.
   Comparison: All changes are new compared to ECG on 4/26/2021.

3. PROCEDURE NOTE:
   Time-out: Performed at 13:00
   Procedure name: Left shoulder reduction
   Indication: Left shoulder dislocation
   Consent: Signed at 12:45
   Time: Started at 13:10
   Medications: Versed 5 mg IV
   Monitoring: Monitored for blood pressure, pulse, and pulse ox
   Details: Traction/countertraction method used
   Stabilizing activities: Shoulder immobilizer placed
   Complications: None
   Results: Good reduction achieved as verified with post-reduction x-ray. Intact axillary nerve and distal neurovascular post procedure

4. PROCEDURE NOTE:
   Procedure name: Laceration repair
   Indication: Left forearm laceration
   Time: 15:35
   Medications: 1% plain lidocaine
   Preparation: Shur Clens
   Details: Two-layer closure. SQ tissue closed with running 5-0 Vicryl suture. Skin closure accomplished with #8 5-0 Ethilon suture. Dressed with bacitracin dressing.
   Complications: None
   Results: Good approximation of edges.

CHAPTER 8

CASE STUDY 8.1 QUESTIONS

1. A chest x-ray (CXR), which is a radiograph
2. The CBC, which was part of the dyspnea panel
3. diazepam
4. Nursing orders
5. PRN, meaning as needed

PRACTICE QUESTIONS

1.
   Name: cyclobenzaprine DAW
   Dose: 10 mg
   Formulation: tab
   Route: po
   Frequency: bid
   Duration: 10 days
   Patient Sig: Take with or without food
   Dispense: 20
2.
   Name: Phenergan
   Dose: 25 mg
   Formulation: Suppository

Route: rectal
Frequency: q4h
Duration: prn
Dispense: 12
3. complete blood count (CBC)
4. basic metabolic panel (BMP)
5. CT scan
6. hepatic panel/liver function testing (LFT)
7. angiography
8. serum toxicology
9. ventilation/perfusion (V/Q) scan
10. electroencephalogram (EEG)
11. c
    Troponin (c) is a heart enzyme that is released when there is injury to heart muscle. A d-dimer (a) measures the breakdown of clots and is a screening test for thrombosis. A sedimentation rate (b) is a nonspecific measure of systemic inflammation. An ANA (d) is an antibody assay used to screen for autoimmune disease.
12. a
13. d
    An ultrasound (d) is routinely used in this manner because there is no risk of injury to the fetus from radiation exposure. Both x-rays (a) and CT (b) put the baby and mother at risk from radiation exposure. MRI (c) is costly, time consuming, and provides an unnecessary amount of detail for the information being sought.
14. D
15. E
16. A
17. F
18. C
19. B
20. symptom
21. diagnosis
22. sign
23. sign
24. clinical impression

CHAPTER 9

CASE STUDY 9.1 QUESTIONS

1. After
2. Oliguria
3. A recording (picture) of the kidney
4. The urinary bladder
5. Between the bladder and the vagina

PRACTICE QUESTIONS

1. b
2. a
3. Discharge of flow of the nose

4. A softening of the bones
5. An eponym

CHAPTER 10

CASE STUDY 10.1 QUESTIONS

1. Vertigo
2. The ear
3. Since is it the distal end of the humerus, it is closer to the elbow.
4. Shallow or more externally located
5. pertinent negatives

PRACTICE QUESTIONS

1. medial; lateral
2. superior; inferior
3. anterior/ventral; posterior/dorsal
4. **Constitutional:** + malaise
   Immunologic/allergic: + fever
   Endocrine: + fatigue
5. **Constitutional:** WDWN male who appears his stated age.

CHAPTER 11

CASE STUDY 11.1 QUESTIONS

1. The patient
2. Pruritic
3. Duration
4. Progressively worsening, especially at night
5. Yes, under family history.

PRACTICE QUESTIONS

1. Melanocytes
2. Sebaceous glands
3. Adipocytes
4. Superficial to deep: epidermis, dermis, hypodermis
5. **Constitutional**: – recent illnesses
   Integumentary: + erythema
   Hematologic/Lymphatic: – bruising
   Immunologic/Allergic: + pruritus and rash
   Note: This patient's positive symptoms could have also been designated by "positive" or "affirms" (alternatively to using "+"), and her negative symptoms could have been designated by "negative" or "denies" (alternatively to using "-").
6. **Constitutional**: Well-developed and well-nourished female.
   Integumentary: Faint urticarial lesions over both arms and upper chest.
   Hematologic/Lymphatic/Immunologic: Residual stippling and bruising near older lesions.
7. Excisional biopsy
8. a

CHAPTER 12

CASE STUDY 12.1 QUESTIONS

1. The patient's daughter, Lynette
2. Answers will vary. One possibility is: The patient's daughter reports that 2 hours ago she fell in the bathroom, developing an immediate constant lumbago (or lower back pain).
3. The patient probably has a diagnosis of osteoporosis.
4. The lower thoracic vertebrae
5. The posterior or back side

PRACTICE QUESTIONS

1. glenohumeral
2. synovial, ball and socket
3. abduction
4. a. cervical (C)
   b. thoracic (T)
   c. lumbar (L)
   d. sacral (S)
   e. coccygeal
5. **Constitutional**: – recent illnesses
   Integumentary: + rashes
   Musculoskeletal: + arthralgias, joint stiffness and swelling
   Immunologic/Allergic: + fever
6. **Constitutional**: Disheveled appearing.
   Integumentary: No rashes.
   Musculoskeletal: Synovitis diffusely in the MCP joints of both hands and the left wrist. There is ulnar deviation bilaterally. Hammertoe deformities are seen in both feet but there is no synovitis. Effusion is noted in the left knee with some loss in range of motion. Range of motion is otherwise intact throughout.
7. Arthrocentesis
8. c
   Rheumatoid arthritis (c) is a systemic inflammatory autoimmune disease that often affects small synovial joints and causes joint pain, swelling, and deformity.
   Ankylosing spondylitis (a) is an inflammatory back disease. Fibromyalgia (b) is a pain hypersensitivity syndrome without another explainable cause. Osteoarthritis (d) is "wear and tear" arthritis.
9. d
   Naproxen (d) is the NSAID. Baclofen (a) is a muscle relaxant. Methotrexate (b) is an immunosuppressant. Prednisone (d) is a steroid (also an immunosuppressant).

CHAPTER 13

CASE STUDY 13.1 QUESTIONS

1. Otalgia
2. Cerumen
3. Over 1 year
4. Otoscope

5. Answers will vary. One possibility is "Q-tips; over-the-counter "ear dry" remedy, likely alcohol-based. Lavage and otic antibiotic about 2 months prior with temporary relief."

PRACTICE QUESTIONS

1. oropharynx
2. immune
3. lingual
4. uvula
5. **Constitutional:** + chills and malaise
   Integumentary: – rashes
   Musculoskeletal: – arthralgias or myalgias
   HEENT: +sore throat, post nasal drainage, congestion, rhinorrhea
   Neurologic: – blurred vision or diplopia
   Immunologic/Allergic: +fever
6. **Constitutional**: Atoxic. Well-developed and well-nourished.
   Integumentary: No rashes.
   Musculoskeletal: Full range of motion in all major joints.
   HEENT: Conjunctiva are clear. Turbinates are swollen and there is scant clear rhinorrhea. Tonsillar enlargement, erythema, and exudates bilaterally. No uvular deviation. Tympanic membranes are pearly white with intact light reflexes.
   Neurologic: PERRL.
   Note: "PERRL" can be placed under "Neurologic" because it is actually a reflex test of two cranial nerves (CN II [input] and CN III [output]).
7. Septoplasty
8. Peritonsillar abscess
9. d
   Azithromycin (a) is another antibiotic. Vitamin C (b) is a vitamin and would not help with this patient's symptoms. Dapsone (c) is an antibiotic.

CHAPTER 14

CASE STUDY 14.1 QUESTIONS

1. Anger outbursts; combativeness
2. These are signs observed by the physician during his physical exam.
3. Paranoia
4. The cerebellum. The findings are suggestive of cerebellar ataxia.
5. This is "Additional history," specifically "Past medical history" PMHx.

PRACTICE QUESTIONS

1. cerebellum
2. autonomic
3. subdural
4. cranial
5. **Constitutional:** - recent falls or traumatic injury
   Musculoskeletal: + back pain and radicular symptoms
   Neurologic: + saddle anesthesias and leg weakness
   Genitourinary: + urinary incontinence
   Immunologic/Allergic: - fevers

6. **Constitutional**: Moderate distress.
   Integumentary: Unremarkable.
   Musculoskeletal: Range of motion is limited in flexion and extension of the low back. There is diffuse low back tenderness in the paraspinal region but no vertebral step off or deformity.
   Neurologic: Motor strength is 5/5 in both arms but 3/5 in both legs. He has symmetric diminished sensation to light touch in the buttocks, inner thighs, and perineal region. Anal reflex is absent. Patellar and Achilles reflexes are diminished.
7. Spinal stenosis
8. Laminectomy
9. a
   Morphine (a) is a narcotic. Naloxone (b) is an opioid antagonist. Amphetamine (c) is a CNS stimulant. Haloperidol (d) is an antipsychotic.

CHAPTER 15

CASE STUDY 15.1 QUESTIONS

1. Hyperlipidemia and hypertension
2. Laboratory testing of lipid levels
3. This is documented as syncope in the ROS under the cardiovascular system.
4. This is dyspnea on exertion (DOE), under the respiratory system in the ROS.
5. Chest pain (a pertinent negative), fatigue, and insomnia
6. Hyperlipidemia

PRACTICE QUESTIONS

1. mitral/bicuspid
2. myocardium
3. pulmonary veins
4. Pulses
5. **Constitutional:** + fall, – chills
   Integumentary: + diaphoresis
   Musculoskeletal: + radiating pain into left arm
   HEENT: - head injury
   Neurologic: + paresthesias
   Psychiatric: + anxiety
   Cardiovascular: + chest pain and syncope
   Respiratory: + dyspnea on exertion
   Immunologic/Allergic: - fevers
6. **Constitutional**: Obese man in moderate distress.
   Integumentary: Diaphoretic with pallor.
   HEENT: Atraumatic.
   Neurologic: No focal neurologic deficits.
   Cardiovascular: Tachycardic with a 2/6 systolic ejection murmur. Pulses are diminished in all four extremities and he has 1+ pitting bilateral lower extremity edema. No jugular venous distension.
7. Coronary artery stenting
8. Hypertension, hyperlipidemia

9. b

Diltiazem (a) is a calcium channel blocker. Enalapril (c) is an ACE inhibitor. Losartan (d) is an ARB (angiotensin receptor blocker).

CHAPTER 16

CASE STUDY 16.1 QUESTIONS

1. The patient is a 21-year-old male with right-sided pleuritic chest pain and shortness of breath.
2. Answers will vary. Procedure note, thoracostomy note, or EKG/ECG note are all plausible.
3. **8 hours ago** (the duration) he had a **sudden** onset (the onset) of **constant** (the timing) dyspnea and pain that has progressively worsened.
4. Mr. Meyer suffered a right-sided pneumothorax and the surgeon performed a thoracostomy.
5. The type and concentration, e.g., 1% plain lidocaine.

PRACTICE QUESTIONS

1. trachea
2. diaphragm
3. pleural fluid
4. Alveoli
5. **Constitutional:** - fever or chills
   Neurologic: - paresthesias
   Cardiovascular: - lightheadedness or syncope
   Respiratory: + dyspnea, wheezing, productive cough
   Immunologic/Allergic: + seasonal allergies
6. **Constitutional**: Mild respiratory distress
   Integumentary: No clubbing or cyanosis.
   HEENT: Clear rhinorrhea and nasal turbinates are swollen. Cobblestoning in the oropharynx.
   Cardiovascular: Tachycardic but no murmurs, gallops, or rubs.
   Respiratory: Tachypneic and oxygen saturation is 91% on room air. No stridor. There is bibasilar expiratory wheezing.
7. Asthma
8. Endotracheal intubation
9. d

   Salmeterol (a) is a preventative inhaler used to treat inflammatory airway disease. Fluticasone (b) is a steroid inhaler. Dextromethorphan (c) is an antitussive.

CHAPTER 17

CASE STUDY 17.1 QUESTIONS

1. + flatulence
   + distension
   + diarrhea
   – reflux
   – hematochezia
2. Over a year

3. About 2 months
4. Palpation
5. Ibuprofen and prednisone
6. Glucocorticoid

PRACTICE QUESTIONS

1. gallbladder
2. pancreas
3. epigastric
4. duodenum
5. **Constitutional:** + anorexia
   Integumentary: – diaphoresis
   Cardiovascular: – chest pain
   Digestive: + abdominal pain, bloating, nausea, vomiting, dyspepsia
   Hematologic/Lymphatic: – hematemesis
6. **Constitutional**: Cachectic and appears older than stated age.
   Integumentary: Generalized jaundice.
   HEENT: Scleral icterus.
   Cardiovascular: Normal rhythm and rate. No murmurs gallops, or rubs. 4+ pitting edema in both lower extremities. Thready pulses in both legs.
   Respiratory: Normal breath sounds.
   Digestive: Hepatomegaly with tenderness in the right upper quadrant and abdominal ascites.
7. Paracentesis
8. Cirrhosis
9. b
   Loperamide (a) is an anti-diarrheal. Ondansetron (c) is an antiemetic. Magnesium citrate (d) is a laxative.

CHAPTER 18

CASE STUDY 18.1 QUESTIONS

1. The patient is a 10-year-old male who presents with hematuria.
2. Oliguria
3. In the ROS under Constitutional as anorexia
4. Well-developed and well-nourished (WDWN). Appears his age of 10. Afebrile.
5. a. + edema *Musculoskeletal (Cardiovascular would be acceptable as well)*
   b. – lymphadenopathy *Hematologic/Lymphatic*
   c. – thyromegaly *Endocrine*
   d. Tender abdomen *Gastrointestinal*
   e. Bilateral flank tenderness *Genitourinary*

PRACTICE QUESTIONS

1. Testes
2. Ovaries
3. Kidneys
4. urethral

5. **Constitutional:** + chills
   Gastrointestinal: + Low midline abdominal pain (or suprapubic pain) with intermittent radiation to the flanks
   Genitourinary: +G2P1A1, dysuria, urinary urgency and frequency, incontinence
   Immunologic/Allergic: + fever
   Hematologic/Lymphatic: - hematuria
   Endocrine: + hot flashes, postmenopausal
6. **Constitutional**: Cachectic appearing.
   Integumentary: Well-healed incision in the lower abdomen.
   Musculoskeletal: Dorsal kyphosis is noted.
   HEENT: Mucous membranes are dry.
   Cardiovascular: A pulsatile mass is present around the umbilicus.
   Respiratory: Normal breath sounds.
   Gastrointestinal: Suprapubic tenderness to palpation.
   Genitourinary: Right CVA tenderness to percussion.
7. Bilateral oophorectomy
8. Pyelonephritis

CHAPTER 19

CASE STUDY 19.1 QUESTIONS

1. The patient is a 35-year-old male who presents with abdominal pain, lymphadenopathy, night sweats, and malaise.
2. Answers will vary. One possibility is:
   The patient reports that several weeks ago he developed a sudden onset of constant malaise and night sweats. He also noticed cervical and axillary lymphadenopathy. The patient also relates abdominal pain. He describes it as vague and rates it as a 3/10. He denies nausea, vomiting, and diarrhea, shortness of breath, or chest pain. The patient has taken Theraflu with little relief.
3. Subjective fever, malaise, night sweats
4. Hematologic/Lymphatic
5. Pancytopenia
6. Lymphoma or leukemia

PRACTICE QUESTIONS

1. B cells
2. Lymph nodes
3. Bone marrow
4. Thrombocytes/platelets
5. **Constitutional:** + recent illness
   Integumentary: + bruising
   HEENT: + epistaxis
   Respiratory: + hemoptysis
   Digestive: + hematochezia
   Immunologic/Allergic: + fever
   Hematologic/Lymphatic: + lymphadenopathy
6. **Constitutional**: Frail appearing
   Integumentary: Bruising in various stages of healing over all four extremities

HEENT: Swollen nasal turbinates, and cobblestoning with erythema of the posterior oropharynx

Cardiovascular: Normal rate and rhythm

Respiratory: Normal breath sounds

Digestive: Soft and nontender

Hematologic/Lymphatic/Immunologic: Lymphadenopathy in the cervical chain bilaterally and of the posterior auricular nodes

7. Bone marrow biopsy
8. Pancytopenia
9. c

Acyclovir (a) is an antiviral. Nystatin (b) is an antifungal. Cetirizine (d) is an antihistamine.

CHAPTER 20

CASE STUDY 20.1 QUESTIONS

1. The patient reports that 3 or 4 weeks ago she developed a sudden onset of polydipsia and polyuria. She states that 4 days ago she began waking up at night with heart palpitations and polydipsia. She affirms lightheadedness, irritability, nausea, and blurred vision. She denies vomiting. The patient states that blurred vision began after snacking.

2. **Eyes:** + blurred vision
   Neurological: lightheadedness
   Psychiatric: + irritability
   Cardiovascular: + palpitations
   Gastrointestinal: + nausea, - vomiting
   Genitourinary: + polyuria
   Endocrine: + polydipsia

3. kidneys
4. clinical impression
5. dehydration

PRACTICE QUESTIONS

1. thyroid
2. pancreas
3. Insulin
4. adrenal
5. **Constitutional:** + weight loss
   Integumentary: + diaphoresis, hair loss, brittle nails
   Musculoskeletal: + myalgias
   Psychiatric: + irritability
   Cardiovascular: + palpitations
   Respiratory: - dyspnea
   Digestive: + polyphagia
   Endocrine: + heat intolerance
6. **Constitutional**: Cachectic appearing.
   Integumentary: Diaphoretic. Hair is thinning in various places and skin is dry and flaky.
   Musculoskeletal: No calf tenderness.
   HEENT: Exophthalmos. Dry mucous membranes.

Nervous: Slight resting tremor in both hands and hyperreflexia is present in both lower extremities.

Psychiatric: Anxious.

Cardiovascular: Irregular and tachycardic.

7. Thyroidectomy
8. Hyperthyroidism
9. a

Glipizide (b) is a diabetic medication. Metformin (c) is also a diabetic medication. Vasopressin (d) decreases water excretion as urine.

CHAPTER 21

PRACTICE QUESTIONS

1. Cholecystitis
2. Abdominal aortic aneurysm dissection
3. Kidney stones (or ureteral calculi)
4. Cirrhosis
5. C
6. B
7. D
8. A
9. E
10. B
11. A
12. F
13. D
14. C

GLOSSARY

abduction: movement away from the body's midline

abortion: the loss of pregnancy secondary to premature expulsion of the fetus from the uterus; an abortion may be spontaneous (miscarriage) or induced (intentionally caused)

abscess: a collection of pus in body tissues

abuse: in healthcare, improper conduct that goes against acceptable business and/or medical practices

accreditation: a status awarded by an independent certifying organization to a healthcare facility that indicates the facility has met the standards for quality

acidosis: an abnormal increase in the acidity of blood and tissues, resulting from an accumulation of an acid or the loss of a base. It is indicated by a blood pH below the normal range (7.35 to 7.45).

acromion process: a bony knob where the scapula articulates with the distal clavicle, forming the acromioclavicular (AC) joint

acronym: a word formed from the initial letters of other words

action verb: the second verb, typically written in past tense, required when writing an HPI. An action verb denotes that something is happening to a historian, usually the development of signs or symptoms.

acuity: in healthcare, the degree or severity of illness

acuity level: the score, based on the Emergency Severity Index (ESI), assigned to a patient presenting to an emergency department that reflects the triage nurse's assessment of the severity of illness or intensity of services thought to be required

adduction: movement toward the body's midline

adenohypophysis: the anterior lobe of the pituitary gland. It secretes growth hormone, thyroid-stimulating hormone, and several other hormones.

admission: the transition of a patient, typically from the emergency department, to a bed in the hospital

adnexa: tissue or structures in the body adjacent to, or near, another, related structure. For example, the ovaries and the fallopian tubes are adnexa of the uterus.

adrenal glands: small, triangular endocrine glands located on the superior portions of the kidneys

adrenaline: a hormone produced by the adrenal glands in times of stress and regulated by the sympathetic nervous system. Also called *epinephrine*.

adrenocorticotropic hormone (ACTH): a hormone produced by the pituitary gland that acts on the adrenal glands

afebrile: the condition of being without a fever

affect: the observable emotional tone

afferent: the nerves that transmit sensory information from the body via the peripheral nervous system to the central nervous system

affirm: to note the presence of a symptom or problem during history taking

against medical advice (AMA): the term for the situation in which a patient leaves an emergency department prior to the completion of the provider's evaluation but after receiving discharge instructions with the safest plan of care, given the circumstances

age-related macular degeneration (ARMD): the degeneration of the macula that causes vision loss

algorithm: a set of rules or calculations for solving a problem in a finite, ordered number of steps

alkalosis: an abnormal condition of body fluids, characterized by a tendency toward a blood pH level greater than 7.45 caused by an excess of alkaline bicarbonate or a deficiency of acid

alopecia: a partial or complete lack of hair resulting from normal aging, an endocrine disorder, a drug reaction, an anticancer medication, or a skin disease

alveoli: the small outpouchings along the walls of the alveolar sacs through which gas exchange between alveolar air and pulmonary capillary blood takes place

Alzheimer disease: a neurodegenerative disease associated with plaques and tangles in the brain that cause memory loss and personality changes

amenorrhea: the absence of menses

amnesia: a loss of memory caused by brain damage or by severe emotional trauma

analgesic: a medication used to reduce pain that does not cause loss of consciousness

anatomic position: the point of view in which the patient is facing the examiner with the arms at the sides and the palms of both hands facing forward

anemia: a decrease in the amount of red blood cells or hemoglobin leading to inadequate tissue oxygenation and frequently symptoms of shortness of breath and fatigue

anesthetic: a medication used to diminish physical pain sensation, with or without loss of consciousness

aneurysm: a bulge in the wall of an artery that may rupture and bleed

angina: chest pain with a cardiac etiology

angiography: an imaging study of certain vessels, typically arteries, using dye and x-rays in "real time," often in conjunction with other procedures

ankylosing spondylitis (AS): an inflammatory back disease that forms bony syndesmoses around the vertebrae, resulting in loss of flexibility and back stiffness

anorexia: a lack or loss of appetite

anorexia nervosa: a disorder characterized by a prolonged refusal to eat, emaciation, amenorrhea in women, emotional disturbance concerning body image, and fear of becoming obese

anterior: a directional term meaning toward the front of the body

antibody: a protein produced by plasma cells that can identify and neutralize pathogens. Also known as *immunoglobulin* (Ig).

antigen: a substance that the immune system recognizes as foreign and mounts an immune response against

antipyretic: a medication used to reduce fever

antiseptic: an agent that destroys or inhibits the growth of microorganisms and can be applied to human skin or mucous membrane

anus: the opening of the rectum lying in the fold between the buttocks

aorta: the main trunk of the systemic arterial circulation, comprising four parts: the ascending aorta, the arch of the aorta, the thoracic portion of the descending aorta, and the abdominal portion of the descending aorta

aortic coarctation: a narrowing of the aorta that can cause cardiac hypertrophy and differences in blood pressure between the extremities

aortic valve: the heart valve that separates the left ventricle from the aorta

apex: the top or uppermost section

aphasia: the inability to express speech

aphtha: a small, shallow, painful ulceration that usually affects the oral mucosa but not underlying bone

apnea: an absence of spontaneous respiration

appendicular skeleton: the appendages of the skeleton, which include everything not classified as axial

appendix: a vestigial organ at the end of the cecum with a debated function

aqueous humor: the clear, watery fluid circulating in the anterior and posterior chambers of the eye

arachnoid mater: the meningeal layer deep to the dura mater

arrhythmia: an irregular heartbeat

artery: one of the large blood vessels carrying blood in a direction away from the heart to the tissues

articulation: the place where two bones are joined by a joint

ascending colon: the first of four segments of the large intestine

ascites: an accumulation of fluid in the peritoneal cavity

aspiration: the inhalation and trapping of foreign materials within the bronchial tree or lungs

assault: a threat of bodily harm that reasonably causes fear of harm in the victim

asterixis: a tremor of the hand when the wrist is extended that indicates a problem with the motor systems in the brain

asthenic: the condition of appearing weak

asthma: a long-term inflammatory disease of the airway that causes bronchial narrowing and difficulty breathing

ataxia: a condition in which muscle movements are poorly coordinated, typically indicative of a cerebellar problem

atherosclerosis: a thickening of the arterial wall due to plaque formation

atlas: another name for cervical vertebra C1

atria (*s. atrium*): the two superior chambers of the heart

atrial fibrillation: an arrhythmia of the atria, typically with a rapid and irregular heartbeat ("irregularly irregular" on physical exam); often designated as being with or without *rapid ventricular response (RVR)*

atrial flutter: an arrhythmia of the atria that manifests as very rapid regular beating, typically 250–400 beats per minute and is inefficient at pumping blood to the ventricles

atrioventricular (AV) node: a component of the heart, located inferiorly to the sinoatrial node on the posterior wall of the right atrium, that receives the electrical signal after its generation in the sinoatrial node and mediates its transmission from the atria to the ventricles

atrophy: the shrinkage and weakening of muscle

attending note: a note that contains the important elements of history and physical, and any discussion that shows that an attending physician was involved and coordinated the care of the patient along with a resident, physician assistant (PA), or nurse practitioner (NP)

audit trail: a record of every individual who accessed an electronic health record and what they did in it

aural: referring to the ear

auricle: the oval-like cartilaginous tissue that most recognize as the ear. Also known as the *pinna*.

auscultation: the technique of listening, usually employing the stethoscope, and describing what is heard which could have diagnostic significance

avascular: a term meaning lacking blood or lymph vessels

avulsion: an injury in which a body structure or skin is forcibly detached

axial skeleton: the centralized components of the skeleton, including the skull, vertebral column, sternum, and ribs

axillary: referring to the armpit

axis: another name for cervical vertebra C2

axis: the direction of electrical flow in the heart

B cell: a type of lymphocyte involved in the production of antibodies against an antigen

Barrett's esophagus: an abnormal condition in which a change in the cell type of the lower esophagus, usually as a result of chronic acid reflux, represents a precancerous state

base: the bottom or inferior section

battery: the unconsented physical contact on another person

benign paroxysmal peripheral vertigo (BPPV): a condition in which small particles become loose in the balance organs of the inner ear

benign prostatic hyperplasia (BPH): a noncancerous enlargement of the prostate, potentially resulting in urinary retention

bicuspid valve: the heart valve that separates the left atrium from the left ventricle. Also called the *mitral valve.*

bilateral: a directional term meaning that something occurs on both sides

billable element: a pertinent aspect of a history that factors into the determination of the history's level of complexity; also known as a descriptor or documentation element

biopsy: the removal of tissue for pathologic analysis

bladder: a hollow, muscular, expandable sac that collects and stores urine before excretion

blood pressure: the pressure exerted by the circulating volume of blood on the walls of the arteries and veins and on the chambers of the heart

blood tonicity: the concentration of solutes in the blood

body temperature: the level of heat produced and sustained by the body processes

bolus: (1) A round mass of solids and semisolids that have been chewed and mixed with saliva in order to be swallowed. (2) A specified amount of medication given over a discrete unit of time, most often but not always through an IV.

bone marrow: the soft, organic, spongelike material in the cavities of bones, the chief function of which is to manufacture erythrocytes, leukocytes, and platelets

bradycardia: a condition in which the heart contracts at a rate less than 60 beats per minute

brain: the most centralized organ of the nervous system, protected within the hard cranial vault of the skull

brainstem: the part of the brain comprised of the midbrain, pons, and medulla, located on the ventral aspect of the cortex, that is responsible for more life dependent functions, such as respiration and heart rate

breach: a break or violation of the security of a patient's protected health information

bronchiole: a small airway of the respiratory system extending from the bronchi into the lobes of the lung

bronchoscopy: the visual examination of the tracheobronchial tree, using a standard rigid, tubular metal bronchoscope or a narrower, flexible fiberoptic bronchoscope

bronchus: any one of several large air passages in the lungs through which pass inhaled air and exhaled air; these are smaller than and branch from the trachea, but larger than and leading to the bronchioles

bruit: an abnormal sound of arterial blood flow due to a partial blockage or other narrowing or kinking of the artery, causing turbulent flow

business associate: a company that works closely with a HIPAA covered entity and, as a result, must comply with HIPAA rules

cachectic: the condition of having generalized bodily wasting

calcaneus: the heel bone of the foot

candidiasis: any infection caused by a species of the fungus *Candida,* usually *Candida albicans*

capillary: a tiny vessel that exchanges nutrients, wastes, and gases with the body's tissues, connecting the arterial and venous systems

carbuncle: a large pustular lesion

cardiac conduction cycle: the cycle of events in the heart, equivalent to one heartbeat, during which an electrical impulse is conducted from the sinus node to the atrioventricular (AV) node, to the AV bundle, to the bundle branches, and to the Purkinje fibers

cardiovascular system: the body system consisting of the heart and the blood vessels

cardioversion: the use of chemicals or electricity to convert an irregular rhythm into normal sinus rhythm

caries: tooth decay. Also called *cavities.*

carpal: one of the small bones of the wrist

cataract: a clouding of the lens in the eye that causes visual loss

cauda equina: a group of nerve roots located in the lumbar region and the terminal point of the spinal cord

cauda equina syndrome: a medical emergency in which compression of the terminal nerve roots of the spinal cord occurs, potentially causing low back pain with numbness in the groin (documented as saddle anesthesias), leg weakness, and urinary or bowel incontinence

caudad: a directional term meaning toward the tail

cecum: the first portion of the ascending colon

celiac disease: an autoimmune hypersensitivity to gluten, which is found in wheat, oats, and barley

Centers for Medicare and Medicaid Services (CMS): a federal agency within the Department of Health and Human Services that administers the Medicare and Medicaid programs

central nervous system (CNS): the division of the nervous system that includes the brain and spinal cord, in which most major neurological functions and decision making occur

cephalad: a directional term meaning toward the head

cephalgia: a sensation of discomfort or pain in any region of the head. Also called "headache."

cerebellum: the part of the brain, located ventrally and posterior to the cortex, with the primary role of motor function, especially involving coordination and balance

cerebral cortex: the outer layer of gray matter in the cerebrum

cerebrospinal fluid (CSF): a fluid produced within the ventricles of the brain that nourishes and protects the entire central nervous system

cerebrovascular accident (CVA): the blockage of the blood supply to a part of the brain, resulting in tissue injury or death. Also called "stroke."

cerebrum: the largest part of the brain, responsible for higher level thought and decision making, interpretation of the senses, and execution of voluntary motor function, among other functions

certification: (1) The process that ensures an individual has been trained, tested, and can be counted on to perform a given job with competence. (2) The designation received by the individual who has completed the process of certification.

cerumen: a yellowish or brownish waxy secretion in the ear. Also called "ear wax."

cervical spine (c-spine): the superior portion of the vertebral column, which comprises the neck and consists of seven vertebrae (C1–C7)

cervix: the part of the uterus that lies partly in the vagina and partly in the pelvic cavity, joining the body of the uterus at a narrow junction termed the isthmus

chief complaint: a short description of a patient's symptom(s), sign(s), or in some instances, diagnosis, that brought the patient to the medical setting

chlamydia: a common sexually transmitted infection known to cause white penile or vaginal discharge, dysuria, and abdominal pain

cholecystectomy: the surgical removal of the gallbladder

chronic obstructive pulmonary disease (COPD): the condition of chronic lung inflammation causing bronchial narrowing, difficulty breathing, and eventually, lung scarring; often but not always associated with a prolonged history of smoking

circumcision: the surgical removal of the male prepuce, or foreskin

cirrhosis: an abnormal condition of liver scarring; often, but not always, caused by alcoholism

claim: a request for reimbursement from a payer for medical services rendered

clavicle: one of a pair of thin narrow bones that cross over the anterior upper chest. Also called the "collar bone."

clinical decision support (CDS): a feature of many electronic health record systems which analyzes the information input into the record to suggest to the provider things to do for the patient

clinical impression: an assessment of the patient's condition, typically after a rapid work-up in the emergency department, based upon their symptoms and results. A clinical impression may or may not be a diagnosis.

clitoris: the vaginal erectile structure of the female

clubbing: a nail deformity frequently, but not always associated with chronic hypoxia related to cardiopulmonary disease

coccyx: the inferior portion of the sacrococcygeal spine. Also called the "tailbone."

cochlea: the auditory portion of the inner ear, resembling a tiny snail shell and containing the sense organ for hearing

coding: the conversion of information into numeric or alphanumeric codes designed to communicate information

colon: the portion of the large intestine extending from the cecum to the rectum; frequently used interchangeably with the term large intestine.

colostomy: the surgical creation of an artificial anus by bringing a part of the large intestine (colon) through an incision in the abdominal wall

combining form: a word root with a vowel

compartment syndrome: a condition in which there is increased pressure within a muscle region (compartment) causing decreased blood flow and death of muscle tissue

complete blood count (CBC): a laboratory test that measures the quantity and size of red blood cells, the quantity and type of white blood cells, and the quantity of platelets

compliance: the adherence to a set of standards

computed tomography (CT): an imaging modality that combines radiographs and computer technology assistance to achieve a rudimentary 3-D view of a portion of the body by creating a cross-sectional view of that area

computerized physician order entry (CPOE): a feature of the electronic health record system that allows the physician or other provider to create and send secure orders

concussion: a brain injury that temporarily affects brain function and may result in headaches and temporary short-term memory loss; also referred to as mild traumatic brain injury

conduction: the way in which electricity is transmitted throughout the heart

confidentiality: the careful safeguarding of the patient's health information

congestion: swelling and/or irritation of the nasal tissues that causes the sensation of not being able to inhale through the nasal cavity

conjunctiva: the membrane that covers the external eye and the internal eyelids. Also called the *conjunctival membrane.*

conjunctivitis: the inflammation of the conjunctiva, caused by bacterial or viral infection, allergy, or environmental factors. Also called "pinkeye."

connective tissue: a type of tissue that supports, forms, and protects the body, and also functions to store and transport substances; mainly consists of bone, ligament, tendon, cartilage and adipose (fatty) tissue.

conscience clause: a legislative provision that relieves a person from compliance or duty based on moral or other personal beliefs

consent: the permission for something to happen

consolidation: a lung area in which air has been replaced by fluid or other material

constitutional: a term used to describe a person's overall health or appearance, including vital signs; it is considered a body system for billing in both review of systems and physical exam

consultant: a provider who evaluates a patient and provides recommendations for an evaluation and/or a treatment plan; generally the consultant makes recommendations relating to a single area of his or her expertise

consultation: a formal request by a physician for the opinion or services of another healthcare professional

continuity of care: the safe and effective delivery of healthcare over time; it implies shared and coordinated information over time and across places of healthcare service

contraindication: an absolute reason why a certain line of treatment should not be utilized

contralateral: a directional term meaning pertaining to the opposite side

contrast medium: a substance that obstructs the x-rays that would normally pass through an organ or structure, allowing less dense tissue to be visualized

controlled substance: any drug defined in the five categories of the federal Controlled Substances Act of 1970

contusion: an injury that does not disrupt the integrity of the skin, caused by a blow to the body and characterized by swelling, discoloration, and pain. Also called a "bruise."

cornea: a transparent thickening of the sclera over the pupil and iris that refracts light as it enters the eye

coronary artery bypass graft (CABG): a procedure in which the heart is put on bypass and a coronary artery graft is placed to restore blood flow

cortisol: a hormone, often produced in times of stress, that affects metabolism and is an immuno-suppressant. Also called the "stress hormone."

costovertebral angle (CVA): one of two angles that outline a space over the kidneys. CVA tenderness to percussion is a common finding in pyelonephritis and other infections of the kidneys and adjacent structures.

cough etiquette: the practice of containing potentially infectious respiratory secretions by covering one's mouth and nose when sneezing or coughing

covered entity: a body that must have appropriate administrative, technical, and physical safeguards to protect the privacy of protected health information; refers to those organizations and businesses that are included in the requirements of HIPAA

cranial nerves: the twelve pairs of nerves that arise from the brain, serving to transmit sensory information from the head and neck to the central nervous system, and motor information from the central nervous system to the head and neck. They also supply sensory organs in the head.

cranial vault: the protective, dome-like structure of the skull which is composed of four bones or bone pairs: frontal, parietal, temporal, and occipital

crepitus: clicking, cracking, or crunching noises

croup: a viral infection affecting the upper airway, resulting in a "barking" cough and sometimes stridor. Also called *laryngotracheobronchitis.*

cryptorchidism: a developmental defect in which one or both testicles fail to descend into the scrotum and are retained in the abdomen or inguinal canal

culture: the process of identifying the organisms in a sample by inoculating a growth medium

Current Procedural Terminology (CPT): the code set used to code services rendered by providers in all settings

cyanosis: the blue or purple discoloration of the skin due to hypoxia

cystic fibrosis: an inherited disorder that causes abnormally thick body secretions leading to problems throughout the body and especially the lungs

cystocele: a herniation or protrusion of the urinary bladder through the wall of the vagina

cystoscopy: endoscopy of the urinary bladder

decubitus ulcer: an inflammation, sore, or ulcer in the skin over a bony prominence, most often caused by prolonged pressure on the skin in those confined to bed or a wheelchair. Also called a *pressure ulcer* or a "bedsore."

deep: a directional term meaning more internally located, as opposed to *superficial*

deep vein thrombosis (DVT): a venous blood clot, usually in the extremities, that is known to cause unilateral leg pain and swelling and can embolize and cause pulmonary embolism

defendant: an individual or entity sued or accused in a court of law

denervation: the condition of being without a nerve supply

deny: to note the absence of a problem during history taking

depolarization: a change in membrane potential between the intracellular and extracellular compartments of the plasma membrane

depression: (1) In body movements, the movement of a part of the body inferiorly, as opposed to *elevation*. (2) In electrocardiography, the location of a line segment in an ECG that is below the expected baseline, as opposed to segment elevation.

dermis: a component of skin, located below the epidermis, that contains many structures, including nerves, vessels, and glands

descending colon: the segment of the colon that extends from the end of the transverse colon to the beginning of the sigmoid colon in the pelvis

descriptor: a pertinent aspect of a history that factors into the provider's assessment of the patient, the subsequent plan of care, and the determination of the history's level of complexity; also known as a documentation element or billable element. Common descriptors include location, quality, severity, duration, timing, context, modifying factors, and associated signs and symptoms.

diabetes insipidus (DI): a metabolic disorder characterized by excessive thirst and secretion of large amounts of urine due to abnormal production or response to vasopressin

diabetes mellitus (DM): a complex disorder characterized by a deficiency or complete lack of insulin secretion by the pancreas, or by resistance to insulin, causing high blood glucose over a prolonged period

diagnosis: a provider's official determination of a patient's injury or illness

diagnostic: a type of procedure or test used to help confirm a diagnosis

diaphoresis: the secretion of sweat, especially the profuse secretion associated with an elevated body temperature, physical exertion, exposure to heat, or mental or emotional stress

diaphragm: a large dome-shaped muscle that separates the thoracic and abdominal cavities

diastole: the instant of maximum cardiac relaxation

differential: a list of possible diagnoses or impressions

dilatation and curettage (D&C): induced expansion of the cervix and removal of uterine contents, sometimes performed after miscarriage or abortion

diplopia: double vision caused by defective function of the extraocular muscles or a disorder of the nerves that innervate the muscles

direct admission: an admission to a hospital that occurs without going through the emergency department first

discharge: the process of sending a patient from a healthcare facility to another setting

disclosure: the communication of private information

disequilibrium: the loss of balance or adjustment, particularly mental or psychological balance

disinfection: the process of destroying microorganisms, typically on an object or surface, using a germicidal agent

dislocation: the condition in which a joint has been removed from normal articulation

dispense as written (DAW): a designation in a prescription that explicitly forbids the pharmacist from filling a trade name drug with a generic equivalent

disposition: the status change at the end of the patient's visit in the emergency department or an inpatient facility; common examples are discharge, admit, and transfer

distal: a directional term meaning further from the center of the body, as opposed to *medial*

distension: the state of being swollen or ballooned out. Also spelled *distention*.

diverticulitis: the inflammation of one or more diverticula in the colon (see diverticulosis)

diverticulosis: the presence of small pouches in the colon wall (diverticulae), particularly the sigmoid colon

documentation element: a pertinent aspect of a history that factors into the provider's assessment of the patient, the subsequent plan of care, and the determination of the history's level of complexity; also known as a billable element or descriptor

don: to put on, as an article of clothing or gear

dorsal: a directional term meaning toward the back of the body, as opposed to *ventral*. Also known as *posterior*, as opposed to *anterior*.

dorsiflexion: the action by which a hand/foot is moved toward the dorsum, as opposed to palmar flexion or *plantarflexion*

dose: the amount of drug to be given

duodenum: the shortest, widest, and most fixed portion of the small intestine

dura mater: the most superficial meningeal layer

duration: the period of time over which a drug should be taken, usually written in number of days

dysmenorrhea: painful menses

dyspepsia: a vague feeling of epigastric discomfort after eating. Also called "indigestion."

dysphagia: difficulty swallowing

dyspnea: a distressful subjective sensation of uncomfortable breathing that may be caused by many disorders, including certain heart and respiratory conditions, strenuous exercise, or anxiety

dysuria: pain with urination, often described as "burning"

ecchymosis: discoloration of the skin from bruising or bleeding internally

echocardiogram: a graphic outline of the movements of heart structures produced by ultrasonography

eclampsia: a potentially life threatening disorder of pregnancy, characterized by hypertension, generalized edema, and proteinuria with seizures

ectopy: a condition in which premature heartbeats arising from the atrium, ventricle, or elsewhere occur

eczema: a general superficial dermatitis of unknown cause

ED contact order: a request for the receptionist to page the hospitalist or another specialist so the emergency medicine provider can discuss the patient's case and confirm the status change; may be termed somewhat differently in different institutions (page order, consultation order, or similar)

edentulous: the condition of being toothless

efferent: a nerve that transmits impulses away or outward from the central nervous system, usually causing a muscle contraction or release of a glandular secretion

ejaculate: (1) The semen discharged in a single emission. (2) A mixture of sperm and nutritional fluids.

ejaculatory duct: the passage formed by the junction of the duct of the seminal vesicles and ductus deferens through which semen enters the urethra

electrocardiogram (ECG): a tracing of the electrical activity of the heart that is recorded as a waveform pattern on grid paper. May also be abbreviated as *EKG*.

electromyogram (EMG): the graphic representation of nerve conduction testing

electronic health record (EHR): a database of patient information that enables information sharing among authorized healthcare professionals, often linked to a knowledge base that can help providers make decisions about patient care

electrophysiology: a cardiac subspeciality in which diseases of the heart's electrical system are evaluated, treated and managed

elevation: (1) In body movements, the movement of a part of the body superiorly, as opposed to *depression*. (2) In electrocardiography, the location of a line segment in an ECG that is above the expected baseline, as opposed to segment depression.

eloping: the term for the situation in which a patient leaves an emergency department before the provider's evaluation is complete and before receiving circumstantial discharge instructions

Emergency Medical Treatment and Active Labor Act (EMTALA): a law enacted in 1986 that requires a facility, usually an emergency department, to perform a medical screening exam and provide stabilizing treatment prior to transfer to another healthcare facility, regardless of the patient's legal status, citizenship, or ability to pay

emergent: arising, often unexpectedly

emesis: vomit or vomiting

endocardium: the innermost, membranous layer or lining of the heart

endocrine: a term used to describe an organ that is glandular in nature

endocrine system: a group of organs and glands that produce hormones, which are chemical messengers that travel through the blood to other parts of the body to exert an effect

endometriosis: an abnormal condition in which endometrial tissue (tissue that is the normal inner lining of the uterus, usually shed monthly during the menstrual cycle or period) grows outside of the uterus

epicardium: the outermost layer of the heart

epidermis: the outermost layer of skin

epididymis: one of a pair of long, tightly coiled ducts that carry sperm from the seminiferous tubules of the testes to the vas deferens

epidural space: the space immediately above and surrounding the dura mater of the brain or spinal cord, beneath the endosteum of the cranium and the spinal column

epiglottis: the cartilaginous structure that covers the opening of the trachea during swallowing, preventing food or foreign objects from entering

epilepsy: a seizure disorder

epistaxis: a nosebleed

eponym: a medical term named after a person

erythema: redness or inflammation of the skin or mucous membranes that is the result of dilation and congestion of superficial capillaries. Also called *rubor*.

erythrocyte: a mature red blood cell

esophageal varices: bleeding veins in the lower part of the esophagus

esophagus: the musculomembranous canal, about 24 cm long, extending from the pharynx to the stomach; the food tube

ethics: a belief system about what behaviors are acceptable

eustachian tube: the structure that connects the middle ear to the nasal cavity and is responsible for equalizing pressure between these two air filled compartments. Also known as the *auditory canal*.

evaluation and management (E/M) code: a CPT code that is used to bill for the provider's level of service (LOS)

eversion: the movement of the heel away from the body's midline, as opposed to *inversion*

exocrine: a term used to describe an organ that secretes substances out onto an epithelial surface, as opposed to endocrine that secrete substances into the blood stream; examples are sweat glands, mammary glands, lacrimal (tear) glands

exophthalmos: the protrusion of the eyes due to excessive thyroid hormone

expiration: (1) Exhalation. (2) Death.

explicit consent: an individual's permission to proceed when clearly presented with an option to agree or disagree or to express a preference or choice, often verbally or in writing

extension: the state in which the angle of a joint is increased, as opposed to *flexion*

external rotation: the rotation of a joint away from the midline, as opposed to *internal rotation*. Also called *lateral rotation*.

extraocular muscles: the six muscles, innervated by three cranial nerves, that work together to move the eye in various directions

exudates: pustular patches sometimes found near the tonsils that can indicate infection by streptococcus or other bacteria

fallopian tube: one of a pair of ducts that serves as the passage through which an ovum is carried to the uterus and through with spermatozoa move out toward the ovary

fatigue: the feeling of being excessively tired

febrile: the condition of being with a fever

felony: a more serious crime punishable by larger fines and/or imprisonment for more than one year or, in some states, death

femur: the long bone of the lower extremity extending from the hip to the knee

fibromyalgia: a condition characterized by hypersensitivity to pain accompanied by excessive fatigue without another explainable cause

fibula: the lateral of the two bones in the foreleg

flank region: the area that lies atop the kidneys, but is a broader region than the costovertebral angle

flexion: the movement in which the angle of a joint is decreased, as opposed to *extension*

foramen magnum: a large hole at the base of the skull through which the spinal cord exits the skull

formulation: the physical form in which the drug is dispensed (e.g., tablet, ointment, aerosol). The formulation is associated with the chemical properties and purpose of the drug.

fracture: a break in a bone

fraud: an intentional act to misrepresent facts or mislead for financial gain

frequency: the number of times that a drug should be administered in the prescribed dose within a period of time (e.g., once daily, at bedtime, as needed)

fundoscopy: the examination of the internal eye structures with an ophthalmoscope

gait: the manner or style of walking, including rhythm, pattern, cadence, and speed

gallbladder: a secretory sac, located on the liver, that stores and concentrates bile

gallop: a third or fourth heart sound, which at certain heart rates sometimes sounds like the gait of a horse. Also called *gallop rhythm*.

general consent: an individual's permission to be medically evaluated

genitourinary system: a combination of both male and female reproductive systems and the renal or urinary system. The genitourinary system is counted as one system together in the review of systems and physical exam for billing.

glans: the head of the penis

Glasgow Coma Scale (GCS): the scale used to score a patient's conscious state that is used to predict morbidity/mortality from neurologic injury. Lower scores represent a more severe neurological problem.

glucagon: a hormone that increases blood glucose when levels are too low

glucocorticoids: a group of hormones that increase the formation of glucose, exert an anti-inflammatory effect, and influence many body functions

gonorrhea: a sexually transmitted infection that can cause green penile or vaginal discharge

gout: a disorder in which uric acid deposits in joints cause pain, swelling, and redness

gravid: the condition of being pregnant

gyri: the folds of the cerebral cortex

habitus: the physique of the body

hair: a sensory organ that can detect touch or movement

hallucination: an occurrence of hearing (auditory) or seeing (visual) things not actually present

hand hygiene: an important infection control measure consisting of handwashing using traditional soap and water, alcohol-based foam or other antiseptic formulation

hard palate: the anterior portion of the muscular partition between the oral and nasal cavities that, together with the posterior soft palate, forms the roof of the mouth

hard-stop: a safeguard mechanism within an electronic health record placed in various workflows to ensure that the user is aware of a significant fact that could detrimentally affect outcomes if missed

Health Insurance Portability and Accountability Act (HIPAA): a federal law that, among other measures, limits the sharing of patient health information without patient authorization

health record: the documentation of all the data about a patient and the care he or she received, including the patient's identifying information, medical history, laboratory results, diagnoses, medications, problems, and procedures and other services. The health record is the cornerstone of the efficient, safe, and effective delivery of healthcare.

heart: a hollow muscular organ which is responsible for pumping blood throughout the vasculature

heart rate: the frequency with which the heart beats

HEENT (head, eyes, ears, nose, throat): a group of organs, many of which are special sensory organs, or body structures, that are often organized together for purposes of efficient documentation

hematemesis: the vomiting of bright red blood, indicating rapid upper gastrointestinal (GI) bleeding

hematochezia: the passage of red blood in the feces

hematology: the scientific study of blood and blood-forming tissues

hematopoietic stem cells: the cells that reside in the bone marrow and give rise to all three classes of cells found within the blood

hematuria: the abnormal presence of blood in the urine

heme: the pigmented iron-containing nonprotein part of the hemoglobin molecule

hemodialysis: the procedure of blood filtration and removal of waste products in a person with renal dysfunction

hemoptysis: coughing up of blood from the respiratory tract

hemorrhoid: a vascular structure in the anal canal that may become swollen, painful, and inflamed

hepatomegaly: enlargement of the liver

hernia: the protrusion of an organ through the wall of the cavity it is normally contained within

hirsutism: the condition of excessive body hair in a masculine distribution pattern as a result of heredity, hormonal dysfunction, porphyria, or medication

historian: the person (often, but not always, the patient) who tells the story of the history of the present illness (HPI)

history and physical (H&P): one of the most common notes, documenting the reason the patient is seeking medical service, the patient's medical history, the provider's findings, and the provider's plans to treat the patient

history of the present illness (HPI): a coherent story, usually chronologic, describing the patient's illness or injury from the first sign or symptom to the present

Holter monitor: a portable device for making prolonged (usually 24 hours) electrocardiograph recordings while the patient conducts normal daily activities

hormone: a chemical messenger that travels through the blood to other parts of the body to exert an effect. Each hormone has a different function and target, and they are regulated in various ways.

hospitalist: an internist who works exclusively within a hospital. The hospitalist will only document on any problem that requires close monitoring or intervention while the patient is hospitalized.

human immunodeficiency virus (HIV): a retrovirus that causes acquired immunodeficiency syndrome (AIDS)

humerus: the long bone of the upper arm

hypermobility: the ability to extend the joint to a greater degree than normal. Also called *joint laxity*.

hyperthyroidism: a condition characterized by hyperactivity of the thyroid gland, resulting in excessive production of thyroid hormone

hypertonic: a state in which muscles have abnormally increased tone or strength

hyperventilation: rapid and inefficient breathing that decreases carbon dioxide

hypodermis: a component of skin, located deep to the dermis, comprised of fat and connective tissue. Also called *subcutaneous tissue*.

hypothalamus: a structure in the brain that makes a connection to and regulates the pituitary gland

hypothyroidism: a condition characterized by decreased activity of the thyroid gland

hypoxia: a state of oxygen deprivation

hysterectomy: the surgical removal of the uterus (partial hysterectomy), or the surgical removal of the uterus, fallopian tubes, and ovaries (complete hysterectomy)

ileum: the lower-third distal portion of the small intestine, extending from the jejunum to the cecum

ileus: a condition of diminished propulsion of intestines causing stagnation of flow of the intestinal contents

ilium: the uppermost of the three bones that make up the innominate bone (hip bone). Also called the "wings" of the pelvis.

illicit drug: any drug that is illegal to make, sell, transport, or use

imaging study: any of a number of tests used to better visualize an interior structure of the body (e.g., x-rays, MRI, ultrasound, nuclear medicine studies)

impetigo: a contagious bacterial skin infection, common in small children, that usually localizes on the face, particularly around the mouth

implied consent: an individual's permission to proceed with evaluation and/or treatment suggested by his or her actions or circumstances. For example, a person who presents herself to the emergency department implies that she wishes to be evaluated and treated without having to expressly state so. A person unconscious from a motor vehicle accident is said to be giving implied consent for treatment because that would be suggested by his condition and circumstances.

indication: a valid reason for the provider to order tests, prescribe medications, or perform procedures, including surgeries

inferior: a directional term meaning lower down or below another structure, as opposed to *superior*

informed consent: in medicine, an individual's signed agreement to a treatment or procedure which the healthcare provider has explained in detail, including the rationale for it, its risks and potential prognoses, and available alternatives

innominate bone: one of two bowl-shaped bones that together form the pelvis. Also called the "hip bone."

insertion: the place of attachment, such as that of a muscle to the bone it moves

inspection: the technique of simply looking at a patient and his or her various anatomical areas and describing what is seen

inspiration: inhalation

insulin: a hormone, secreted by the pancreas in response to increased blood glucose, which acts to promote transport of glucose into muscle cells and other tissues

intensive care unit (ICU): a unit of a hospital intended for the delivery of critical care

intercapping: the capitalization of letters within a drug name

International Classification of Diseases, 10th Edition, Clinic Modification (ICD-10-CM): the code set used to record patient problems and diagnoses in all types of medical settings

interstitium: the space between cells in a tissue

interval: the time between events on an ECG

interventional cardiology: a cardiac subspecialty in which catherization procedures are performed

interventional radiology: a radiology subspecialty in which imaging-guided minimally invasive diagnostic or therapeutic procedures are performed

intolerance: a condition characterized by inability to absorb or metabolize a nutrient or medication, and in which exposure to the substance may cause an adverse reaction. Often used in counter distinction to an allergy.

introitus: an entrance or orifice in a cavity or a hollow tubular structure of the body, such as the vaginal introitus

intubation: the placement of a tube in the trachea to help with respiration

inversion: the movement of the heel of the foot toward the body's midline, as opposed to *eversion*

ipsilateral: a directional term meaning pertaining to the same side, as opposed to *contralateral*

iris: the colored portion of the eye, which is a muscle that adjusts the size of the pupil depending on levels of ambient light

irritable bowel syndrome (IBS): a chronic condition of unknown origin in which the small and large intestines are abnormally motile, usually accompanied by diarrhea

ischium: the curved bone inferior to the ilium and behind the pubis. The ischium is one of the three bones that comprise one half of the pelvis.

isolation: the placement away from other patients of a patient known or suspected of having certain types of infection. Different types of isolation are recognized based on transmissibility of the pathogen (infectious agent), some requiring respiratory isolation, others contact isolation for example.

jejunum: the middle of the three portions of the small intestine

joint laxity: the ability to extend the joint to a greater degree than normal. Also called *hypermobility*.

keratin: a protein that is responsible for the skin's protective function

kickback: a payment or other incentive to an entity or individual to facilitate an action, especially illicitly

kidney: one of a pair of urinary organs, located on each side of the vertebral column, responsible for filtering the blood and eliminating wastes in the urine

kyphosis: the excessive convex curvature of the thoracic spine

labia majora: the two long lips of skin, one of which is located on each side of the vaginal opening

labia minora: the two thin folds of skin between the labia majora

laparoscopy: a technique to examine the abdominal cavity with a laparoscope (a long thin fiber-optic instrument with camera attached) through one or more small incisions in the abdominal wall, usually at the umbilicus

laryngopharynx: the most inferior of the three anatomical divisions of the pharynx and the one that contains the vocal cords

laryngotracheobronchitis: a viral infection affecting the upper airway, resulting in a "barking" cough and sometimes stridor. Also called *croup*.

lateral: a directional term meaning away from the midline, as opposed to *medial*

lateral rotation: the rotation of a joint away from the midline, as opposed to *medial rotation*. Also called *external rotation*, as opposed to *internal rotation*.

laterality: the indication of the affected side (left, right, or both) of a pair of body parts

lavage: the washing out, or irrigation, of a body cavity, such as the ear canal or nose

leave without being seen (LWBS): the term for the situation in which a patient checks into an emergency department but leaves before being brought to a room or seen by a provider

lens: the part of the eye, located deep to the iris, responsible for the ability to adjust between looking at near versus far objects

lesion: an alteration in body tissue caused by illness or injury

lethargy: a condition of excessive fatigue and inactivity, suggesting difficulty arousing and inability to be alert

leukemia: a group of cancers of the blood/bone marrow characterized by proliferation of abnormally developed and malfunctional white blood cells

leukocyte: a blood cell that participates in immunity and inflammation. Also called white blood cell.

leukocytosis: an abnormally elevated total peripheral white blood cell count, often associated with bacterial infection

leukorrhea: a white or yellow vaginal discharge

level of service (LOS): the intensity and extensiveness of a history and physical exam, as well as medical decision making. Levels of service, from simplest to most complex, are problem focused, expanded problem focused, detailed, and comprehensive.

ligament: connective tissue that connects two bones together, typically across a joint, providing stability to the joint

lithotripsy: the destruction of kidney stones with lasers, ultrasound waves, or mechanically

litigation: a legal dispute

liver: the largest gland of the body and one of its most complex organs, responsible for metabolism of wastes and toxins, participation in metabolic cycles, the processing of nutrients absorbed during digestion, and the synthesis of cholesterol and blood-clotting proteins

lordosis: the excessive concave curvature of the lumbar/cervical spine

lumbar puncture: a procedure in which the subarachnoid space is accessed with a needle for the collection of cerebrospinal fluid for analysis. Also called a "spinal tap."

lumbar spine: the portion of the vertebral column that comprises the lower back and consists of five vertebrae (L1–L5)

lung: one of a pair of light, spongy organs in the thorax, constituting the main component of the respiratory system

lymph node: one of the many small oval structures that filter the lymph and fight infection and in which lymphocytes, monocytes, and plasma cells are formed

lymphadenopathy: a swelling of the lymph nodes

lymphangitis: an inflammation of one or more lymphatic vessels, usually resulting from an acute streptococcal infection of one of the extremities, resulting in red streaking; sometimes colloquially referred to as blood poisoning

lymphatic fluid: the name for the interstitial fluid collected by the lymphatic vessels after it enters the lymphatic system

lymphatic vessels: fine, thin walled, transparent valved channels, distributed through most tissues, that terminate in open-ended tubes in the interstitium

lymphocyte: the functional unit of the adaptive immune system that circulates in blood, lymph, and peripheral lymphatic tissues. Lymphocytes are categorized as B and T lymphocytes and natural killer cells. Also called *lymph cell*.

lymphoma: a type of cancer of lymphoid tissue

macrophage: a phagocyte that recognizes and engulfs foreign materials and presents fragments on their membranes to initiate an immune response

macula lutea: the area of highest visual acuity of the retina

magnetic resonance imaging (MRI): an imaging modality that uses radio waves and a magnetic field to make a 3D reconstruction of a region of the body

malaise: a feeling of being unwell

malleolus: a rounded bony process, such as the protuberance on each side of the ankle

malodorous: foul-smelling

malpractice: an act of negligence that describes an improper or illegal professional activity or treatment, often used in regard to a healthcare professional causing an injury to a patient

mandible: the lower bone of the jaw

mania: a period of abnormally elevated mood and activity

maxilla: the upper bone of the jaw

medial: a directional term meaning toward the midline, as opposed to *distal* or *lateral*

medial rotation: the rotation of a joint toward the midline, as opposed to *lateral rotation*. Also known as *internal rotation*.

Medicaid: a healthcare coverage program for low-income adults and children funded jointly by states and the federal government

medical decision making (MDM): the part of the documentation that is the provider's domain to document their evolving thought processes during the patient's visit

medical necessity: the justification, often required by third-party payers, that an order is warranted by the patient's condition

medical scribe: a documentation assistant to the medical provider (most commonly a physician)

Medicare: the federal health insurance program for people aged 65 and over, certain younger people with disabilities, and people with end-stage renal disease (ESRD)

melanin: a pigment, produced by melanocytes, that protects the skin from harmful ultraviolet (UV) radiation

melanoma: skin cancer of melanocytes

melena: abnormal black tarry stool that has a distinctive odor and contains digested blood

meninges: the three membranes enclosing the brain and the spinal cord, comprising the dura mater, the pia mater, and the arachnoid membrane

meningismus: a condition in which the patient shows signs of meningeal irritation, such as neck stiffness, and headache, suggesting a likelihood of central nervous system pathology

meningitis: the inflammation of the meninges often due to infection from a virus or bacteria

meniscus: a curved, fibrous cartilage in the knees and other joints

mesentery: a broad fan-shaped fold of peritoneum suspending the jejunum and the ileum from the dorsal wall of the abdomen

metacarpal: one of five bones of the hand, not including the fingers

metatarsal: one of five bones of the foot, not including the toes

misdemeanor: a lesser crime, usually punishable by monetary fines established by the state

mitral valve: the heart valve that separates the left atrium from the left ventricle. Also called the *bicuspid valve*.

monocyte: a leukocyte essential for phagocytosis and proteolysis, and part of the innate immune system

motor neuron: a neuron that innervates muscles and glands

multigravida: the term for a pregnant woman who has had at least one prior pregnancy

multiparous: the condition of having birthed more than one child

multiple sclerosis (MS): a demyelinating disease damaging the neuronal insulating covers and affecting the transmission of neuronal signal

murmur: an abnormal heart sound caused by turbulent blood flow

myocardial infarction (MI): the necrosis of a portion of cardiac muscle caused by an obstruction in a coronary artery resulting from atherosclerosis, a thrombus, or a spasm. Also called "heart attack."

myocarditis: inflammation of the heart muscle

myocardium: the middle, muscular layer of the heart

myringotomy: a small incision in the tympanic membrane to relieve fluid accumulation that causes increased pressure

nail: a keratinous appendage of the skin, visible above the epidermis at the tips of the fingers and toes

nail bed: the area underneath the nail

naris: one of two external openings of the nose. Also called the *nostril*.

nasal turbinate: a bony structure located on the lateral walls of the nasal cavity that directs airflow into the nasopharynx. Also known as *concha*.

nasopharynx: the most superior region of the pharynx, located posterior to the nasal cavity

National Provider Identifier (NPI): a unique numerical identifier assigned to every provider by the Centers for Medicare and Medicaid Services (CMS)

natural killer (NK) cell: a large lymphocyte primarily involved in attacking tumor cells or virally infected cells

nature of the presenting problem: a barometer to measure the risk of the patient not receiving care. There are five severity levels to this component of the note: minimal; self-limited or minor; low severity; moderate severity; or high severity.

navicular: a small bone located on the radial aspect of the wrist. Also called the *scaphoid*.

negligence: a tort that does not require a specific intent to harm someone and is not a deliberate action, but is the result of an individual or party failing to act in a reasonable way where a duty was owed

nerve block: a method of anesthesia that uses a local anesthetic injected around a nerve to numb the region supplied by that nerve

neurohypophysis: the posterior lobe of the pituitary gland that is the release point of antidiuretic hormone (ADH) and oxytocin. The neurohypophysis is part of the nervous system.

neuron: a specialized cell found in the nervous system

neurotransmitters: chemical messengers that assist in the transmission of signal between neurons, or between a neuron and its target

neutrophil: a leukocyte essential for phagocytosis and proteolysis, and part of the innate immune system

noradrenaline: a hormone that acts to increase blood pressure by vasoconstriction but does not affect cardiac output. Also called *norepinephrine*.

norepinephrine: a hormone that acts to increase blood pressure by vasoconstriction but does not affect cardiac output. Also called *noradrenaline*.

normal sinus rhythm (NSR): an orderly regular progression of heartbeats

normocephaly: the condition of normal development in a head

nuchal rigidity: an inability to flex the neck

nulligravida: the term for a woman having had no pregnancies

nulliparous: the condition of having birthed no children

nystagmus: involuntary rapid eye movement with a variety of causes

objective: the quality of being able to be measured or observed by anyone else besides the person experiencing it

observable element: a portion of the physical exam that may be obtained by carefully watching the patient's movement, appearance, speech, and affect

observation: an alternative to inpatient status, in which a patient stays in the hospital for a short time (usually less than 24 hours) and undergoes brief workups and monitoring

obsessive compulsive disorder (OCD): a disorder in which compulsions are carried out in an attempt to alleviate obsessive thoughts and anxiety

obstructive sleep apnea (OSA): a form of sleep apnea involving a physical obstruction in the upper airways, most commonly the glottis

Office of the Inspector General (OIG): a government agency tasked with protecting the integrity of Health and Human Services (HHS) programs, such as Medicare

oliguria: a diminished capacity to form and pass urine

operative note: a very specific type of procedure note that describes the surgery that a patient has undergone

ophthalmoscope: a handheld device equipped with a light and magnification to examine the internal components of the eye

optic disc: the point at which the optic nerve (CN II) enters the eye

optic nerve: the cranial nerve (CN II) that transmits impulses from the eye to the brain

oral: referring to the mouth

oral cavity: the space within the mouth that contains the tongue and teeth

order: the provider's electronic or written instructions for therapies such as medications, testing such as labs or imaging, or communications that are meant for other healthcare workers

order panel: a predetermined set of orders for frequently ordered tests for certain complaints

origin: an attachment site where the muscle begins

oropharynx: one of the three anatomical divisions of the pharynx that lies posterior to the oral cavity

orthopnea: an abnormal condition in which a person must sit or stand to breathe deeply or comfortably

osteoarthritis: a degenerative joint disease that causes joint pain and deformity

osteopenia: the condition of low bone mineral density, but not to the point of osteoporosis

osteoporosis: the condition of decreased bone mineral density that significantly increases risk of fracture

otalgia: a pain in the ear

otitis media: inflammation of the middle ear

otoscope: an instrument used to look inside the ear canal

outcome: the result of the treatment

ova: the secondary oocytes extruded from the ovary at ovulation. Also called "egg."

ovary: one of the paired female gonads found on each side of the lower abdomen beside the uterus. The ovaries produce ova.

pack-year: a quantification of an individual's degree of tobacco exposure, calculated by multiplying the number of packs a person smokes per day by the number of years the person has smoked

pallor: an unnatural paleness or absence of color in the skin

palpation: the physical exam technique of using the hands with their sense of touch and then describing what is found

palpitations: heartbeats that are abnormal, such as beats that are irregular, hard, racing, fast, or skipped

pancreas: an elongated organ in the abdominal cavity that secretes various substances, such as digestive enzymes, insulin, and glucagon, considered both an endocrine and an exocrine organ

pancytopenia: the simultaneous reduction in red blood cell, white blood cell, and platelet counts

paracentesis: the procedure of collecting peritoneal fluid

paranoia: a state of suspicion or mistrust that can be unrealistic or unwarranted

parathyroid gland: a set of four small glands, located behind the thyroid gland in the neck, that produce parathyroid hormone

parathyroid hormone: a hormone produced by the parathyroid gland that regulates levels of serum calcium and phosphate

paresthesia: a tingling sensation that is usually due to nerve injury, often described as "pins and needles"

parietal pleura: the delicate membrane which lines the chest wall and covers the diaphragm

Parkinson disease: a degenerative brain disease that causes a dopamine deficiency manifested as muscle rigidity and tremor

paronychia: a bacterial or fungal infection where the nail and skin meet, causing redness, swelling, and pain

parous: the condition of having children

patella: a sesamoid bone that lies atop the knee joint and is the attachment point of the quadriceps tendon superiorly. Also called "kneecap."

pathogen: a microorganism that causes disease

Patient Self-Determination Act (PDSA): a law that requires that adult patients be informed of their right to accept or decline any medical or surgical treatment, and to be advised of their right to have an advance directive in place in the event they become incapacitated

pelvic girdle: a bony ring formed by the hip bones, the sacrum, and the coccyx

percussion: the technique of tapping on the body to elicit a sound that suggests wellness or pathology in the patient

pericardiocentesis: a procedure in which a long thin needle is advanced into the pericardial sac to drain excessive fluid

pericardium: the fibrous sac that surrounds the entire heart. Also called the *pericardial sac.*

peripheral nervous system (PNS): the division of the nervous system that includes any nervous tissue that is not part of the central nervous system

peristalsis: the coordinated, rhythmic serial contraction of smooth muscle that forces food through the digestive tract

peritoneal dialysis: a technique of cleansing the blood of impurities in a patient with poorly functioning kidneys. It involves running fluid into the patient's abdominal cavity and then draining it out to allow impurities to slowly leech out of the blood into this fluid and then be removed. This is an alternative to the more common blood cleansing technique that involves filtering the blood more directly using a dialysis machine.

peritoneum: an extensive membrane that lines the entire abdominal wall of the body and is reflected over the contained viscera

PERRL (pupils are equal, round, and reactive to light): the acronym used to indicate a normal result to the pupillary light reflex test

personal protective equipment (PPE): the gear, including gloves, masks, eye protection, respirators, and gowns, that may be worn when using standard precautions while administering to an infected or contaminated patient

pertinent negative: a problem a patient denies having during history taking

pertinent positive: a problem a patient affirms having during history taking

petechiae: tiny spots in an erythematous rash often caused by superficial capillaries under the skin that rupture and bleed

phalanx (*pl. phalanges*): one of the most distal bones of the upper extremity. The phalanges comprise the fingers.

pharynx: the muscular tube, extending from the base of the skull to the esophagus, that serves as a passageway for the respiratory and digestive tracts. Also called the "throat."

physical exam (PE): the provider's physical findings and observations of the patient's body during the patient encounter

pia mater: the meningeal layer, located deep to the arachnoid mater, directly adherent to the brain and spinal cord

pinna: the oval-like cartilaginous tissue that most recognize as the ear. Also known as the *auricle.*

pituitary gland: a gland comprised of two functionally different components, the adenohypophysis and the neurohypophysis, that produces hormones that influence nearly every part of the body

plaintiff: the individual or entity that brings a legal action against another. Sometimes referred to as the complainant.

plantarflexion: the movement of the foot toward the plantar surface (toes down), as opposed to *dorsiflexion*

pleural cavity: the space within the thorax that contains the lungs

pneumothorax: the presence of air or gas in the pleural space, often suggesting a hole or leak in the lung and potentially causing a lung to collapse

polydipsia: excessive thirst

polyphagia: excessive hunger

polyuria: the excretion of an abnormally large quantity of urine

posterior: a directional term meaning toward the back of the body, as opposed to *anterior*. Also called *dorsal*.

pre-charting: the process of reviewing old records for additional information and populating a new note with prior elements that may be relevant before initiating the current patient encounter

precordium: the portion of the chest over the heart

preeclampsia: an abnormal condition of pregnancy characterized by the onset of acute hypertension after the 24th week of gestation. The classic triad of preeclampsia is hypertension, proteinuria, and edema.

prefix: a word part that appears at the beginning of a word

prepuce: a fold of skin that forms a retractable cover, such as the foreskin of the penis or the fold around the clitoris

prescription: a provider's order to be fulfilled at a later time. Most commonly, it is used to dispense a drug to a patient.

pressure ulcer: an inflammation, sore, or ulcer in the skin over a bony prominence, most often caused by prolonged pressure on the skin in those confined to bed or a wheelchair. Also called a *decubitus ulcer* or a "bedsore."

primary care: an area of medicine considered to be the first point of contact for the patient in caring for their general needs

primigravida: the term for a woman having her first pregnancy

privacy: the characteristic of keeping health information concealed

Privacy Rule: a HIPAA rule prohibiting unauthorized disclosure of protected health information (PHI), and giving patients an array of rights with respect to that information

problem list: a listing of a patient's known active medical problems, including any combination of diagnoses, symptoms and signs, or clinical impressions

problem-oriented charting: a specific approach to documentation in the patient record that breaks down the note into sections that are reflective of the patient's problems from their problem list. Also known as the *problem-oriented medical record (POMR)*.

procedure: an umbrella term used to describe a variety of activities related to patient care, ranging from taking vital signs to suturing a laceration

progress note: a note written each day, or as indicated by the patient's condition, on a patient who is admitted to the hospital or seen in an office

pronation: the movement of the palms of the hands downward, as opposed to *supination*

prostate gland: a gland in men that surrounds the neck of the bladder and the proximal part of the urethra and produces a fluid that becomes part of semen

protected health information (PHI): any health information that can be linked to an individual

protraction: the extension of a part of the body, as opposed to *retraction*

provider: a professional who is understood to have the education, experience, and demonstrated competency to practice medicine, meaning that they can recommend and perform treatments to cure a health problem or maintain health

provider note: any note created in the health record by a medical provider

proximal: a directional term meaning closest to the center of the body, as opposed to *distal*

pruritis: the sensation of itchiness

psychosis: a psychological state in which one has lost contact with reality

pubic symphysis: the cartilaginous joint of the anterior pelvis, formed by the articulation of the right and left pubic bones at the midline

pubis: the forwardmost of the three bones that comprise the pelvis

pulmonary artery: a blood vessel that exits the right ventricle of the heart and transports blood to the lungs for reoxygenation. The pulmonary arteries are the only arteries within the body that normally carry deoxygenated blood.

pulmonary embolism: the blockage of a pulmonary artery by fat, air, tumor tissue, or a blood clot that usually arises from a peripheral vein

pulmonary hypertension: abnormally high blood pressure within the pulmonary circulation

pulmonary vein: a blood vessel that carries oxygenated blood from the lungs to the left atrium of the heart. The pulmonary veins are the only veins in the body that normally carry oxygenated blood.

pulmonic (pulmonary) valve: the heart valve that separates the right ventricle from the pulmonary artery

pulse: the regular, recurrent expansion and contraction of an artery, produced by waves of pressure caused by the ejection of blood from the left ventricle of the heart as it contracts

pupil: in the eye, an adjustable aperture through which light enters to project to the retina

pupillary light reflex: a test used to test the integrity of the optic nerve (CN II) and the oculomotor nerve (CN III)

purpura: any of several bleeding disorders characterized by hemorrhage into the tissues, particularly beneath the skin or mucous membranes, producing an itchy, purple rash

pyrexia: a fever

quality: the rendering of services that follow the most current medical knowledge to achieve health in patients

radiograph: an image created by directing x-rays through part of the body onto a detector

radius: one of two bones of the forearm; the other is the ulna

rales: the crackling, rattling, or clicking noises heard during inspiration caused by small airway collapse. This finding often indicates abnormal presence of fluid in alveoli.

range of motion: the plane or degree of movement of a joint

rate: of the heart, the average number of beats per minute

rectal: referring to the rectum

rectum: the lower part of the large intestine

reflex: an involuntary response to a stimulus in which the input is not sent to the brain for interpretation before an output is generated

reflux: an abnormal backward or return flow of a fluid

regurgitation: the backward flow of blood through a defective heart valve

reimbursement: the payment for healthcare services

release of information (ROI): the administrative function of disclosing protected health information (PHI) to an outside individual or entity

renal system: the body system comprised of the pair of kidneys connected to a series of tubes which ultimately terminate outside the body. Also called the *urinary system*.

renin-angiotensin-aldosterone system (RAAS): the body's regulatory system that plays a role in sodium balance, fluid volume, and blood pressure

repolarization: the process by which the membrane potential of a neuron or muscle cell is restored to the cell's resting potential

respirator: an air filtration mask that may be required as a part of the personal protective equipment in some cases

respiratory rate: the rate of breathing

resuscitation: the process of sustaining the vital functions of a person in respiratory or cardiac failure while reviving him or her

retina: the most posterior structure of the eye, containing rods and cones

retinal subluxation: a condition in which the retina separates from surrounding support tissues. Also called *retinal detachment*.

retraction: the withdrawal of a body part, as opposed to *protraction*

revenue cycle: a series of processes used to file claims and obtain payment from payers

review of systems (ROS): a list of the patient's symptoms organized by body system

rheumatoid arthritis: an inflammatory autoimmune disease that typically affects smaller synovial joints, resulting in joint destruction manifested as joint pain, swelling, and deformity

rhinorrhea: the free discharge of a thin, watery nasal fluid. Also called "runny nose."

rhonchi: the rattling noises caused by secretions within the bronchi

rhythm: the regularity with which the heart is beating

ribs: bones of the axial skeleton that articulate with the thoracic spine and curve around the body to form the thoracic cage and protect its contents

route: the manner in which a drug should be administered (e.g., oral, intranasal, topical). The route is based on factors such as drug metabolism, duration of action, dose, and patient condition.

rule out: to eliminate from consideration a cause of a patient's symptoms or signs

sacrum: the superior portion of the sacrococcygeal spine, which articulates with the fifth lumbar vertebra superiorly

sanitization: the use of water and mechanical action with or without detergents to remove foreign substances, such as soil, organic material and germs, from objects. Also called "cleaning."

sarcoidosis: a chronic disorder of unknown origin characterized by the formation of inflammatory granulomatous tissue in the lungs and other organs

scaphoid: a small bone located on the radial aspect of the wrist. Also called the *navicular*.

scapula: one of a pair of flat bones located over the posterior upper thorax. Also called the "shoulder blade."

schizophrenia: any one of a large group of psychotic disorders characterized by gross distortion of reality, disturbances of language and cognitive function, withdrawal from social interaction, disorganization and fragmentation of thought, altered perception, and emotional reaction.

sclera: the area of the eye surrounding the iris. Also called the "white" of the eye.

scleral icterus: the yellow discoloration of the conjunctiva that is caused by jaundice

scoliosis: a lateral curvature of the spine

scrotum: the pouch that holds the testicles

sebaceous gland: a type of gland that produces sebum, which is secreted into hair follicles

sebum: a lubricant, produced by sebaceous glands, that is secreted into hair follicles

Security Rule: a HIPAA rule that requires all covered entities to enact all reasonable measures, both technical and nontechnical, to protect the confidentiality of patient health data against any potential violation that could be anticipated

segment: a portion of an ECG that does not include any waveform within its duration; the time between waveforms, as opposed to intervals which may include waveforms.

semen: the thick, whitish secretion of the male reproductive organs discharged from the urethra during ejaculation. Also called *sperm* or *seminal fluid*.

semicircular canal: any of three bony fluid-filled loops in the osseous labyrinth of the internal ear, associated with the sense of balance

seminal vesicle: either of the paired saclike glandular structures of the male that produce a fluid that is added to the secretion of the testes and other glands to form semen

serum: the liquid portion of a blood sample after it has been spun in a centrifuge

sesamoid: any one of numerous small round bony masses embedded in certain tendons that may be subjected to compression and tension (e.g., the patella, which is embedded in the tendon of the quadriceps femoris at the knee)

sick sinus syndrome (SSS): the term used to describe malfunction of the heart's internal pacemaker, the SA node (sinoatrial node). This condition results in sporadic changes in the patient's rhythm and frequently leads to placing of an artificial pacemaker to control the rhythm.

sigmoid colon: the part of the colon that extends from the descending colon in the pelvis to the juncture of the rectum

sign: an objective, measurable finding recorded in the physical examination

signatura (Sig.): a component of a prescription for medication that includes specifications describing how a patient should take the drug and often under what circumstances a patient should take it

sinoatrial (SA) node: a component of the heart, located in the right atrium near the entrance point of the superior vena cava, where electrical activity is generated, and which is the main determinant of heart rate. Also known as the "internal pacemaker" of the heart.

slit lamp: a device used to magnify and examine both the external eye and the anterior portion of the internal eye

small intestine: the longest part of the digestive tract, divided into the duodenum, jejunum, and ileum. It is the major organ of absorption of food.

SOAP note: an acronym standing for Subjective, Objective, Assessment, and Plan. This note is often used in daily rounds on the floor of a hospital, or in an office setting for a patient's regular follow-up visits

soft palate: the posterior portion of the partition between the oral and nasal cavities that, together with the anterior hard palate, forms the roof of the mouth

somnolence: the overwhelming feeling of sleepiness

speaking verb: the first verb, written in the present tense, required when constructing a history. The speaking verb denotes that the historian is actively saying something.

special sensory: the term for an organ that participates in collecting special sensory information, such as sight (eyes), hearing and balance (ears), smell (nose), and taste (taste buds in the mouth and throat)

specialty medicine: an area of medicine with in-depth focus on one specific body system (e.g., cardiology)

sperm: the male reproductive cell formed in the testes and secreted in the semen or seminal fluid during ejaculation

spinal cord: a major component of the central nervous system, contained within the spinal canal and enclosed by three protective membranes

spinal stenosis: a narrowing of the vertebral foramen that may cause nerve compression

spirometry: a pulmonary function test of the ability to move air through the respiratory system

spleen: a soft, highly vascular organ, located in the left upper quadrant of the abdominal cavity, comparable to a large lymph node. It also filters the blood to screen for foreign antigens.

splenectomy: the removal of the spleen

splenomegaly: an abnormal enlargement of the spleen

sprain: a condition in which ligaments are overextended and partially or completely tear

standard of care: the type and level of care an ordinary, prudent, healthcare professional, with the same training and experience, would provide under similar circumstances

standard precautions: the infection control measures, used with all patients, based on the underlying assumption that all patients are carrying bloodborne pathogens and are therefore treated as such. Formerly called universal precautions.

stenosis: an abnormal condition characterized by the constriction or narrowing of an opening or passageway in a body structure, commonly used to describe heart valve and vessel abnormalities

sterile: the state of being free of all microorganisms

sterile field: a microorganism-free area that may be created around a patient prior to a procedure to prevent subsequent infection

sterile technique: the methods used to destroy all microorganisms and keep them away from the exposed surgical site

sterilization: the process of destroying all microorganisms and their spores with chemicals or intense heat and pressure, such as in an autoclave

sternum: the flat bone in the center of the anterior chest; also known as the breastbone

stomach: the food reservoir and first major site of digestion, located just under the diaphragm and divided into a body and pylorus

strabismus: an inability to direct both eyes toward the same point simultaneously

stratified squamous epithelium: a flat cell found in the epidermis that makes the skin protective, and is often layered for extra protection

streptococcal infection: a bacterial infection caused by the streptococcus bacteria, causing infection in any number of areas of the body. Often it causes infection of the tonsils in which case it can produce a sore throat, fever and malaise. Also called "strep throat."

stridor: a high pitched sound heard during inspiration, usually caused by upper airway obstruction or narrowing

subarachnoid space: the area between the arachnoid mater and the pia mater, through which cerebrospinal fluid circulates through the spinal canal

subcutaneous tissue: a component of skin, located deep to the dermis, comprised of fat and connective tissue. Also called the *hypodermis.*

subdural space: the area between the dura mater and the arachnoid mater

subjective: the quality of being felt or valued by the individual experiencing it, and not able to be measured or observed by anyone else

suffix: a word part the appears at the end of a word

suicidal ideation: thinking or planning to kill oneself

sulci: the grooves of the cerebral cortex

superficial: a directional term meaning more externally located, as opposed to *deep*

superior: a directional term meaning higher or above a more inferior structure, as opposed to *inferior*

supination: the movement of the palms of the hands to face upward, as opposed to *pronation*

surgical: pertaining to a type of procedure that alters or repairs the body

suture: (1) *n.*, A border or joint, such as between the bones of the cranium. (2) *v.*, To stitch together cut or torn edges of tissue with suture material. (3) *n.*, A surgical stitch taken to repair an incision, tear, or wound. (4) *n.*, Material used for surgical stitches, including absorbable or nonabsorbable types such as silk, catgut, wire, or synthetic material

symptom: a subjective element of disease, often recorded in the chief complaint, history of present illness, and review of systems

synapse: an electrochemical junction at which signal is transmitted between neurons, or between a neuron and its target

syncope: a brief loss of consciousness. Also called "fainting" or "passing out."

synovial fluid: the substance within a joint capsule that nourishes the joint and provides lubrication

systemic: a term meaning overall. For example, a systemic disease affects the entire body rather than just one small area or a single system.

systemic lupus erythematosus (SLE): an inflammatory autoimmune disease that affects multiple organ systems, including the joints, where it manifests as joint pain, stiffness, and swelling

systole: the contraction of the heart, driving blood into the aorta and pulmonary arteries

T cell: a lymphocyte with activation and destruction capabilities

tachycardia: a condition in which the heart contracts at a rate greater than 100 beats per minute

tachypnea: an abnormally rapid rate of breathing (more than 20 breaths per minute in adults)

tall-man letters: a safety precaution in the electronic medical record used to distinguish between similar-sounding drugs

tarsal: pertaining to the seven bones that comprise the hindfoot and ankle

telangiectasia: a collection of dilated capillaries and venules near the surface of the skin and mucous membranes

telemetry: a monitored bed in a hospital

temporal: referring to the sides of the head in the area of "temple" where the temporal bones are located

temporomandibular joint (TMJ): a synovial joint between the temporal bone and the mandible

tendon: any one of many white, glistening bands of dense fibrous connective tissue that attach muscle to bone

testicle: one of the pair of male gonads that produces sperm and testosterone. Also called *testis*.

The Joint Commission (TJC): one of several accrediting agencies approved by CMS for reviewing and certifying hospitals as well as many other healthcare settings

therapeutic: a type of procedure that is part of a patient's treatment plan

therapy: treatment intended to relieve or heal a disorder

third-party payer: an entity that pays the provider for all or part of the services rendered on behalf of the patient

thoracentesis: a procedure in which a hollow needle is inserted into the thorax to remove fluid or pus from the pleural space

thoracic spine: the portion of the vertebral column that comprises the upper back and consists of twelve vertebrae (T1–T12)

thoracostomy: a procedure in which a small incision/opening is created in the chest wall for draining the pleural cavity of abnormal collections of air, fluid or pus, usually accomplished with a thoracostomy tube

thrombocyte: a cell that participates in the clotting cascade, which prevents abnormal bleeding. Also called a *platelet*.

thrombocytopenia: a deficiency in platelets that affects the ability of the body to form blood clots

thrush: a fungal infection, or candidiasis, of the mouth and tongue due to yeast

thyroid gland: a butterfly-shaped gland in the anterior neck that produces the thyroid hormones triiodothyronine (T3) and thyroxine (T4)

thyroid stimulating hormone (TSH): a hormone secreted by the anterior lobe of the pituitary gland that controls the release of thyroid hormone and is necessary for the growth and function of the thyroid gland. Also called *thyrotropin*.

thyroid storm: a crisis of uncontrolled overproduction of T3 and T4 which can cause a dangerous increase in metabolism

thyromegaly: enlargement of the thyroid gland. Also called *goiter*.

thyroxine (T4): a hormone of the thyroid gland that stimulates metabolic rate

tibia: the medial of the two bones of the foreleg. The tibia is a weight-bearing bone of the body.

tinea corporis: a superficial fungal infection. Also called "ringworm."

tinnitus: a condition in which sound is heard when none is present, often described as "ringing in the ears."

tonsils: small, rounded masses of immune tissues in the oral cavity

tort: a wrongdoing or violation of civil law

toxic appearance: the condition of appearing severely ill

trachea: a nearly cylindrical tube in the neck, composed of C-shaped cartilage, membrane, and muscle, that conveys air to the lungs

transfer: the transition of a patient from one facility to a bed in another facility

transmission-based precautions: the infection control measures used in addition to standard precautions when in the vicinity of patients known or suspected to have certain types of infections

transverse colon: the segment of the colon that extends from the end of the ascending colon to the beginning of the descending colon

trauma note: a note including trauma-specific considerations, often in addition to elements of a tradition history and physical

treatment plan: the provider's instructions for how to care for the patient

trichomoniasis: a sexually-transmitted infection that can cause malodorous yellow/green frothy vaginal discharge, itching, and burning

tricuspid valve: the heart valve that separates the right atrium and the right ventricle

triiodothyronine (T3): a hormone that helps regulate growth and development, helps control metabolism and body temperature, and, by a negative-feedback system, acts to inhibit the secretion of thyrotropin by the pituitary gland

tripod position: a position in which a patient is leaning forward with hands on a support (e.g., bed, legs), using accessory muscles to breath. This position may be observed when the patient is in respiratory distress.

true allergy: a hypersensitivity of the immune system to an innocuous antigen that results in a reaction to the antigen as if it were pathogenic as opposed to a sensitivity or intolerance

tubal ligation: a procedure in which the fallopian tubes are tied off to prevent eggs from reaching the uterus. Tubal ligation is an effective way to prevent pregnancy.

turgor: the expected resiliency of the skin caused by the outward pressure of the cells and interstitial fluid. Also called *elasticity*.

tympanic: referring to the eardrum

tympanic membrane (TM): the terminal point of the auditory canal, which separates the external ear from the middle ear, known as the eardrum

ulcerative colitis (UC): a chronic, episodic, inflammatory disease of the large intestine and rectum, characterized by profuse watery diarrhea containing varying amounts of blood, mucus, and pus

ulna: one of two bones of the forearm; the other is the radius

ultrasound (US): an imaging modality that uses sound waves of various frequencies to construct an image of an organ or structure

unilateral: a directional term meaning pertaining to only one side of the body, as opposed to *bilateral*

upcoding: billing for a higher level of service than that provided

ureter: one of a pair of tubes that carries urine from the kidney into the bladder

urethra: a small tubular structure that drains urine externally from the bladder

urethral meatus: the opening of the urethra

urinalysis: a laboratory test that measures the appearance and amount of protein, bacteria, cells, and other characteristics of the urine

urinary system: the body system comprised of the pair of kidneys connected to a series of tubes which ultimately terminate outside the body. Also called the *renal system*.

urine: the fluid secreted by the kidneys, transported by the ureters, stored in the bladder, and voided through the urethra

urticaria: a welt-like rash, notable for red, raised, pruritic bumps, that is often due to an allergen. Also called "hives."

uterus: the hollow, pear-shaped internal female organ of reproduction in which the fertilized ovum is implanted and the fetus develops

uvea: a layer beneath the sclera, comprising the choroid (at the posterior), the iris, and the ciliary body

uvula: a muscular tissue that dangles from the soft palate and plays a role in the gag reflex

vaginal canal: the potential space of the female genitalia represented by the area that extends from the vaginal opening to the uterine cervix

vaginal fornix: a recess in the upper part of the vagina caused by the protrusion of the uterine cervix into the vagina

vaginal vault: the enlargement of the internal end of the vagina

value-based purchasing: an initiative that rewards hospitals with incentive payments for what the government deems to be quality care for Medicare patients

varicose vein: a vein that has become enlarged and tortuous. The condition can increase susceptibility to thrombophlebitis, blood clots in the veins.

vas deferens: the extension of the epididymis that ascends from the scrotum into the abdominal cavity and joins the seminal vesicle to form the ejaculatory duct

vasculature: the network of veins and arteries in an organ or tissue

vasectomy: a procedure in which the vas deferens is severed to prevent sperm from being ejaculated. Vasectomy is an effective way to prevent pregnancy.

vasoconstriction: the narrowing of blood vessels

vasodilation: the widening of blood vessels

vein: a blood vessel that carries deoxygenated blood to the heart

vena cava: a major vein that directs deoxygenated blood from the body to the right atrium

ventilation perfusion (VQ) scan: an imaging modality that examines pulmonary air and blood flow to identify a possible disturbance of the normal circulation or airflow

ventral: a directional term meaning toward the front of the body, as opposed to *dorsal*. Also called *anterior*.

ventricles: in neurology, compartments within the brain that produce cerebrospinal fluid; in cardiology, the two chambers of the heart located inferiorly to the atria

ventricular hypertrophy: the abnormal enlargement of the heart caused by enlargement of the myocardium. It is often caused by hypertension, a valvular disease, or heart failure.

ventriculoperitoneal (VP) shunting: the placement of a drainage tube (shunt) between the ventricles of the brain and abdominal cavity to drain excessive fluid in the brain

vertebral column: the structure that protects the spinal cord and helps provide support to stand upright and walk bipedally

vertebral disc: a cartilaginous disc, located between each vertebra, that reduces the transmission of force between vertebrae and protects the bony structures of the vertebral column

vertebral foramen: a large hole within the center of each vertebrae through which the spinal cord passes

vertigo: the sensation that the room is spinning

vestibulocochlear nerve: a branch of the eighth cranial nerve associated with the sense of equilibrium

visceral pleura: the delicate membrane which covers the lung, dipping into the fissures between the lobes

vital sign: an external sign that may indicate the functional state of the body. Recorded vital signs typically include temperature, blood pressure, pulse, and respiratory rate, and sometimes blood oxygenation and subjective pain.

vitiligo: a benign acquired skin disease of unknown cause, consisting of irregular patches of various sizes totally lacking in pigment and often having hyperpigmented borders

vitreous humor: a transparent, semigelatinous substance contained in a thin hyoid membrane and filling the cavity behind the crystalline lens of the eye

vocal cords: a pair of strong bands of elastic tissue in the larynx participatory in the generation of sound and voice. Also called *vocal folds*.

vocal folds: a pair of strong bands of elastic tissue in the larynx participatory in the generation of sound and voice. Also called *vocal cords*.

wheezing: an abnormal usually expiratory breath sound, characterized by a high-pitched or low-pitched musical quality, caused by narrowing of the lower airway

whistleblower: an individual who provides the government with information about fraud in the medical professions

Note: Page numbers followed by *f* indicate figures, *t* tables, *b* boxes.